D1200601

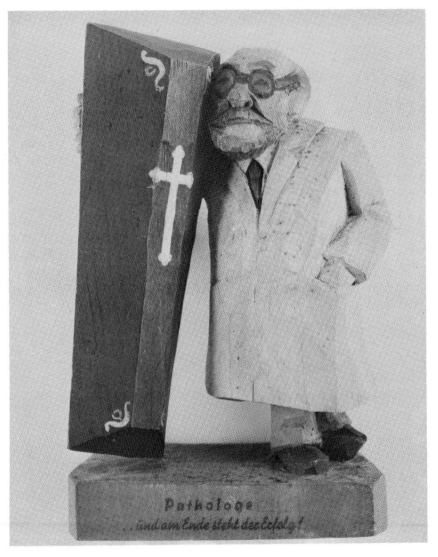

Pathologist

. . . and in the end comes success!

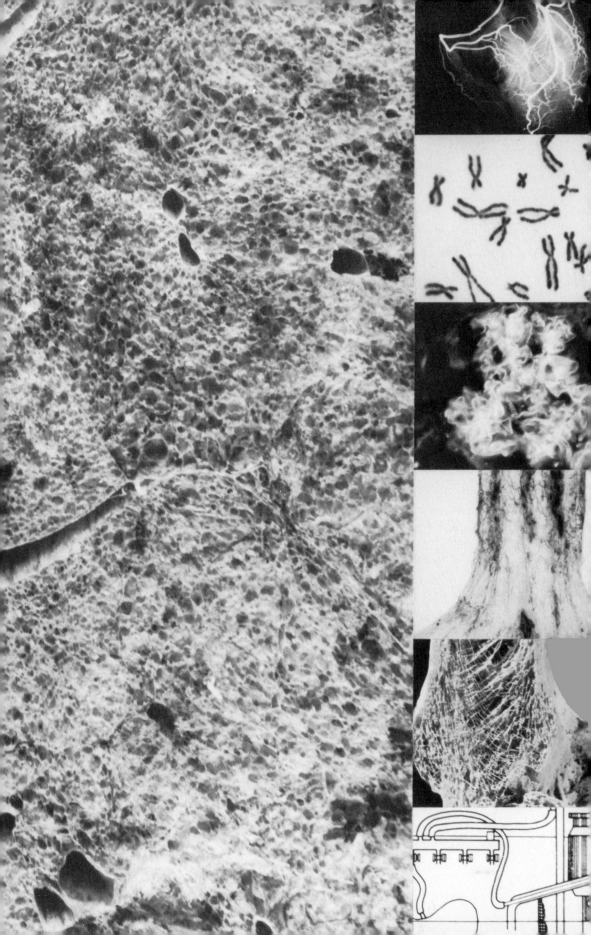

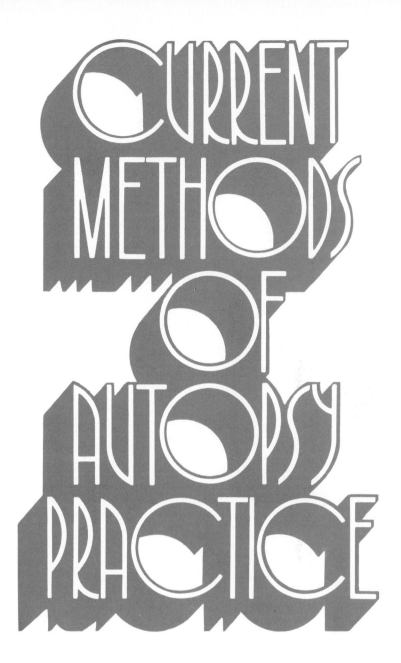

JURGEN LUDWIG, M.D.

Department of Experimental and Anatomic Pathology,
Mayo Clinic,
Rochester, Minnesota

1972
W. B. SAUNDERS COMPANY Philadelphia London Toronto

W. B. Saunders Company: West Washington Square
Philadelphia, Pa. 19105

12 Dyott Street
London, WC1A   1DB

833 Oxford Street
Toronto 18, Ontario

Current Methods of Autopsy Practice   ISBN   0-7216-5803-2

Print No.: 9   8   7   6   5   4   3   2   1

To Marianne

LIST OF CONTRIBUTORS

ROBERT C. BAHN,   M.D., Ph.D. (Pathology)

Department of Experimental and Anatomic Pathology, Mayo Clinic;
Professor of Pathology, Mayo Graduate School of Medicine
(University of Minnesota), Rochester, Minnesota.

ARNOLD L. BROWN, Jr.,   M.D.

Department of Experimental and Anatomic Pathology, Mayo Clinic;
Professor of Pathology, Mayo Graduate School of Medicine
(University of Minnesota), Rochester, Minnesota.

C. TERRENCE DOLAN,   M.D.

Section of Clinical Microbiology, Mayo Clinic; Instructor in
Microbiology, Mayo Graduate School of Medicine (University of
Minnesota), Rochester, Minnesota.

JAUW T. LIE,   M.B., B.S. (Melbourne)

Fellow in Pathology, Mayo Graduate School of Medicine
(University of Minnesota), Rochester, Minnesota.
Presently: Department of Pathology, Royal Melbourne Hospital,
Victoria 3050, Australia.

HARUO OKAZAKI,   M.D.

Department of Experimental and Anatomic Pathology, Mayo Clinic;
Assistant Professor of Pathology, Mayo Graduate School of
Medicine (University of Minnesota), Rochester, Minnesota.

ALAN L. ORVIS,   M.S. (Physics), Ph.D. (Physics)

Department of Therapeutic Radiology, Mayo Clinic; Associate
Professor of Biophysics, Mayo Graduate School of Medicine
(University of Minnesota), Rochester, Minnesota.

GREGG ORWOLL,   LL.B.

Legal Counsel, Department of Administration,
Mayo Clinic, Rochester, Minnesota.

DOZ. DR. MED. HABIL. RAINER THIERBACH

Oberarzt, Pathologisches Institut der Martin Luther Universität,
Halle/Saale, Deutsche Demokratische Republik.

JACK L. TITUS,   M.D., Ph.D. (Pathology)

Department of Experimental and Anatomic Pathology, Mayo Clinic;
Associate Professor of Pathology, Mayo Graduate School of
Medicine (University of Minnesota), Rochester, Minnesota.

PREFACE

This book was written to serve two purposes. The first is to provide quick orientation on autopsy techniques or policies in various conditions. The second is to assist pathologists who wish to extend their autopsy services and facilities and who have to determine what can be done and what is needed.

Of the techniques to be presented herein, some may seem too specialized and others, too pedestrian. Most basic dissection methods are merely touched on—they are best taught by preceptors, and instructive books on them are plentiful. Although my coauthors and I have drawn heavily on the experiences of others, most of the techniques in this book have been tested in our morgue and laboratories; some methods have been witnessed in other institutions, and a few were chosen from the literature. References have been selected not only to document sources but also to provide the reader with alternative approaches. Of course, variations of autopsy techniques are unlimited, and adaptations to local conditions are often required. Besides, technical procedures, no matter how sophisticated, cannot replace interest, open-mindedness, knowledge, and enthusiasm. If the desired information is gained, the methods by which this is accomplished become quite unimportant.

Traditional autopsy procedures will remain as the basis of our work, but they must be supplemented by newer techniques and facilities if we want to remain in step with future teaching obligations and with the advancement of research. The methods of microbiology, roentgenology, biochemistry, tissue culture, and other special fields, as well as refined dissection, preservation, and documentation methods, will be needed in many autopsy services. It is hoped that this book will assist in this endeavor.

Much of the technical work which has been described and illustrated in this book was carried out by the supervisors of our autopsy laboratory, Mr. William H. Mayo (retired) and Mr. Robert V. Mieras, and by their co-workers. The support from our autopsy technicians is greatly appreciated and has been a continued source of satisfaction for my colleagues and myself.

My secretaries, Mrs. Constance McNallan and Mrs. Teresa A. Hughes, were of great help during the preparation of the original manuscript. I also want to thank the members of our Division of Instructional Media, especially Mr. Reignold V. Yule and Mr. Leo O. Johnson. It is a pleasure to acknowledge the help of Miss Joyce E. Morrel who did much of the art work.

I wish to express my thanks especially to Dr. Bernard K. Forscher and his associates in our Section of Publications. Dr. Forscher provided expert editing of this text, Mrs. Nancy Nelson did the proofreading, and Mrs. Betty Calkins prepared the final manuscript. The friendly cooperation of our publisher, the W. B. Saunders Company, is very much appreciated. Acknowledgments to specific journals and authors for permission to use their illustrations are made in the legends of the appropriate figures.

JURGEN LUDWIG
Rochester, Minnesota

CONTENTS

CHAPTER 1

PRINCIPLES OF AUTOPSY TECHNIQUES   1

CHAPTER 2

MEDICOLEGAL AUTOPSIES AND AUTOPSY TOXICOLOGY .   11
    with Jauw T. Lie

CHAPTER 3

HEART AND VASCULAR SYSTEM   51
    with Jack L. Titus

CHAPTER 4

TRACHEOBRONCHIAL TREE AND LUNGS   93

CHAPTER 5

ESOPHAGUS AND ABDOMINAL VISCERA   129

CHAPTER 6

NERVOUS SYSTEM   157
    by Haruo Okazaki

CHAPTER 7

SKELETAL SYSTEM   195

CHAPTER 8

SPECIAL METHODS   207

    Autopsy Microbiology   207

    with C. Terrence Dolan

    Electron Microscopy of Autopsy Tissues   216

    Arnold L. Brown, Jr.

    Chromosome Study of Autopsy Tissues   217

    with Jack L. Titus

CHAPTER 9

AUTOPSY LABORATORY PROCEDURES   229

CHAPTER 10

AUTOPSY OF BODIES CONTAINING RADIOACTIVE
    ISOTOPES   245

    with Alan L. Orvis

CHAPTER 11

MUSEUM TECHNIQUES   253

CHAPTER 12

AUTOPSY PROTOCOLS, DEATH CERTIFICATES, AND
    INTERVIEWS   263

CHAPTER 13

ORGANIZATION OF THE AUTOPSY SERVICE AND TISSUE
    REGISTRY AND METHODS OF DATA RETRIEVAL . .   275

    with R. Thierbach and Robert C. Bahn

CHAPTER 14

MEDICOLEGAL CONSIDERATIONS   297

    with Gregg Orwoll

CHAPTER 15

AUTOPSIES — PAST, PRESENT, AND FUTURE   307

APPENDIX

NORMAL WEIGHTS AND MEASUREMENTS   315

INDEX   349

CHAPTER 1

PRINCIPLES OF AUTOPSY TECHNIQUES

CLASSICAL AUTOPSY TECHNIQUES

References. The most comprehensive text on classical autopsy techniques and their variations and combinations was written by Rössle,[21] in German. The techniques of Albrecht, Fischer, Ghon, Heller, Letulle, Nauwerck, Rokitansky, Virchow, and Zenker, among others, are described. For detailed English descriptions and illustrations of the techniques which are presently used in most institutions the reader is referred to the *Autopsy Manual*[25] of the Armed Forces Institute of Pathology, and the textbooks by Baker,[1] Mallory,[13] and Saphir.[22]

A series of films entitled "Autopsy Dissection Technique—A Cinematographic Atlas" is available for free loan (16 mm only) from:

National Medical Audiovisual Center
Station K
Atlanta, Georgia 30324

These films also can be purchased, as 16 mm, regular 8 mm, or "Super" 8 mm, from:

General Services Administration
National Audiovisual Center
National Archives & Records Service
Washington, D.C. 20409
Attn.: Government Film Sales

The available film titles with price lists and order numbers (National Audiovisual Center Catalogue No.) are available from these centers.

Principal Techniques. The autopsy techniques used in most centers at present differ little in their end results if they are properly executed. Therefore, the pathologist is well advised to depend on the method he masters best. The less experience he has, the closer he should adhere to his scheme. On the other hand, informative specimens cannot be prepared without some technical versatility. Virchow[26] made the following comment on variations of his technique:

> It is scarcely necessary to point out that there are many cases in which deviations from this method are not merely allowable, but also absolutely necessary. The individuality of the case must often determine the plan of the examination. But we must not begin with individualizing, nor make a rule of the exceptions. The expert may allow himself to make alterations, supposing that they are well grounded, but he must be able to remember his motive for so doing, and also to state it.

Most autopsy techniques differ from each other in the order in which the organs are removed, in the planes and lines of sectioning, and, most important, as to whether single organs or intact organ systems are removed from the body.

Technique of R. Virchow.   Organs are removed one by one. This method[13,25,26] has been most widely used, often with some modifications.* Originally, the first step was to expose the cranial cavity and, from the back, the spinal cord, followed by the thoracic, cervical, and abdominal organs, in that order.

Technique of C. Rokitansky.   This technique is characterized by in situ dissection, in part combined with en bloc removal. Only "second-hand" descriptions are available.[13,14,18] The term "Rokitansky's technique" is used erroneously by many pathologists to designate the "en masse" or "en bloc" removal techniques which are referred to in the following two paragraphs.

Technique of A. Ghon.   Thoracic and cervical organs, abdominal organs, and, separately, the urogenital system are removed as organ blocks.[13] Modifications of Ghon's "en bloc" removal technique are now widely used.

Technique of M. Letulle.   Thoracic, cervical, abdominal, and pelvic organs are removed en masse and subsequently dissected into organ blocks.[11,13,22] The steps for dissecting the organ mass are described by Saphir.[22] This technique is probably the best for routine inspection and preservation of connections between organs and organ systems. Another advantage is that the body can be made available to the undertaker in less than 30 minutes without having to rush the dissection. It sometimes may be better to save the whole organ block in a refrigerator rather than to obscure findings or to destroy important specimens by a hasty dissection. Unfortunately, the organ mass is often awkward to handle.

ADULT AUTOPSIES

A detailed description of routine autopsy techniques in adults is beyond the scope of this book. This is a general program for the sequence of suggested procedures:

> External description, including body weight and length; roentgen-

---

* See references 2-7, 27, 30.

ographic examination; Y-shaped primary incision; removal of material from abdomen for microbiologic study; collection of abdominal effusions and exudates; recording of height of diaphragm and level of liver edge; search for herniae; incision of anterior abdominal musculature and breasts; search for pneumothorax; cutting of lower ribs so that chest plate can be lifted and pleural effusion or exudates can be collected; removal of chest plate; removal of thymus fat pad; collection of pericardial contents; removal of heart or peripheral blood for microbiologic and biochemical studies; identification of carotid, subclavian, and femoral arteries for embalmer.

At this point the technique may be varied according to the type of lesion. En masse removal is used when pathologic lesions are expected to involve or pass through the diaphragmatic level, such as dissecting aortic aneurysms. The dissection is then carried out from the posterior aspect of the organ mass.[22] Organ blocks[13] are removed routinely or only when pathologic processes make the preservation of vascular supplies desirable. In all other cases Virchow's technique can be followed.

The central nervous system, peripheral nerves, muscles, bones, and joints usually are exposed at the end of the autopsy, often after embalming.

PEDIATRIC AUTOPSIES

There are numerous descriptions of pediatric autopsy techniques in the older literature.* Most pathologists currently follow the technique described by Potter.[20] Langley[10] has recently published a technique for perinatal postmortem examination.

The external examination, particularly of fetuses and newborns, has to concentrate on the search for malformations such as cleft palate, choanal atresia, or stenosis and atresia of the anus or vagina. Face, ears, or hands may show characteristic changes—for instance, in Down's syndrome, renal agenesis, or gargoylism. The placenta and umbilical cord must be studied in all autopsies of fetuses and newborns.

There is a difference from adult autopsies in the way in which the skull is opened in fetuses and newborns. Usually, windows are cut into the parietal bone ("Beneke technique," see page 160).

In infants, the whole chest cavity can be opened under water in order to demonstrate a pneumothorax. In fetuses and infants, the en masse removal (after Letulle) is the preferable technique in most cases so that certain rare malformations can be properly preserved—for example, anomalous pulmonary venous connections.

Potter[20] lists both lungs, liver, kidney, thymus, and brain as the organs of which histologic sections should be taken as a minimal requirement. In fetuses and newborns, placenta and umbilical cord should be added to this list.

---

* See references 2-7, 13, 21, 22, 26, 27.

POSTOPERATIVE AUTOPSIES

Few autopsies offer more difficulties than postoperative cases. The pathologist often has to evaluate problems with possible medicolegal implications, such as complications of surgical intervention, anesthesia, or drug administration. The following rules are helpful.

1. If several pathologists are available, the most experienced one should perform postoperative autopsies. The help of an assistant pathologist is desirable.

2. The pathologist should insist that the surgeon attend the autopsy or, if this cannot be arranged, that one of the surgeon's assistants who actually participated in the operation is present.

3. Before starting the autopsy the pathologist should thoroughly familiarize himself with the surgical report, the case history, and the results of roentgenographic and laboratory studies. The pathologist should delay the autopsy rather than start working without the benefit of all the necessary information.

4. The autopsy technique should be changed as necessary for the individual case. Incisions should not be carried through operative wounds; these wounds should be viewed from their outer and inner aspects before they are opened and inspected, particularly for suture abscesses. No tension should be applied to sutures. To determine whether a dehiscence developed before or after death, the sutured region should be widely excised and fixed for preparation of properly oriented histologic sections for evaluation of vital tissue reactions. In all cases, air embolism (page 20) must be ruled out, and chest roentgenograms or other appropriate tests for pneumothorax should be performed.[12]

Fistulas should be filled with a stained contrast medium, such as green-stained ethiodized oil (Ethiodol) or diatrizoate (Hypaque), and their course should be demonstrated by roentgenograms and dissection. Drains should not be removed before their precise location has been established, always from an incision distant from the site of the drain. At repeated and appropriate intervals, material for microbiologic examination should be removed. This may be of considerable help in determining the source of an infection.

5. Instructive views of all decisive phases of the autopsy should be documented by photographs.

6. Protocols of postoperative autopsies should be dictated during the actual inspection and dissection of organs. At a later time, surgically significant findings often cannot be recalled and described accurately.

The volume of free fluid should be measured in milliliters. Scars, wounds, and all other significant lesions should be measured in centimeters; weights should be recorded in grams.

7. During the autopsy, the pathologist should describe his findings but not interpret or comment on them. Many pathologists have learned to regret statements they made during the autopsy, only to be proved wrong by later findings.

At the end of the autopsy the pathologist should point out which findings need histologic confirmation.

RESTRICTED AUTOPSIES

Restriction of Skin Incision.   An autopsy permission may specify that only an abdominal incision is to be made. If appropriate consent is given, all thoracic, cervical, and abdominal organs may be removed through such an incision, either organ by organ, en bloc, or en masse.[4,6,16] It seems doubtful that Mallory[13] was correct when he stated that even without special permission it is legitimate for pathologists to remove more than the organs of the body cavity which had been incised.

Autopsies Through Surgical Wounds.   Such an autopsy is done when the autopsy permission is restricted to the reopening of a surgical wound.[19] Techniques and legal implications are similar to those of autopsies through restricted skin incisions.

Autopsies Through Anus and Vagina.   This approach is only of historic interest.[4,6]

Needle Autopsies.   If all efforts to obtain permission for a regular autopsy fail, the next of kin sometimes will agree to multiple sampling by needle.[28] The autopsy permission may specify the organ which is to be studied, or permission may be granted for unlimited study. Vim-Silverman needles are recommended. Terry[24] suggested using a 15-cm-long needle with a bore of 3 mm and fitted to a 20-ml syringe. A trocar on the piston projects 1 cm beyond the needle. The trocar is flattened along one side; the point of the needle is notched and sharpened.

For the less experienced, the yield of "needle autopsies" was found[28] to be best for liver, followed by heart, lung, and kidneys. Motivation also seemed to play a role. In a study[28] of 394 consecutive needle autopsy cases, meaningful pathologic alterations were found in more than 77%. However, in another paper,[29] discrepancies between the results of needle autopsies and subsequent complete autopsies were found in 52% of the cases.

SPECIAL PROBLEMS

Adhesions.   Extensive adhesions, particularly between intestinal loops, can be demonstrated best by en bloc removal and fixation of the organs involved. Subsequently, sections may be cut through the whole organ block in such a manner that the slices remain connected to each other posteriorly.[23] If pleural adhesions cannot be severed, extrapleural separation of the lungs must be carried out.

Hernias.   Peritoneal hernias are diagnosed by careful palpation, through the abdominal incision, of all potential hernia sites.

A sliding hiatus hernia is best demonstrated by the method of Melcher.[15] The stomach is opened in situ so that the mucosal fold overlying the sling muscle fibers of the esophagus can be identified. An artery forceps is applied to the mucosal fold or sling muscle fibers, and then the thoracic esophagus is pulled upward. If this maneuver moves the tip of the forceps above the diaphragm, a potential sliding hiatus hernia is present.

Lesions of Face, Arms, or Hands.   The face is essentially "off limits" for the autopsy pathologist. Small specimens of facial skin tumors occasionally can be taken, particularly when the tumor is large enough to cover the defect. Extensive lesions of the subcutaneous and deep tissues of the face or facial bones may be removed only with special permission. Reconstruction is difficult. A positive plaster of Paris cast is made from a negative mold. Such a negative mold may be prepared from a dried but still moist mixture of agar (100 parts), oil soap (100 parts), magnesium sulfate (40 parts), absorbent cellulose wadding (12 parts), and water (700 to 800 parts).[17] For final restoration, the embalmed skin of the face is placed into the death mask. The plaster of Paris mask is used to recast the facial features. I have never seen this procedure performed.

Accidental iatrogenic lesions of the face may occur—for instance, when the autopsy knife pierces the lips during the removal of the floor of the mouth. The nose may be deformed when the skin of the chest is placed on the face, particularly when breasts and subcutaneous tissue are heavy.

Tissues of the arms and hands should be examined only with special permission. It is suggested that the skin be cut completely around the upper arm and then inverted and rolled downward until the arm lesions are exposed. If bones, joints, or soft tissues of the hands are to be removed, the incisions should be placed at the volar surfaces. An adequate prosthesis must be provided (see page 199).

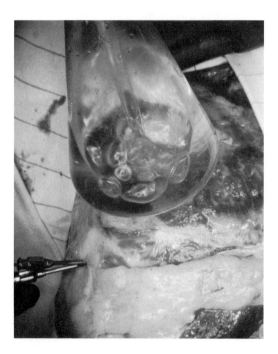

Figure 1–1. Tension pneumothorax. Skin has been dissected off right side of chest, and needle is inserted into chest wall. Rubber hose connects needle with glass tube. Note gas bubbles emerging from tip of glass tube at bottom of water-filled flask.

Pneumothorax, Pneumomediastinum, Subcutaneous Emphysema, and Free Air in the Abdomen.   The simplest qualitative method for the diagnosis of pneumothorax is to incise the thorax at the base of a water-filled skin pocket.[2] Infants can be totally submerged under water before the chest cavity is incised. One also can inspect the chest cavity through the parietal pleura after the intercostal muscles have been scraped off,[9] and one can aspirate gas from a pneumothorax with a water- or oil-filled syringe. It is more reliable to insert a needle into the chest wall and to test whether gas bubbles appear in an attached water-filled flask (Fig. 1–1).

A combined qualitative and quantitative method[8] has been used for the demonstration of air embolism (see page 23) and probably could be adjusted to the gas volumes encountered in ordinary or tension pneumothorax.

Postmortem chest roentgenograms[12] are valuable for the diagnosis of a pneumothorax (Fig. 1–2). Chest roentgenography should be carried out in all cases in which routine aspiration techniques indicate the presence of gas

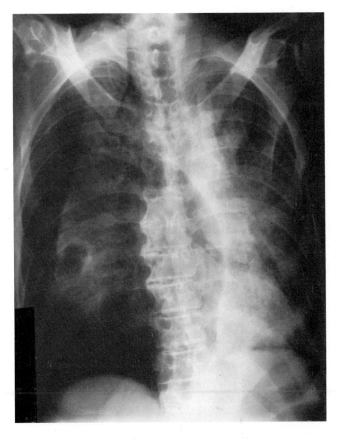

Figure 1–2. Tension pneumothorax in postmortem chest roentgenogram on right side, with marked shift of mediastinum to left. There is some consolidation and a 5-cm cavity in lateral midportion of right lung. (From Ludwig J, Miller WE, Sessler AD: Clinically unsuspected pneumothorax: a postmortem roentgenographic study. Arch Pathol 90:274–277, 1970. By permission of the American Medical Association.)

in the pleural cavity. Roentgenography is the only method to evaluate reliably the extent of the pneumothorax and its main complication, mediastinal shift. Roentgenograms also provide a permanent record.

Pneumomediastinum and subcutaneous emphysema can be diagnosed by inspection, palpation, and roentgenography. Free air in the abdomen can be diagnosed only by roentgenography. Therefore, most clinically unsuspected cases will escape detection at autopsy.

REFERENCES

1. Baker RD: Postmortem Examination: Specific Methods and Procedures. Philadelphia, W. B. Saunders Company, 1967
2. Box CR: Post-mortem Manual: A Handbook of Morbid Anatomy and Post-mortem Technique. London, J. & A. Churchill, Ltd., 1910
3. Busse O: Das Obduktionsprotokoll. Fourth edition. Berlin, Richard Schoetz-Verlag, 1911
4. Cattell HW: Postmortem Pathology: A Manual of the Technic of Post-mortem Examinations and the Interpretations To Be Drawn Therefrom; a Practical Treatise for Students and Practitioners. Third edition. Philadelphia, J. B. Lippincott Company, 1906
5. Delafield F: A Hand-Book of Post-mortem Examinations and of Morbid Anatomy. New York, W. Wood & Co., 1872
6. Farber S: The Postmortem Examination. Springfield, Illinois, Charles C Thomas, Publisher, 1937
7. Hektoen L: The Technique of Post-mortem Examination. Chicago, The W. S. Keener Co., 1894
8. Kulka W: Laboratory methods and technical notes: a practical device for demonstrating air embolism. Arch Pathol *48*:366–369, 1949
9. Kurtz DM: Pneumothorax at Autopsy. *In* Summary Report (Issue No. 86). Vol VI, No. 62. Chicago, ASCP Commission on Continuing Education, September, 1969
10. Langley FA: The perinatal postmortem examination. J Clin Pathol *24*:159–169, 1971
11. Letulle M: Cited by Baker RD[1]
12. Ludwig J, Miller WE, Sessler AD: Clinically unsuspected pneumothorax: a postmortem roentgenographic study. Arch Pathol *90*:274–277, 1970
13. Mallory FB: Pathological Technique: A Practical Manual for Workers in Pathological Histology, Including Directions for the Performance of Autopsies and Microphotography. Philadelphia, W. B. Saunders Company, 1938
14. Maresch R, Chiari H: Anleitung zur Vornahme von Leichenöffnungen. Wien, Urban & Schwarzenberg, 1933
15. Melcher DH: The anatomy and post-mortem diagnosis of sliding hiatus hernia. Proceedings of the Pathological Society of Great Britain and Ireland, July, 1968
16. Menon TB: A technique for making a more or less complete post-mortem examination through an incision in the upper abdomen. Indian J Med Res *15*:907–908, 1928
17. Moritz AR: Repair of the body after autopsy. Hospitals *12*:78–81 (June) 1938
18. Nauwerck C: Sektionstechnik fur Studierende und Aerzte. Sixth edition. Jena, Gustav Fischer Verlag, 1921
19. Polayes SH: Complete postmortem examinations through surgical wounds. J Lab Clin Med *22*:87–88, 1936
20. Potter EL: Pathology of the Fetus and Infant. Second edition. Chicago, Year Book Medical Publishers, Inc., 1961, pp 71–81
21. Rössle R: Technik der Obduktion mit Einschluss der Massmethoden an Leichenorganen. *In* Handbuch der Biologischen Arbeitsmethoden. Vol VIII, part 1 (2). Edited by E Abderhalden. Berlin, Urban & Schwarzenberg, 1935, pp 1093–1246
22. Saphir O: Autopsy Diagnosis and Technic. Fourth edition. New York, Paul B. Hoeber, Inc., 1958
23. Schorr G: Die Forderungen der Thanatologie an die moderne Leichenuntersuchungsmethodik. Virchows Arch [Pathol Anat] *264*:19–30, 1927
24. Terry R: Needle necropsy. J Clin Pathol *8*:38–41, 1955
25. US Department of Defense. Army Department: Autopsy Manual, Washington DC, US Government Printing Office, 1960

26. Virchow R: Post-mortem Examinations With Especial Reference to Medico-legal Practice. Fourth German Edition. (English translation by TP Smith) Philadelphia, P. Blakiston, Son & Co., 1885, p 15
27. Warthin AS: Practical Pathology: A Manual of Autopsy and Laboratory Technique for Students and Physicians. Second edition. Ann Arbor, Michigan, George Wahr, Publisher, 1928
28. Wellmann KF: The needle autopsy: a retrospective evaluation of 394 consecutive cases. Am J Clin Pathol 52:441–444, 1969
29. West M, Chomet B: An evaluation of needle necropsies. Am J Med Sci 234:554–560, 1957
30. Zilgien H: Manuel théorique et pratique des autopsies. Second edition. Paris, A. Maloine, 1911

CHAPTER 2

MEDICOLEGAL AUTOPSIES AND AUTOPSY TOXICOLOGY

With Jauw T. Lie

MEDICOLEGAL AUTOPSIES

Medicolegal autopsies should be carried out by certified forensic pathologists. Unfortunately, the critical shortage in this country of members of this profession will force general pathologists to perform medicolegal autopsies for years to come. A conservative estimate indicates that two thirds of the population of the United States live in areas without any kind of solid program in forensic pathology. In 1970, there were 164 physicians certified by the American Board of Pathology in the subspecialty of Forensic Pathology, but only 30 to 40 qualified forensic pathologists were in actual full-time practice in this country, clustered in a few large metropolitan areas.[22] The next decade will see increasing demands on our already overburdened medicolegal system; violent deaths are likely to increase in number. Causes of unnatural deaths, particularly those associated with drug abuse or overdosage, become more difficult to determine because of the multiplicity of drugs available. Furthermore, medicolegal work is becoming more taxing because of the distrust and hostility toward the American system of justice and law enforcement.[23]

In his Ward Burdick Award Address, Moritz[83] spoke, from his vast experience, of the frequency with which mistakes are made by good general pathologists in performing medicolegal autopsies. He also pointed out that in many instances a seemingly trivial error turns out to have disastrous consequences. Every would-be or "substitute" forensic pathologist should benefit enormously by reading and rereading Moritz' classic paper.

The technical aspects of medicolegal autopsies are well dealt with in several textbooks.[50,124,127]

A medical practitioner called to examine a person presumed to be dead must first ascertain that death has in fact occurred. Failure to do this has on occasions led to serious embarrassments and repercussions. A brief recapitulation of some facets of the early changes of death is pertinent here.

1. Cessation of respiration. As death approaches, the person frequently breathes in gasps. These apneic periods rarely last for more than 30 seconds and can be ruled out by extending the examination over a 10-minute period.

2. Cessation of circulation. A lack of peripheral pulse does not imply cardiac arrest, and the heart beat does not necessarily cease as soon as breathing stops. In the case of a legal hanging, the heart beat might persist for 10 to 15 minutes after the drop.[26]

3. Eye changes. Funduscopic examination has been used to assess the state of retinal circulation after death. The blood in the retinal veins breaks up into segments within seconds after circulatory stagnation, and the segments become stationary in the ensuing 10 to 20 minutes.[66]

Deaths From Natural Causes. Not all medicolegal autopsies deal with violent or unnatural deaths. Over half of all deaths investigated by the Office of the Chief Medical Examiner in New York were deaths from natural causes occurring suddenly, unexpectedly, or in an unusual manner. Arteriosclerotic cardiovascular disease and respiratory infection were the commonest causes, and the greatest incidence was in persons between 45 and 54 years of age.[50] The experiences of forensic pathologists working in other cities of the world have been similar. Table 2–1 presents a convenient checklist of the more common causes of natural deaths and their possible medicolegal implications.

Evaluation of Circumstances of Death. Investigation of the scene where the body was found may be most conclusive, particularly when a crime is suspected.[111] The physician at the scene of a violent death should see to it, whenever possible, that nothing is disturbed before the arrival of police officers. Masterly inactivity is the keynote at this stage of investigation. The position of the body, the distribution of blood lost by the victim or the assailant, or objects in the neighborhood of the body may offer important clues for the reconstruction of the fatal events. This type of investigation also may yield clues as to the approximate time of death (see below) and the interval that may have elapsed between injury and death. Remember, if you are not a specialist in the field of criminal investigation you should try to secure all the help you can get from law enforcement agencies. If the pathologist does not see the site where the body was found, he has to rely on the written report of the circumstances of death with photographs or illustrating sketches which should be available in all medicolegal cases.

The Forensic Autopsy Protocol. A standard autopsy protocol for forensic and accident pathology has been developed by the Registry of Accident Pathology (Armed Forces Institute of Pathology, Washington, D.C.). This autopsy report form (1) permits a checklist-recording of medicolegal data

TABLE 2–1. SOME COMMON CAUSES OF NONVIOLENT DEATHS AND THEIR POSSIBLE MEDICOLEGAL IMPLICATIONS

Condition	Possible Medicolegal Implication
Central nervous system	
Meningitis; cerebral abscess	Fractured skull, jaw, facial bones; injuries to middle ear, nasopharynx, air sinuses; infection introduced by surgical, anesthetic, roentgenologic, chemotherapeutic, diagnostic procedures
Cerebral hemorrhage; subarachnoid hemorrhage; subdural hematoma	Trauma
Meningioma	Trauma (?)
Arteriovenous fistula	Trauma
Cardiovascular system	
Coronary artery insufficiency	Emotional or strenuous physical effort related to occupation
Ruptured heart valve; aortic aneurysm	Trauma; strenuous physical effort
Congenital anomalies	Teratogenic drugs
"Vasovagal attacks"	Trauma; shock; fright
Respiratory system	
Upper airway obstruction	Foreign bodies; trauma; accidental, suicidal, or homicidal asphyxia
Pneumothorax; subcutaneous and mediastinal emphysema; hemopneumothorax	Trauma; strenuous physical effort; surgical, anesthetic, roentgenologic, chemotherapeutic, diagnostic procedures
Pneumonia; pulmonary embolism	Trauma; immobilization
Pulmonary fibrosis; mesothelioma; pneumoconiosis	Exposure to radiation; drugs; asbestosis; industrial exposure
Alimentary system	
Ruptured viscus; perforated ulcer; peritonitis; intestinal obstruction	Trauma; burns; strenuous physical effort; foreign bodies; diagnostic or therapeutic endoscopy; paracentesis; peritoneal dialysis
Acute pancreatitis; bleeding varices; cirrhosis of liver; alcoholic hepatitis	Alcoholic intoxication, acute or chronic
Fulminant toxic hepatitis; massive hepatic necrosis	Exposure to drugs, poisons, anesthetic agents, pesticides; shock
Genitourinary system	
Renal tubular necrosis; papillary necrosis	Poisons; drugs; heavy metals; burns; shock; dehydration
Cystitis, pyelonephritis; ruptured bladder; ruptured uterus; ruptured ectopic pregnancy	Trauma; abortion; injudicious instrumentation
Hematopoietic & reticuloendothelial system	
Hemolytic anemia	Incompatible blood transfusion
Aplastic anemia; agranulocytosis; thrombocytopenia; leukemia	Drugs; poisons; pesticides; industrial and laboratory chemicals; antibiotics
Miscellaneous	
Malnutrition; failure to thrive	Negligence; parental cruelty; eccentric or unusual religious beliefs
"Crib death"	Accidental or homicidal suffocation
"Sudden sniffing death" syndrome	?

in detail and (2) allows the placement of all data into a computer for automatic data processing. The form has 15 pages and is reproduced in the *Proceedings of the 1968 International Conference on Accident Pathology.*[9] There also are 17 pages of anatomic diagrams for optional use.

In order to ensure utmost accuracy, the protocol ideally should be dictated concurrently with the progress of the autopsy. All details must be painstakingly verified so that the value of the protocol is not jeopardized by minor errors. The subjective and objective sections of the protocol should not be confused.[83] Identifying features must be carefully recorded (see below).

Measurements are given in centimeters, grams, and milliliters (see Conversion Tables in Appendix). For legal documents, lay terms such as "teaspoonful" are used, and measurements are given in inches, pounds, and pints. Estimations and hazy terminology such as "extreme" or "large" are to be avoided. "Normal" may be used for organ descriptions.

The protocols should be extensively supplemented by diagrams, sketches, roentgenograms, and photographs. There should always be a metric scale on each picture near the photographed object, and the protocol should include exposure time and other technical photographic data. Casts should be initialed.

The Chain of Custody.   In medicolegal cases the chain of custody of the body must be documented by a record in which each person in charge is identified, including when the body came into his custody and when the period of custody ended. At all times, care must be taken that no one tampers with the body without properly recorded authorization. It is advisable to put a lock on the refrigerator or on the room in which the body is kept.

There also must be a record of chain of custody for other physical evidence such as toxicologic material or bullets. Such material should be saved in sealed containers, each labeled with all significant data and numbered with the corresponding description in the protocol—for instance, to indicate the exact site from which the foreign body had been removed. Confusion is avoided if each specimen is bottled, labeled, and sealed with sealing wax right after it is removed. The pathologist who seals the container should impress his fingerprint on the seal while it is still warm.

Identification of the Body.   All identifying features must be entered into the autopsy protocol. Overall and close-up photographs of the face are important. For the identification of dismembered, decomposed, or burned bodies or parts of bodies, assistance of the State Crime Bureau should be requested—for example, for proper fingerprinting or for serologic studies to differentiate between human and animal tissues. Head hair and pubic hair should be saved for identification purposes; fingernail scrapings should be saved, particularly in homicide cases. Blood typing should be carried out. Roentgenograms may permit positive identification when compared with roentgenograms taken during life.[89] They may also help in determinations of sex, age, and race.

Dentures, teeth, and jawbones may permit reliable identification by dentists and forensic odontologists,[45,52] who also will evaluate roentgeno-grams, photographs, and plaster molds.

Sex determination can be attempted from the contours of the pelvis and skull, size and contour of long bones, and physical or chemical analysis of teeth.[11,45]

Age determination can be based on evaluation of epiphyses, laryngeal and sternocostal cartilages, sacral, hyoid, and cranial bone sutures, and the condition of joints and teeth.[11,28]

Stature is reconstructed by anthropologic methods. Long bones can be used for this purpose by applying Pearson's formula.[85]

Estimation of Time of Death. The ideal method for accurate estimation of the time of death remains to be described. Reliance should not be placed on a single sign as evidence of the time of death. There are exceptions to the development of even well-defined postmortem changes. In most cases, after all available information has been considered, only an approximate time of death can be given, and the pathologist should clearly state this when asked to give his opinion.

Association Method. The time of death is estimated by circumstantial evidence. For instance, when, after a rainy night, the ground under the body was found to be dry, death probably occurred before the onset of rain.

Rate Methods for Short Postmortem Intervals. The time of death is estimated from physical or chemical measurements of values whose rate of postmortem change has been found empirically to be fairly constant. Unfortunately, these methods are not very useful and most seem to be applicable only to short postmortem intervals.

1. The postmortem temperature regression is roughly 1 C/hr in the axilla and in the rectum; it is somewhat faster in the cisterna magna. Estimations of the postmortem interval are most reliable when the outside temperature is constant, when the body temperature is measured repeatedly in 30-minute intervals for 2 to 3 hours, and when the postmortem interval is not longer than about 4 hours.[107] Clothing, body build, and overheating prior to death, as in some cases of cerebral hemorrhage or asphyxia, may affect the reliability of the calculations. The formulas for calculating the time of death reported in the literature were reviewed by Marshall.[78] It must be noted that the accuracy obtained under experimental conditions cannot be assumed to extend to practical situations in which the investigator has to contend with errors which will affect the results of any temperature formula no matter how accurate it is. Two of the better known methods will be given here.

The formula of Moritz,[82]

$$\text{Postmortem interval (hours)} = \frac{98.6 - \text{rectal temperature (F)}}{1.5}$$

or

$$= \frac{37 - \text{rectal temperature (C)}}{0.83},$$

applies to the idealistic situation of an adult of average body build and nutrition and wearing indoor clothing who is found in a room with an environmental temperature between 50 and 70 F (10 and 21 C).

The method of Fiddes and Patten[38] is based on the "virtual cooling time." To use this method, one needs to know the prevailing atmospheric temperature where the body lies and the rectal temperature of the body (1) soon after the body was found and (2) at an interval of 3 to 4 hours later. The authors give the following practical example which best explains the principle and the application of this method.

> The body of a dead man is found in a house at 11:30 a.m. Rectal temperature is determined first at 12 noon and again at 3:00 p.m.
> Presumed rectal temperature at time of death = 99 F
> Prevailing atmospheric temperature in the room = 52 F
> Temperature difference at the time of death = 47 F
> Rectal temperature at noon = 83 F,
>   a decrease of 16 F = 34% temperature difference
> Rectal temperature at 3:00 p.m. = 79 F
>   a decrease of 20 F = 42.6% temperature difference
> From Figure 2–1 it is seen that a decrease through the first 34% of the temperature difference occupies 23.5% of the virtual cooling time and a decrease through the first 42.6% of the temperature difference occupies 31% of the virtual cooling time. Therefore, in this case, 7.5% (31 − 23.5) of the virtual cooling time = 3 hours (12 noon to 3:00 p.m.) and thus the virtual cooling time is 40 hours. At noon, 23.5% of the virtual cooling time had already elapsed—that is, 9.4 hours. Therefore, the time of death was approximately 2:30 a.m.

2. Chemical postmortem changes also can be used. Amino acids, xanthine, and hypoxanthine in cerebrospinal fluid and creatine in serum

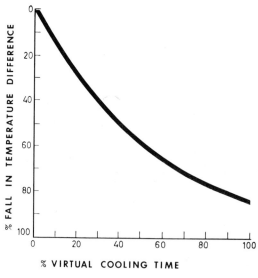

Figure 2–1. Virtual cooling time, per cent. (Redrawn from Fiddes FS, Patten TD: A percentage method for representing the fall in body temperature after death: its use in estimating the time of death. J Forensic Med 5:2–15, 1958.)

or cerebrospinal fluid seem to be of some value in estimating the post-mortem interval.[107]

Amino acid concentrations increase after death in approximately linear fashion. If the amino acid nitrogen in cerebrospinal fluid is less than 14 mg/100 ml, death may be presumed to have occurred less than 10 hours previously.

The concentration of xanthine plus hypoxanthine in spinal fluid increases during the first 8 hours after death, at a fairly constant rate.[99] There is much fluctuation after 8 hours.

A serum creatine value of less than 11 mg/100 ml indicates a post-mortem interval of less than 28 hours. Values less than 5 mg/100 ml indicate a postmortem interval of less than 12 hours. Cerebrospinal fluid creatine values less than 10 mg/100 ml indicate a postmortem interval of less than 30 hours; values less than 5 mg/100 ml indicate a postmortem interval of less than 10 hours.[35] However, creatine measurements for the estimation of the postmortem interval can only be used when antemortem azotemia can be ruled out.

Inorganic serum phosphorus in a concentration greater than 15 mg/100 ml usually indicates a postmortem interval of more than 10 hours.[35]

3. A great number of physical[107] and chemical[29,35,76,107] postmortem changes have been found to be unsuitable for the determination of post-mortem intervals. Postmortem functions, such as muscle excitability or sweat gland activity, have not yet been sufficiently studied to be helpful.

Rate Methods for Long Postmortem Intervals. The potassium concentration in vitreous humor permits fairly reliable prediction of postmortem intervals of more than 24 hours but less than 95 hours.[71] Two to 3 ml of vitreous humor of one or both eyes is gently aspirated from the lateral angle of the eye with a 10-ml sterile syringe (Fig. 2–2). The tip of the needle should lie near the center of the eyeball. Forceful aspiration must be avoided because it may detach retinal cells which cloud the specimen and give spuriously high potassium values. Before dilution, the specimen must be inverted more than 10 or 12 times to ensure thorough mixing. The vitreous humor may be stored refrigerated (4 C) for up to 48 hours. The potassium concentration may be determined by flame photometry or atomic absorption spectrophotometry. The postmortem interval is calculated[71] from the formula of Sturner:

Postmortem interval (hours) = (7.14 × K⁺ concentration [mEq/liter]) − 39.1.

Longer postmortem intervals can be estimated roughly from post-mortem autolysis, rigor mortis,[46] and livor mortis. Muscular rigidity begins after 2 to 4 hours and disappears after 24 to 84 hours. The dark line of gravitating blood reaches its maximum after 8 to 12 hours. Putrefaction is very slow in newborns; it may be rapid in persons with infectious diseases, congestive heart failure, or malignant tumors involving the intestinal tract. Extreme cold or dryness may delay putrefaction indefinitely whereas, in a moist, warm environment, putrefaction may occur in a very short time after death.

The presence of maggots or insect larvae may be helpful in deter-

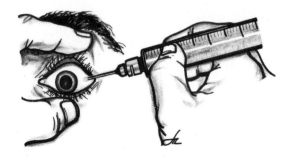

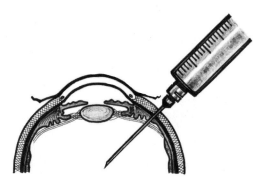

Figure 2–2. *Upper,* Aspiration of vitreous humor from lateral angle of eye. *Lower,* Correct position of aspirating needle.

mining the time of death. Certain insects lay eggs or deposit living larvae only during certain phases of the postmortem period. Adipocere formation requires weeks or months and occurs most often in a moist atmosphere.[98]

Embalming.   Embalming must never be allowed prior to medicolegal autopsies. Not only do the induced changes of color and consistency make proper evaluation impossible but also bacteriologic, most toxicologic, and many other laboratory tests become useless after the embalming procedure.

Cyanide reacts chemically with formaldehyde so that it is no longer identifiable. Many embalming fluids contain methyl or ethyl alcohol or both, so that analysis for these substances is meaningless. Prior fixation of tissues with formalin solution also makes them more resistant to extraction of nonvolatile organic compounds, and thus recovery of these substances is falsely low.[40]

The Examination.   *External.*   Clothing must be carefully examined. In many instances, such as firearm injuries, clothing must be saved as important evidence. Attention is directed to weight, height, complexion, age (estimated if unknown), color of hair and eyes, scars, tattoo marks, bite marks, puncture marks of hypodermic needles, wounds (bruises, lacerations, mutilations), appearance and content of body orifices, and appearance of hands and feet (in particular, of the fingernails). Most identifying features will be recorded during this phase of the autopsy. It is obvious that the external examination in medicolegal autopsies must be much more thorough and therefore more time-consuming than in ordinary autopsies.

Internal. The examination must be complete. Virchow's technique should be followed for the dissection of the thoracic, cervical, and abdominal organs. The first step should be the removal of cerebrospinal fluid. Roentgenograms should be prepared, ideally of all parts of the body but at least of areas of suspected trauma and foreign bodies. The primary incision should be modified in some cases by carrying the midline incision all the way up to the tip of the chin. This permits careful removal of the neck organs, particularly in cases of suspected strangling. Tests for pneumothorax are carried out as described in chapter 1. Tests for the presence of air embolism (see below) are particularly important in cases of abortion or trauma or postoperatively. In order to avoid laceration of the upper thoracic veins, only the lower three fourths of the chest plate should be removed. The heart chambers are punctured under water. The volume of the escaping gas must be recorded. Heart blood, peripheral blood, bile, and urine are collected in properly labeled containers for chemical and toxicologic examination (see Autopsy Toxicology). If a test for air embolism had been carried out and the pericardial sac was filled with water, care must be taken not to let it mix with the heart blood which is to be analyzed. In general, the remainder of the internal examination will not differ significantly from a routine autopsy. Certain conditions may require special procedures. Some are discussed below.

Special Procedures. *Abortion.* Examination of genital organs must include the pelvic veins. Fetal parts, foreign bodies, instrument marks, and perforations are especially looked for. The age of the fetus should be estimated. Breast tissue is studied histologically. Tests for air embolism (see below) must be carried out in all cases. Because water with antiseptics or soap solution may have been introduced into the uterus, osmium fixation of lung tissue for electron microscopy has been recommended. This will help to identify embolized soap or other solutions.[15] Bacteriologic studies of blood, lung tissue, and other organs are particularly important in later stages when septicemia may be expected to occur.

Vehicular Accidents. Numerous important aspects of modern practice and research in accident pathology have been published in the *Proceedings of the 1968 International Conference on Accident Pathology.*[9] Inspection of the scene of the accident may be essential for its reconstruction and for the interpretation of wounds and the mode of dying.[101] Drag marks may indicate that the victim had crawled from the car and was not ejected. The presence or absence of restraint systems and whether they had been in use must be recorded. The victim's injuries may yield valuable information regarding the mechanism of the accident. Spitz[113] pointed out that not every injury can be interpreted and that patterned injuries should primarily be considered, such as the imprint of a door knob, which is known by experience to be caused in a specific way. Incisions should be made into soft tissues to reveal injuries which may be accompanied by minimal or no injuries of the overlying skin and which may help to locate the points of impact. Evidence of preexisting disease or physical disability must be looked for, although this seems rarely to be responsible for the crash.[3]

Some vehicular accidents are suicidal. This should be suspected particularly when the circumstances of the accident seem obscure. Occasionally, suicide notes will be found. Rarely, premeditated homicide may be disguised as an accident. Suspicion arises when the accident cannot be reconstructed. Mechanical failure is another important consideration in vehicular accidents. The help of an experienced automobile mechanic may be required.

Wounds of accident victims, particularly those in hit and run accidents, should be excised to permit search for paint and glass fragments. Specimens should be saved for toxicologic examination, primarily for alcohol. Narcotics, hallucinogens, stimulants,[32] and depressants (see Autopsy Toxicology) also may be responsible for fatal traffic accidents, although this seems to be rare.[128]

Aircraft Accidents. Most principles of automobile accident investigation apply here also. Proper recording should include notes as to the site and the circumstances of the accident and the site and the position in which the bodies were found. Special autopsy guides are available.[65,115,124,125] The sudden influx of bodies following an aircraft accident and the request for speedy identification and autopsy of the victims overburden most institutions. Handling such a disaster requires an efficient organization, and it seems advisable to work out a plan before the necessity arises. It has been found practical to deal first with those bodies which seem the easiest to identify, so as to narrow the field for the more difficult cases. For the latter, dental records seem to offer the most certain method of identification.[123]

Photographs should document the more important autopsy findings. Roentgenograms of each victim should be prepared, both for identification purposes and because they may help to reconstruct the accident—for instance, when a bullet is found in the chest of the pilot. Material for chemical and toxicologic examination must be saved for the diagnosis of alcohol or carbon monoxide intoxication, drowning, or hypoxia (see below). The autopsy may not only reveal evidence of assault, burning, or sudden decompression but it also may indicate a natural cause of death—for instance, coronary occlusion. Histologic studies are essential to differentiate between antemortem and postmortem lesions.

Air Embolism. Air embolism may occur after injuries to large veins (especially in the neck, skull, or uterus), crush injuries of the chest, induction of artificial pneumothorax, insufflation of fallopian tubes (particularly in pregnancy or during the menstrual period), or criminal abortion. Air embolism also may occur as a complication of subclavian vein catheterization in the semi-Fowler position,[37] following blood transfusion when the bottle has emptied unnoticed (particularly when the pressure in the bottle has been artificially increased or when a pump is used),[100] or as a complication of positive-pressure ventilation in newborn infants.[51] The volume of air needed to cause death in adults is probably in the range of 100 ml.[109] In general, large volumes can enter the pulmonary circulation without being fatal, but a very small amount entering the systemic circulation may cause death within minutes.[100] Delayed air embolism with fatal outcome also may occur.[109]

If air embolism is suspected, the autopsy should be performed as soon after death as possible. Decomposition gases may be produced within a few hours. Roentgenography of the whole body may detect large quantities of air, and the roentgenograms may serve as a guide to the most advantageous way of dissection.[122]

Air embolism can be diagnosed if one succeeds in demonstrating, with an ophthalmoscope, air bubbles in the retinal arteries. This should be done as a first step of the autopsy in all cases in which this diagnosis is entertained. The cornea must be moistened with isotonic saline[66] so that opaqueness of it cannot interfere with this method of diagnosing air embolism.

After the ophthalmoscopic examination, the prosector opens the thoracic cavity, lifts the bony chest plate, clamps the internal mammary vessels below the sternoclavicular joint, and cuts across the sternum distal to these clamped vessels so that the sternoclavicular joint area remains intact. The pericardial sac is carefully opened. Large fatal pulmonary air embolism is readily apparent. The right atrium and ventricle are distended with fine, frothy, bright-red blood which also may distend the pulmonary arteries and large systemic veins. The blood is fluid throughout the body,

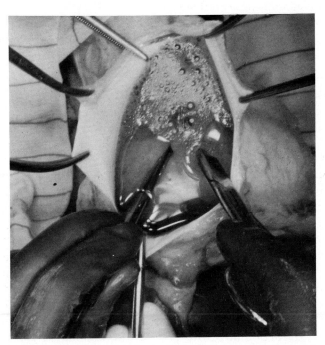

Figure 2–3. Gas-forming bacteria simulating air embolism. The pericardial sac is opened and filled with water. The heart is kept submerged with a pair of scissors. The coronary arteries have been incised with a scalpel. Note gas bubbles and foam on the water surface. No discoloration of 2% pyrogallol was noted. Blood cultures were positive for organisms of the enterococcus group. Microscopically, gram-negative rods were found in most tissues.

the viscera are congested, and petechiae are present in the serous surfaces and in the white matter of the brain. Microbiologic examination of blood and pericardial sac contents will help to rule out the presence of gas-forming bacteria which may simulate air embolism (Fig. 2–3). However, the differentiation between air and decomposition gases should be done at the autopsy table with the pyrogallol test.

> A 2% pyrogallol solution is prepared (it should be water-clear). Two 10-ml syringes (syringe A and syringe B) are loaded with 4 ml of the pyrogallol solution in each, without permitting any air to enter the system. Immediately before the solution is used, 4 drops of 0.5N NaOH are aspirated through the needle of syringe A to adjust the pH to about 8 (1 drop per 1 ml of solution); the mixture will turn faint yellow. Six milliliters of gas is then aspirated from the heart or blood vessels. The needle is immediately sealed with a cork or replaced by a cap, and the syringe is vigorously shaken for about 1 minute. In the presence of air, the pyrogallol solution will turn brown. If the solution remains clear, decomposition gases were present. In the latter instance, 4 drops of 0.5N NaOH and 6 ml of room air should be aspirated into syringe B which is then also sealed and shaken for 1 minute. The mixture should turn brown, thus serving as a control that pyrogallol solution had been properly prepared. Syringe B may also serve as a reserve. If only one syringe is used, the decomposition gas can be expelled and room air can be aspirated for the control test.
>
> If only small amounts of gas can be aspirated the volume of the pyrogallol solution should be decreased so that the gas-fluid volume ratio is at least 3:2.

If no bacterial gas formation is present, the edges of the pericardial incision are elevated and the pericardial sac is filled with water. Clamping of the ascending aorta and venae cavae prevents the escape of gas into these vessels. The heart is held under water while the coronary arteries are incised, and the escape of gas bubbles is observed. When the right coronary artery is opened, care must be taken that the right atrium is not incised. Air in the coronary arteries indicates systemic embolism. The heart chambers are then incised.

When there is gas in any of the arteries or heart chambers, gas bubbles rise to the surface of the water in the pericardial sac. Sometimes the vessels have to be somewhat compressed in order to cause the gas to escape. Large amounts of air or other gases cause the heart to float, so that it must be kept submerged before the vessels and chambers are incised. Basically the same procedure is used for demonstrating gas in the superior or inferior vena cava and the pelvic veins (for example, in cases of criminal abortion). In this situation the abdominal cavity is filled with water and the inferior vena cava and its tributaries are incised.

For the diagnosis of systemic air embolism, the skull vault should be removed without puncturing the meninges, so that the meningeal vessels can be inspected for gas bubbles. The demonstration of gas bubbles in the meningeal vessels and in the circle of Willis is only meaningful when the neck vessels are still intact and the internal carotid artery and the basilar artery have been clamped before the brain is removed. In acute cases, gas bubbles will be visible within the cerebral vessels. They are released under water when the clamps are taken off and the vessels are slightly compressed.

For the collection of gas from blood vessels or cavities, a system of little quantitative reliability is an air-tight, water-filled glass syringe with a needle. The needle is inserted into the vessel or cavity in question and gas is carefully aspirated.

A combined quantitative and qualitative method has been described by Kulka.[69] He devised an apparatus for gas collection and described it as follows (the letters refer to those shown in Fig. 2–4):

A. One wide-mouth glass bottle (2 to 3 ounces; 60 to 90 ml) fitted tightly with a two-hole rubber stopper.

B. Two sections of glass tubing, approximately 3 mm inside diame-

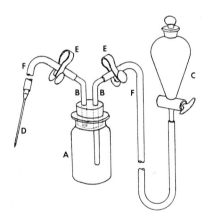

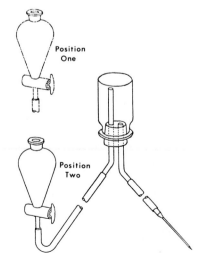

Figure 2–4. Apparatus for demonstration of air embolism. *Upper,* Apparatus. *Lower,* Positions of separatory funnel during test. (Redrawn after Kulka W: Laboratory methods and technical notes: a practical device for demonstrating air embolism. Arch Pathol 48:366–369, 1949.)

ter, each bent at an angle of 120°. One of these sections should be longer than the other. The shorter one should reach just through and be even with the inner surface of the stopper. The longer one should reach to within 1 or 1.5 cm of the bottom of the bottle. Both tubes should fit tightly into the holes of the stopper.

C. One separatory funnel (60 to 100 ml, pear-shaped) connected to the longer section of bent glass tubing by rubber tubing 100 cm in length (F). An amber, pure gum rubber tubing, such as is used on blood diluting pipets, has proved satisfactory.

D. One transfusion needle, 14- or 15-gauge and 4 to 5 cm long, connected to the shorter glass tube by a short (<5 cm) section of rubber tubing (F).

E. Two pinchcocks, one for each length of tubing. They may be of the spring type or of the household syringe type. The latter will prove advantageous if the gas collected is to be transported for analysis.

The entire system is filled with mineral oil so that, when the funnel is level with the upright bottle, the oil fills only about half of the funnel. In operation, the funnel is first raised to a position 30 to 40 cm above the level of the upright bottle. All the cocks are opened and the position is held until every trace of gas has been driven from the system through the needle which is thereby coated on the inside by a film of oil. After all air has been expelled, the cocks are closed and the funnel is lowered to its original position.

As a precautionary measure and control, the air-tightness of the whole system should be tested before operation. This is done by inserting the needle into musculature or skin and attempting aspiration in the manner described in the next paragraph.

To make the test, the bottle is inverted and the needle is inserted into the cavity in question. When the needle is in position, all cocks are opened. The funnel is lowered about 70 to 90 cm, or until adequate suction is created. This aspirates the contents of the cavity, which may consist of air or other gases, either pure or mixed with blood or other liquid. Any gas or liquid entering this system may be observed through the wall of the short bent glass tubing. In a positive test, gas bubbles will collect in the bottle above the level of the oil. If desired this gas can be saved for further examination by closing all the cocks and returning the bottle to its upright position.

Anesthesia-Associated Deaths.   There are a great many causes of anesthesia-associated deaths which are not drug-related. Some of the complications are characteristically linked to a specific phase of the anesthesia,[10] and many cannot be proved morphologically. The autopsy has to rule out airway obstruction by external compression, aspiration, tumors, or inflammatory processes.

The most important step in these autopsies is the gathering of information concerning drugs and chemical agents which had been administered or to which the victim might have had access. Some nonmedical chemicals and many drugs are known to affect anesthesia.[103] Drugs and their metabolic products, additives, stabilizers, impurities, and deterioration products also can be identified in postmortem tissues.[2] Therefore, all appropriate body fluids, particularly bile, and organs (see Autopsy Toxicology) should be submitted for toxicologic examination. If the anesthetic had been injected into or near the spinal canal, spinal fluid should be withdrawn from above the injection site, preferably from the suboccipital cysterna; 250 mg of sodium fluoride should be added per 30 ml of fluid. If the anesthetic was injected locally, tissue should be excised around the needle puncture marks, at a radius of 2 to 4 cm. Serial postmortem analysis of specimens may permit extrapolation to tissue concentration at the time of death.[103] The time interval between drug administration and death sometimes can be calculated from the distribution and ratio of administered drugs and their metabolic products.[92]

Assault. Blood should be scraped from clothing and body surfaces. Occasionally, the blood of the assailant can be identified. Toxicologic examination, particularly for alcohol, is indicated. Knife wounds are documented in the same way as bullet tracks.

Decompression Sickness. There are no diagnostic findings at autopsy unless gas bubbles are found in blood vessels. Cerebral edema, pulmonary congestion, and, less frequently, ischemic infarcts, fat embolism, fatty liver, Tardieu's spots, and pleural effusions may be present.[125] Roentgenograms of chest, elbows, hips, and knees will help to identify aseptic necroses of bones.[13]

Drowning. In investigating deaths from drowning, it is well to remember that death may have occurred before immersion and that the immersion may have been in shallow water (unconscious persons can drown in a puddle or ditch of shallow water if the mouth and nose of the victim are covered).

TABLE 2–2. DEATHS FROM DROWNING*

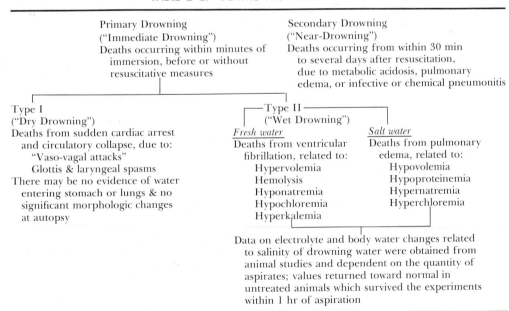

Primary Drowning ("Immediate Drowning") Deaths occurring within minutes of immersion, before or without resuscitative measures	Secondary Drowning ("Near-Drowning") Deaths occurring from within 30 min to several days after resuscitation, due to metabolic acidosis, pulmonary edema, or infective or chemical pneumonitis

Type I ("Dry Drowning") Deaths from sudden cardiac arrest and circulatory collapse, due to: "Vaso-vagal attacks" Glottis & laryngeal spasms There may be no evidence of water entering stomach or lungs & no significant morphologic changes at autopsy	Type II ("Wet Drowning") *Fresh water* Deaths from ventricular fibrillation, related to: Hypervolemia Hemolysis Hyponatremia Hypochloremia Hyperkalemia	*Salt water* Deaths from pulmonary edema, related to: Hypovolemia Hypoproteinemia Hypernatremia Hyperchloremia

Data on electrolyte and body water changes related to salinity of drowning water were obtained from animal studies and dependent on the quantity of aspirates; values returned toward normal in untreated animals which survived the experiments within 1 hr of aspiration

* Compiled from references 12,43,79–81,90,104,114,118,119.

Different types of death can be caused by immersion, depending on the circumstances (Table 2–2). Although much emphasis has been placed on the differentiation between salt-water drowning and fresh-water drowning, with special reference to serum biochemical and hematologic values in animals,[118,119] it appears that these bear little relationship to the type of drowning in humans.[43,80,104] The common denominator in all drowning deaths, in animals and humans, regardless of the composition or volume of fluid aspirated, appeared to be acute asphyxia with persistent arterial hypoxemia and acidosis.[79,80]

In autopsies in drowning cases, 10 ml of blood is withdrawn from the right chambers of the heart and from the left chambers for sodium chloride determinations. The surfaces of the heart and the needles and syringes must be absolutely dry. The difference in salt concentration is most significant in recent salt-water drowning but less helpful in fresh-water drowning.[125] The Gettler test[47] for sodium chloride concentration will become inconclusive when atrial or ventricular septal defects are present or when drowning occurred in brackish water with a sodium chloride concentration similar to that of blood. The test will be negative when death occurred from other causes and before water was aspirated in amounts large enough to affect the sodium concentration of the heart blood. The test is positive (indicates drowning) if the difference in sodium chloride concentration between the two sides of the heart is more than 25 mg/100 ml. In all cases of drowning, blood also should be analyzed for alcohol.

Another chemical test useful in drowning is determination of the blood magnesium concentration.[81] The principles are the same as those of the sodium chloride test. This test is considered superior in sea-water drowning and when postmortem decomposition has already set in. Blood magnesium seems to change less rapidly after death.

The freezing point of plasma is said to be decreased in cases of drowning.[125]

A sample of the water from which the body was recovered should be saved. This may help to determine where the actual drowning had occurred. Water samples also may help in evaluating the significance of the sodium chloride concentrations. The degree of chlorination in the fresh water of swimming pools may be significant because of its capability to induce fulminant pulmonary edema.

Stomach contents and mud, algae, or other material in the tracheobronchial tree are saved because they may offer important clues as to the circumstances of death. Liver, spleen, kidneys, and bone marrow are saved for diatom recovery. However, the recovery of diatoms in the liver and in other organs of individuals dying from causes other than drowning casts doubt on the specificity of this method in the diagnosis of drowning deaths.[114] The ubiquity of diatoms has been known to geologists for many years.

For diatom detection,[14] 2 to 5 gm of tissue is boiled for 10 to 15 minutes in 10 ml of concentrated nitric acid and 0.5 ml of concentrated sulfuric acid. Then, sodium nitrate is added in small quantities until the black color of the charred organic matter has been dispelled. It may be necessary to warm the acid-digested material with weak sodium hydroxide, but the material must soon be washed free from alkali so as to not dissolve the diatoms. The diatoms are washed, concentrated, and stored in distilled water. For examination, a drop of the concentrate is allowed to evaporate on a slide and then mounted in a resin of high refractive index. All equipment must be well cleaned, and distilled water must be used for all solutions. There are several variations and adaptations of this method.

The usual morphologic findings in drowning are common knowledge. Of particular importance is inspection of the middle ear and the mastoid air spaces for hemorrhages. The presence of such hemorrhages is strong evidence of drowning.[87,90,106] "Cutis anserina" and the "washerwoman" changes of the hands and feet are well-known external signs of immersion but are of little value in determining the cause of death. Another sign of drowning commonly mentioned, the presence of foam at the mouth or nostrils, is also inconclusive and is seen in cases of strangulation or status epilepticus, to mention only two conditions.

Exposure to Cold. Exposure to cold leads to hypothermia which is defined as an oral or axillary temperature less than 35 C (95 F). Death from hypothermia may occur in temperate or cold climates, especially at the extremes of life; neonates are particularly susceptible to cold.[75] Myxedema and cerebral infarcts or hemorrhages are natural disease states predisposing to the development of hypothermia. However, deaths from hypothermia usually are accidental. The changes seen at autopsy have been attributed to stagnation of blood as a result of hemoconcentration and sludging.[27,68,77] In these cases one finds generalized edema, red discoloration of the face and extremities due to the lack of oxygen dissociation of the blood, and abdominal distention due to paralytic ileus. The viscera are congested. Histologically, hemorrhagic pancreatitis, gastric and intestinal mucosal ulcerations, pulmonary hemorrhages, fat necrosis, and fatty degeneration of the liver, renal tubules, and myocardium may be found. There are perivascular hemorrhages in the region of the third ventricle of the brain.

There are no diagnostic chemical findings. Toxicologic sampling must be carried out in all cases, in particular for alcohol and narcotic drugs.

Gunshot Injuries. Roentgenograms of all parts of the body should be prepared. This occasionally will lead to the detection of bullets or fragments in unsuspected locations. One may also discover a bullet with an obscure entrance wound, particularly in severely decomposed bodies.[7] Photographs of all layers of clothing, particularly those in bullet tracks, and of all entrance and exit wounds should be taken with a ruler placed nearby. Diagrams should be prepared. The clothing is best examined with a hand lens or dissecting microscope. The dry clothing may then be saved as evidence and for possible test firing, nitrite tests, or stain analysis. For identification purposes the face should be photographed (full-face, profile, and oblique), blood should be typed and fingerprinting carried out. Scalp and pubic hair is saved. Bullet tracks should be numbered and described individually. Photographs are best prepared in black and white and in color. The examination with the hand lens or with the dissecting microscope also should include the skin and hair surrounding bullet wounds. Whenever feasible these wounds are then widely excised and saved for analysis—for instance, for metal traces by neutron activation or for carboxymyoglobin. Powder marks on the hands must be looked for. A "paraffin test"[50] may be helpful. This may be important evidence in cases of suspected suicide.

In all cases of gunshot injuries, body fluids and tissues for toxicologic studies should be saved. Analysis may reveal alcohol intoxication or drug addiction. In women proper tests should be carried out to rule out rape (see page 30).

Bullets or bullet fragments should not be handled with a forceps or other sharp instruments which may produce artifactual markings and thus hamper proper identification. Accidental loss of bullets or bullet fragments must be prevented by protecting all drains of the autopsy table by wire meshes. In cases of gunshot wounds of the head, a tray should be placed under the skull so that blood, sawdust, and tissue fragments can be collected and later rinsed through a sieve. Bullets and bullet fragments should be saved in properly labeled and sealed containers. The chain of custody must be preserved.

For reconstruction in cases of close-range rifle or shotgun wounds, the protocol should state the distance between the entrance wound and the trigger and the distance between the entrance wound and the forefinger.

The determination of the distance from which a shot had been fired may be difficult. Shotgun wound patterns frequently permit more accurate range estimates than do those from hand weapons, especially for ranges beyond 1 foot.[8] Constant development of firearms and ammunition may cause variations in wound patterns[93] which only specialists will be able to analyze. Many techniques, including spectrographic and polarographic methods, are available.[108] The main task of the general pathologist will be the documentation and preservation of the evidence. Figure 2–5 shows schematic drawings which permit estimation of the distance between the muzzle and the entrance wound.

Foreign Bodies. The same rules for the handling of bullets and bullet fragments pertain here, including the chain of custody. Roentgenograms may also be useful.

Hypoxia. It is difficult if not impossible to establish hypoxia as a cause of death.[74] Cyanosis, dark blood, vacuolated hepatic cells, and so-called Tardieu's spots are unreliable signs. Increased lactic acid levels in the central nervous system have been considered a valuable sign of antemortem hypoxia, but normal values do not rule out death by hypoxia. Unfortunately, in drowning, suffocation, shock, and hyperventilation, hyperglycemia may also cause increased lactic acid values. Lactic acid levels of more than 200 mg/100 ml in the central nervous system indicate hypoxia if other factors can be excluded.[125]

Central nervous system tissue can be shipped to special laboratories for lactic acid determination (see page 242). If the determination is to be

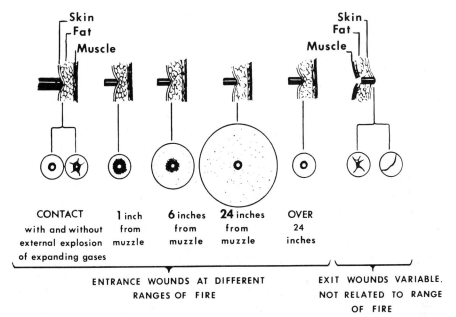

CONTACT | 1 inch | 6 inches | 24 inches | OVER
with and without | from | from | from | 24
external explosion | muzzle | muzzle | muzzle | inches
of expanding gases

ENTRANCE WOUNDS AT DIFFERENT
RANGES OF FIRE

EXIT WOUNDS VARIABLE.
NOT RELATED TO RANGE
OF FIRE

Figure 2–5. Bullet wounds. Differences in the appearance of cutaneous wounds of entrance and of exit and differences in wounds of entrance according to the distance between muzzle and skin at the moment of fire. Entrance wounds invariably differ from exit wounds in that the former are surrounded by a narrow zone of abrasion and discoloration produced by the nose of the bullet. If the muzzle of the gun is in close contact with the skin at the moment of fire, the combustion products will be blown into the wound and will not be visible on the surface. The stippling of the skin around the wound, produced by particles of burned and unburned powder, becomes progressively more dispersed as the range of fire increases and is ordinarily not perceptible if the range has been greater than 24 inches (61 cm). In addition to showing no marginal abrasion and no powder stippling, exit wounds are characteristically larger and more irregular than entrance wounds. (From Moritz AR, Morris CR: Handbook of Legal Medicine. Third edition. St. Louis, C. V. Mosby Company, 1970. By permission.)

carried out by the Armed Forces Institute of Pathology, the director should be notified.

In cases of asphyxia from mechanical obstruction of the airways, petechial hemorrhages are found not only on the serosal surfaces of the chest but also on the mucosa of the middle ear.[106]

Infanticide. The main objective of many of these autopsies is to decide whether the infant was born alive or whether a stillborn baby had been disposed of.

The hydrostatic lung test is still the most widely used. The trachea must be tied before the lung block is removed. When the intact lungs and fragments of both lungs are placed in water, they will sink if they had not been aerated. However, the presence of gas in the lungs does not rule out stillbirth. After death, air can be introduced into the lungs, or putrefaction gases might be present. Air artificially introduced after death will not distend the alveoli and can be squeezed out,[50] while this does not seem to be the case after active ventilation.

Histologic examination of the lungs, the presence of extraneous material in the air passages, the presence of milk in the stomach, or changes in the attachment of the umbilical cord also may help to determine whether an infant was born alive.[98]

In infants born alive but dying shortly thereafter, the location of air in the intestinal tract can be used for the determination of how long life lasted.[60] The propulsion of gas along the gastrointestinal tract proceeds at the same speed in full-term infants as in premature ones. The stomach is reached after 15 minutes, the small intestine after 1 to 2 hours, the colon after 5 to 6 hours, and the rectum after 12 hours. Bacterial gas production is a source of error, and resuscitation attempts may also lead to the accumulation of large amounts of air in the stomach and intestine.

If there is suspicion that one is dealing with a battered child, the coroner and the police should be notified. Pictures should be taken before the clothing is removed and at several stages during the removal of the clothing. Whole-body roentgenograms are essential.[16] Bruises and any other abnormal findings on the skin and mucous membranes should be described and photographed. The autopsy follows the principles of forensic autopsies. Blood should be collected for grouping, which may be required if paternity problems arise. Hair from scalp and eyebrows is saved for future comparison.[16]

Rape. The internal genital organs should be removed together with the widely excised vulva. If spermatic fluid (semen) can be detected internally or externally, it is saved for microscopic, chemical, microbiologic, and serologic examination.

Intravaginal spermatic fluid is aspirated, swabbed, or washed from the posterior fornix. Wet smears and gram-stained material are examined to identify spermatozoa. Gram stains will also demonstrate *Neisseria gonorrhoeae.* Other samples are used for quantitative acid phosphatase analysis[105] and serologic identification and grouping. Procedures usually applied to living assault victims also may be useful after death because of their medicolegal implications. These include the removal of blood for serologic tests for syphilis, urine for pregnancy tests, and cultures of spermatic fluid for *N. gonorrhoeae.*[56]

The morphologic survival time of spermatozoa in the vagina is probably about 24 hours.[6] Blood, hair, urine, or saliva on the body or clothing of the victim may be the assailant's and should be saved for identification.[129]

Stains (for example, on clothing) suspected of being seminal should be examined as soon as possible because bacterial action may make identification of spermatozoa impossible. The Florence test is widely used as a preliminary means of identifying seminal stains.[5]

A 0.5-cm square of cloth is cut from the suspected stain. This is soaked in 0.3 ml of a 1:1,000 solution of 85% aerosol OT (the dioctyl ester of sodium sulfosuccinate, American Cyanamid & Chemical Corporation) in water for 1 hour on a microscopic slide; the slide is covered with a Petri dish to prevent evaporation. The cloth is teased and the fluid is wrung out of it with forceps; 0.1 ml of this extract is placed on a separate slide, and one drop of the Florence reagent (potassium iodide, 5%, and iodine, 8% in aqueous solution) is added. A positive reaction is indicated by the formation of brown rhomboid crystals which show parallel extinction between crossed Nichol prisms. The original extract is stained with methylene blue, and spermatozoa or parts thereof may be identified in the wet mount.

The Florence test is extremely sensitive; extracts of seminal stains in which spermatozoa can no longer be identified will give a strongly positive reaction. The typical crystalline material has not been observed with aqueous extracts of tissue, lipoids from liver and kidney, dried milk, dried egg yolk or egg white, old lecithin, nasal and vaginal mucus, serum, sweat, gonorrheal pus, or wine, whisky, beer, or ice cream residues.[5] However, in the medicolegal examination of seminal stains, a positive Florence test preferably should be supported by the demonstration of spermatozoa.

For a detailed discussion on the investigation of semen and seminal stains, see the exhaustive review by Pollak.[97]

Exhumation. The examination of exhumed bodies is done too rarely by general pathologists to deserve detailed description here. We have had no personal experience with it. The legal and technical aspects of exhumations have been discussed in detail by Gonzales et al[50] and Curry.[24] The degree of decomposition will depend on the length of the postmortem interval, the weather at the time of death, and the nature of the coffin and the surrounding soil.[91] For the study of mummies or old bones, the carbon-14 method and other special techniques can be used.[34]

AUTOPSY TOXICOLOGY

Most toxicologic autopsies are also medicolegal autopsies. Therefore, the pathologist should never ask or permit a funeral director to remove tissues or body fluids for him. When the autopsy is done in mortuaries, the pathologist should use his own instruments and containers. Cleanliness is of utmost importance in these cases.

The techniques of toxicologic analysis are beyond the scope of this book. Several excellent pertinent publications[20,24,49,116,117] are available.

Request for Toxicologic Examination. Table 2–3 shows the type of information that should be supplied with a request for toxicologic examination in cases of sudden death. It is clear that such a request cannot be completed without information gathered from next of kin, police officers, attending physicians, or other persons who had contact with the deceased. Less elaborate requests will suffice if the nature of the incriminated toxic substance is known—for example, a request for blood alcohol determination—and the information on the label of the container will be sufficient. Of particular interest is the time interval between the alleged intake of the poison and the death of the patient.[86] Figure 2–6 shows that this time interval may be too long or too short to make death from a specific poison likely.

Containers. Glass containers should be treated with sulfuric acid-

Police Force:		Name of Deceased:		Date:
Sex:	Age of Deceased:		Approx. Weight of Deceased:	

1. On what date and at approximately what time was the deceased last seen to have been in his usual state of health?
2. Time and date of death, if known.
3. If the time of death is not accurately known, when was the deceased found to be dead?
4. If deceased died suddenly give details and time of last known meal.
5. Was the deceased admitted to hospital while still alive? If so, on what day and at what time?
6. Give details of the type and quantity of the substance thought to have been the cause of death.
7. Did the deceased take any medicine, pills, etc., in the three days prior to death? If so, give details.
8. Name of any medicine, pills, antibiotics, etc., given to deceased in hospital or elsewhere. If possible give quantities and times administered.
9. Please put a tick against any of the following symptoms that apply:

Diarrhoea	Constipation	Loss of weight	Eye pupils contracted
Vomiting	Blue tinge to the skin (Cyanosis)	Shivering	Delirium
		Hallucinations	Drunkenness
Thirst	Jaundice	Convulsions	Sweating
Blindness		Eye pupils dilated	Unconsciousness

10. When giving dates and times please be as exact as possible.
11. It would be appreciated if the pathologist could inform the laboratory of the findings of his post-mortem.
12. Name and address of Coroner.

* From Curry A: Poison Detection in Human Organs. Second edition. Springfield, Illinois, Charles C Thomas, Publisher, 1969. By permission.

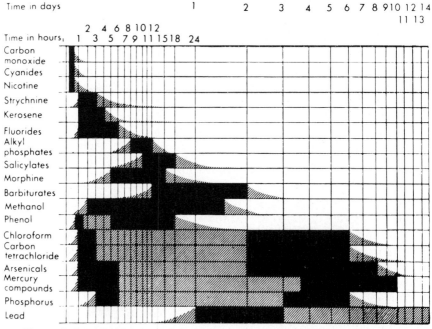

Figure 2-6. Average time of death after ingestion or inhalation of fatal dose of poison. Solid regions indicate interval in which most deaths occur. Shaded regions indicate intervals in which death occurs occasionally but less commonly. (From Moritz AR, Morris CR: Handbook of Legal Medicine. Third edition. St. Louis, C. V. Mosby Company, 1970. By permission.)

dichromate cleaning solution, rinsed with distilled water, dried, and stored in a place protected from dust. Rubber inserts should not be used. Polyethylene bags or containers are widely used and are preferable in many situations. However, volatile poisons may diffuse through plastic. Therefore, polyethylene bags should not be used when the type of poison is unknown or is suspected to be volatile. Several kits should be ready in the autopsy room at all times, each containing at least four large and two medium-sized glass jars (1 liter), and six smaller bottles for heart blood, peripheral blood, urine, bile, and hair. Containers for material from cases of suspected lead poisoning need special preparation (see below).

The description of each container should state: the date and hour when the toxicologic material was secured; the full name, age, weight, and clinic and autopsy numbers of the victim; exhibit number; nature (for instance, "blood," "liver," or "cerebrospinal fluid"); origin (for instance, "blood from right iliac vein"); quantity and appearance of toxicologic material; type and quantity of preservative; size of container and type of cap or sealing (screw cap, cork, Bakelite, heat-sealed plastic bag); and identification of submitting person and institution. The actual label on the container may be a transcript of the description, or it might only state the full name and clinic and autopsy numbers of the victim, exhibit number, nature of toxicologic material and preservative, and name, address, institution, and phone number of the submitter or whoever should be contacted for further information. If the content of the container is infectious, a clearly visible warning should be put on the label.

The continuity of custody of the specimen has to be documented. A blank space on the toxicologic report form can be used for this purpose. All persons who had been in charge of the specimen should sign and state the precise times at which the custody periods began and ended. Samples should be kept in a locked refrigerator or freezer.

Routine Sampling of Toxicologic Material. The highest concentrations of toxic substances may be found in the dialysis and lavage fluids which had been used in the hospital. The following samples are recommended[36] for routine sampling and storage in medicolegal and toxicologic autopsies, particularly when the nature of the toxic substance is unknown. In all cases, a variety of body fluids and tissues should be sampled. A common misconception is that it is only necessary to analyze gastric contents in order to establish whether poisoning has occurred in a given case. It should be pointed out that the gastrointestinal tract is not the only route of entry of poisons into the body. Furthermore, if any significant period (4 to 6 hours) elapses from the time of ingestion until death or treatment, the poison will have passed out of the stomach. Poison also could have been introduced into the stomach after death to mask a homicidal act.[40] The knowledge of the postmortem distribution of a toxic agent in different body fluids and tissues enables the forensic pathologist to distinguish inhalation poisoning from ingestion poisoning, a distinction of vital importance from the medicolegal standpoint.[39] Table 2–4 summarizes the suggested types and sizes of samples.

Blood, bile, and urine should be kept refrigerated. Sodium fluoride

TABLE 2–4.   ROUTINE SAMPLING OF TISSUES AND FLUIDS*

Tissue or Fluid	Sample	Jar
Brain	500 gm or whole organ after histologic sampling; frontal lobes usually least important for neuropathologist	Large
Liver	500 gm or whole organ after histologic sampling	Large
Lung	One lung or each lung separately after histologic sampling	Large
Kidneys	Each kidney separately after histologic sampling	Medium
Stomach	Entire with contents or contents separately; vomitus if available	Medium
Intestine	Separately tied portions of intestinal tract with contents	Large
Cerebrospinal fluid	As much as can be withdrawn	Small
Heart blood	100 ml with preservative and 100 ml without preservative	Small
Peripheral blood	30 ml	Small
Bile	All	Small
Urine	All	Small
Muscle	200-gm aliquots	Medium
Fat	200-gm aliquots	Medium
Hair	} 10 gm	Small
Fingernails		Small

* Compiled from references 24,36.

may be added as a preservative to some samples (250 mg/30 ml of fluid). If tissues had been stored in a fixative, it is essential to submit both tissues and fixative to the toxicologist. For longer storage periods, toxicologic material is best kept in a deep freeze.

Cerebrospinal Fluid.   Cerebrospinal fluid is removed by suboccipital or lumbar puncture. This is preferably done before the internal examination is begun. The technique does not differ from the one used under clinical conditions. The preservative is sodium fluoride, 250 mg/30 ml of fluid.

Vitreous Humor.   Vitreous humor can be used for determination of alcohol and possibly for other toxicologic studies, particularly when other body fluids are not readily available. Removal of vitreous humor has been described previously (page 17).

Blood.   Blood is removed under sterile conditions from the right atrium and from a peripheral vein (we usually use an iliac vein). Anaerobic technique is important in order to avoid evaporation of volatile substances.[112] Therefore, care must be taken that very little air remains between the surface of the blood and the lid of the container. If the heart blood is clotted, the venae cavae or the aorta should be punctured. If peripheral blood cannot be obtained, samples from the right and left sides of the heart should be collected separately. In cases of drowning, 10 ml of blood is removed from each side of the heart for separate sodium chloride or magnesium determinations. In barbiturate and ethanol poisoning, toxicologic examination of portal vein blood may be of interest. Any anticoagulant other than heparin may be used. The preservative is sodium fluoride, 250 mg/30 ml of fluid.

Bile.   Bile is best removed by puncturing the gallbladder in situ.

Gastrointestinal Tract.   The stomach can be saved with its contents by placing ligatures around the lower end of the esophagus and the upper end of the duodenum. The organ is then placed in a jar and the tox-icologist is asked to describe the contents of the stomach at the time he opens the organ. Others[24] prefer to open the ligated stomach at the time of the autopsy so that the stomach contents and walls can be inspected and described and tablets or other solid material can be removed. After material for histologic examination of the gastric wall has been saved, the stomach is submitted for toxicologic examination, together with its contents. This latter method seems preferable except in cases of suspected poisoning with yellow phosphorus. The presence of a fatty liver may alert the pathologist. In such a case, the stomach has to be opened under nitrogen, just before analysis.

Several portions of small and large bowel, each about 60 cm long,[130] are tied by double ligatures. The separate portions are labeled and submitted unopened for toxicologic examination.

Hair. Hair should be pulled from the scalp, not cut. A large sample, about 10 gm, should be collected and tied in locks with cotton. This should be done in a manner which identifies the ends where the hair roots are.

Skin. If it is suspected that a poisonous substance had been injected, the skin around the needle puncture mark is excised at a radius of 2 to 4 cm from the injection site. If a poisonous substance might have been taken up by absorption, the skin is excised in the area where the absorption is thought to have occurred, and in a distant, preferably contralateral, area as a control specimen.

Urine. Urine is best collected with a sterile needle and syringe through the dome of the bladder. The sterilized wall is stretched between two hemostats and then punctured. Urine may be of utmost importance for toxicologic examinations, and every effort should be made to collect it. When the urinary bladder appears to be empty, the urethra should be tied or clamped and the dome of the bladder widely incised between hemostats which then are used to hold the bladder open. Often, with this technique, a few drops of urine can be collected from between the trabeculae of the wall or at the internal urethral orifice. Urine should be saved in 50-ml aliquots.[130] The preservative is sodium fluoride, 250 mg/30 ml of fluid.

Sampling for Specific Toxicologic Substances.   The suggested procedures indicate the most important tissues and body fluids to save and some orienting tests. These supplement rather than replace routine sampling.

Alcohols. 1. Ethyl alcohol (ethanol). Blood, urine, and cerebrospinal fluid are collected as described above and sodium fluoride preservative is added. Brain tissue analysis is also suggested.[130] Vitreous humor should be saved if blood and brain tissue are not available.[21] The containers should be filled to just under the lid so that evaporation is minimal. Toxicologic examination for drugs such as barbiturates should be considered. Experimental and actual medicolegal case studies have demonstrated the fatal synergistic effect of sublethal doses of alcohol and phenobarbital when ingested together.[63] One should also search for conditions that might have caused tissue hypoxia, including carbon monoxide poisoning. In the presence of certain concomitant poisons such as carbon tetrachloride, even small amounts of alcohol may be fatal. Further details, particularly concerning the interpretation of alcohol values, are discussed below.

2. Methyl alcohol (wood alcohol; methanol) and isopropyl alcohol (rubbing alcohol; propanol). The same sampling procedures are required. These poisons give nonspecific autopsy findings; visceral congestion, pulmonary edema, and cerebral edema are the predominant changes.

3. Glycols (ethylene glycol; antifreeze). These substances may cause acute poisoning characterized by pulmonary and cerebral edema. Chronic poisoning may result from exposure to ethylene glycol vapors and causes severe renal tubular necrosis with masses of calcium oxalate crystals. These crystals are light yellow, are birefringent when examined by polarized light, and are arranged as sheaves, rhomboids, or prisms. Central hydropic degeneration and fatty metamorphosis of the liver with focal necrosis also are common findings in ethylene glycol poisoning.[41,53]

Alkaloids.   Brain tissue is best for analysis (500 gm or entire brain).[130] The diagnosis of digitalis toxicity has recently become amenable to postmortem verification by analysis of myocardial tissue.[62] This method employs methanol extraction, alumina column purification, a solvent partition procedure, thin layer chromatography, and fluorometric assay. Certain drugs seem to interfere with proper determination.

Arsenic.   About 10 gm of hair should be pulled, not cut, from the scalp and tied in locks with cotton. The ends where the hair roots are should be identified. Some fingernails should be collected.

Barbiturates.   Sampling for toxicologic examination should include a search for tablets or gritty residues of unabsorbed substances in the esophagus or among the stomach contents and vomitus. Barbiturates should be determined together with the total volume of the stomach contents. This may permit a quantitative estimation of the barbiturates still in the stomach. Stomach contents should also be analyzed for alcohol.[17]

Of special interest are the barbiturate concentrations in liver and cerebral tissues and in portal vein and peripheral blood. Camps[17] suggested that, in addition, bile should be analyzed, total urine volume and urine pH should be determined, and evidence of proteinuria, glucosuria, ketone bodies, and drugs should be searched for in the urine.

Death from barbiturate poisoning may occur at levels only slightly above the lowest level needed to produce unconsciousness, at least if no treatment had been given.[48] Interpretation of toxicologic findings in acute poisoning is discussed below.

Bromides.   Blood is best for bromide determination.[130]

Carbon Monoxide.   A quick qualitative test for carbon monoxide should be carried out whenever there is appropriate circumstantial evidence or when cherry red blood, bullous edema of the skin, and hemorrhagic necrosis of the basal ganglia suggest the diagnosis of carbon monoxide poisoning. In a completely unsuspected case, the failure of tissue to turn gray quickly in formalin solution is a clue to the possibility of carbon monoxide poisoning. Toxicologic examination can be carried out on blood or any tissue from which hemoglobin can be extracted.[88] Hemoglobin concentration of the blood should be determined in all cases.[120]

Blood can be tested quickly for the presence of carboxyhemoglobin (carbon monoxide hemoglobin) by viewing the pattern of absorption in a hand spectroscope. The blood is diluted with water. In a more elaborate test, this solution is examined in the visible range of a recording spectrophotometer.[120]

> One or two drops of blood in water gives a solution which reads "on scale" with absorption peaks near 575 and 537 mμ for both carboxyhemoglobin and oxyhemoglobin. After this curve is recorded, a few crystals of sodium dithionide are added to the cuvette. The persistence of two absorption peaks indicates the presence of carboxyhemoglobin. In the absence of it, the 556-mμ peak of reduced hemoglobin will appear.

Another test is based on the ability of carboxyhemoglobin to resist the effects of tannic acid: it remains cherry red while oxyhemoglobin turns deep brown. This technique is said to be applicable even after embalming.[120]

The Hoppe-Seyler or alkali test of blood is also a commonly used simple screening method.[13,50]

> In a porcelain evaporating dish, mix several drops of blood (may be diluted in water) with 5 to 10% NaOH. Normal blood turns greenish brown due to the formation of alkaline hematin. Blood containing carboxyhemoglobin is unaffected by the alkali and the solution remains cherry red.

The test will give a positive result if the blood is more than 10 to 15% saturated with carbon monoxide. However, because fetal hemoglobin (Hb F) is alkali-resistant, the test is misleading when used on the blood of a newborn or a very young infant.[58] Similarly, the test also is unsuitable for blood from adults with high-fetal-hemoglobin hemoglobinopathies (thalassemias and other forms of anemia[72]).

The best quantitative methods are based on freeing the carbon monoxide from the hemoglobin with acid in a closed system and identifying it by gas chromatography.

Although many methods of carbon monoxide determination have been described[120,125] and reliable values are available, in postmortem samples the carbon monoxide content may be difficult to interpret. If only tissue is available for carbon monoxide determination, as is often the case in aircraft accidents, it is best to use water to extract blood from liver, spleen, kidneys, lungs, or other organs and to determine the carbon monoxide content and binding capacity of this mixture. The method is not accurate for values less than 10% saturation.

If the victim survived the carbon monoxide poisoning for several hours, postmortem blood samples usually will fail to show carboxyhemoglobin. Blood drawn at the time of admission to the hospital—for instance, for crossmatching—may still be available and may yield positive results.[120]

Cyanides and Hydrocyanic Acids.   Speed is essential because the poison is highly volatile. Stomach contents, blood and other body fluids, tissues, and containers from which the poison might have been ingested should be submitted for examination. An orienting test in the autopsy room can be carried out with filter paper dipped into normal blood. This filter paper is then treated with potassium chlorate, whereupon brown methemoglobin forms. This preparation is now placed into the fluid suspected to contain cyanide. If bright-red cyanmethemoglobin forms, the reaction is positive.[49] Minimal cyanide levels are supposed to be present occasionally in decomposed bodies.

DDT and Related Compounds.   Fat and muscle tissue are best for the determination of these insecticides. Routine determination of insecticides and pollutants, such as mercury, in autopsy tissues might become an important public health activity of the future.

Fluoride.   Stomach contents, liver, bone, kidneys, and urine are preserved for analysis.

Narcotics, Hallucinogens, Stimulants, and Depressants.   The mortality among illicit drug users has increased alarmingly during the past decade.[30,57,73] Narcotics[30] are the main offenders, but hallucinogens,[31] stimulants, and depressants[32] also are involved. Drugs may be the immediate cause of death, or death may be due to an infection, particularly when narcotics have been used intravenously. Drugs also may be a contributory cause of death — for instance, in suicides or in traffic accidents after the use of hallucinogens. However, the majority of fatalities are due to an acute reaction to the intravenous injection of a mixture containing heroin. Death may occur with such speed that the bodies are found with needles and syringes in the veins or clenched in the hands.[57] The character of the sudden collapse and death suggests a hypersensitivity or other type of reaction to an adulterant such as quinine or strychnine rather than an actual overdose of the narcotic itself. Lactose, sucrose, procaine, magnesium silicate, and mannitol are other adulterants which are often found in "street" narcotics.[18] Hard-core addicts subject themselves to more than 1,000 intravenous injections each year and thus are exposed repeatedly to possible antigens in the crude heroin or its adulterants.[1]

Collapse after intravenous injection of hashish (crude marihuana) has been reported to be associated with thrombocytopenia. The cause is unknown. Some suggest a direct effect of marihuana on platelets;[67] others attribute it to disseminated intravascular coagulation.[59]

In evaluating suspected drug-related deaths, one should take into consideration the conclusions which Irey[61] reached from studying 500 cases of drug-related disease: (1) histologic patterns in tissue reactions to drugs may point to classes of drugs but are rarely if ever specific for a single drug; (2) supplemental historical, clinical, and laboratory data, with emphasis on time-related drug and disease information, are almost always required in establishing the agent responsible for drug-induced pathologic changes, regardless of the degree of sophistication of later studies on the tissues; and (3) before attributing a reaction to a drug, it is necessary to consider and rule out other factors.

The autopsy findings in drug-associated deaths may be inconclusive. The many potentially fatal medical complications of drug abuse, particularly of intravenous narcotics, include hepatitis, endocarditis, thrombophlebitis, sepsis, pulmonary talc granulomatosis, tetanus, malaria,[18,57,73] and necrotizing angiitis.[19] Tissues with evidence of chronic inflammation and granulomas should be studied by polarizing microscopy.

Needle marks must be searched for in all cases of suspected drug-associated deaths. The needle marks may be hidden under tattoos or cigarette burns, or the needle may still be in place. Subcutaneous or perivenous hemorrhages or scarring may be present at the injection sites.

Foam may exude from the nostrils. There is pulmonary edema and congestion in the acute stages, sometimes associated with aspiration. The pulmonary vessels may reveal embolized material which can be analyzed.[64] Later, a diffuse lobular pneumonia with macrophages and polymorphonuclear leukocytes may develop. The histologic appearance of the lungs conforms roughly to one of four progressive patterns which can be correlated with the time interval between the injection and death.[110]

Periportal lymph nodes are enlarged and inflamed. Neuropathologic complications include bilateral symmetric necrosis of the globus pallidus, transverse myelitis, brain abscess, and meningitis.[30]

Helpful information as to the nature of the drug may be obtained from witnesses. Narcotic paraphernalia may be found at the scene. Qualified agents of the Bureau of Dangerous Narcotics and Drugs* may carry out field tests. If the drug is known only by a slang name, Table 2–5 may help in its identification. Of course, the slang terms may imply different compounds in years to come, or their meanings may vary from place to place.

The biologic material submitted for toxicologic examination should include gastric and intestinal contents, parenchymatous organs, brain, fat, and muscle tissue, blood, bile, and urine.

In d-lysergic acid diethylamide (LSD) poisoning, lung blood is supposed to show the highest levels of the drug.[24] The determination of LSD in biologic tissues is extremely difficult. The doses involved are in the range of 75 to 100 μg.[31]

Morphine is not found in blood but accumulates in bile.

Heroin is metabolized to morphine. Needle marks should be excised in all cases, together with the surrounding skin and underlying tissues, and submitted for analysis. For screening purposes, urine is used.

Blood alcohol determination should be carried out in all cases.

Gases. Carbon monoxide poisoning and volatile substances capable of causing "sniffing" death are discussed elsewhere in this section. For other gases or volatile substances, including volatile anesthetics, the following procedures are suggested. Lungs, with bronchi ligated, should be submitted in air-tight containers not made of plastic. Gases from cavities,

---

* For information and expert analysis of solid prescribed material, contact: The Bureau of Dangerous Narcotics and Drugs, 1405 I St. NW, Washington D.C. 20537. Phone 382-4437.

TABLE 2–5. SLANG TERMS OF COMMONLY ABUSED DRUGS*

Slang Term	Generic Name	Trade Name
Barbiturate hypnotics (goof balls, fool pills, downs)		
Blue heavens	Amobarbital	Amytal
Tooies, rainbows, Christmas trees	Amobarbital + secobarbital	Tuinal
Yellow jackets	Pentobarbital	Nembutal
Purple hearts	Phenobarbital	Luminal
Reds, red birds, red devils	Secobarbital	Seconal
Nonbarbiturate hypnotic		
Cibas	Glutethimide	Doriden
Amphetamines (ups)		
Bennies, splash, peaches	Amphetamine	Benzedrine
Dexies, co-pilots, oranges	Dextroamphetamine	Dexedrine
Footballs	Dextroamphetamine + amphetamine	Biphetamine
Crystal, meth, speed	Methamphetamine	Methedrine or Desoxyn
Amphetamine-like		
DET	Diethyltryptamine	
DMT	Dimethyltryptamine	
STP or DOM	2,5-Dimethyl-4-methylamphetamine	
DPT	Dipropyltryptamine	
Cocaine		
Cake, snow, big, candy, girl, Charlie	Cocaine	
Psychomimetics		
Acid	d-Lysergic acid diethylamide (LSD)	
Grass, hemp, hash, pot, weed, hashish	Marihuana	
White light, blue caps, pink wedge	Mescaline	
Anticholinergic		
Jimson seed, Jimson weed, thornapple	Datura plant (atropine, scopolamine, hyoscyamine)	
Mixtures		
Speedball	Heroin + cocaine	
Bombita	Heroin + amphetamine + Tuinal	
Speedball	Methamphetamine + LSD	

* Modified after DeGross J: Emergency treatment of drug abuse and poison ingestion. Resident Staff Physician *16*:43–51, 1970.

heart, or vessels should be removed by the method of Kulka[69] (see above) or with a mercury-sealed syringe. Another method[103] is to fill the body cavities with water and to use a rubber dam to trap the gases before cutting the organs. Samples from various organs should be transferred into hermetically sealed, nonplastic containers or into the analyzing solutions. These specimens should be taken at timed intervals. Blood should be submitted in the mercury-sealed syringe with which it was drawn.

Lead. Blood is drawn with a lead-free syringe and needle and stored in lead-free polyethylene containers. Urine is collected and stored for coproporphyrin studies. Also, a sample, of at least 10 gm, of bone should be submitted for examination. In fluids intended for lead analysis, anticoagulants or preservatives must *not* be added. If glass containers are to be used, they should be rinsed first in water, then in hot 10% nitric acid, and, finally, repeatedly in double-distilled water. The glassware should be dried in an oven so that it remains protected from lead-containing dust. If acute poisoning is suspected, blood, small and large bowel, the entire liver, and both kidneys separately are the most important organs to be analyzed. In cases of chronic exposure, liver, kidneys, brain, soft tissues, and bone should be submitted for toxicologic examination.

Volatile Substances ("Sniffing Death" or "Spray Death"). Trichloroethane, fluorinated refrigerants, and other volatile hydrocarbons are most commonly involved in the "sudden sniffing death" syndrome.[4] No anatomic abnormalities are noted at autopsy. Among the toxic agents in "glue sniffing" are benzene and toluene; these are fat soluble and accumulate chiefly in the brain.[131] Also present in various glues are acetone, hexane, cyclohexane, aliphatic acetates, isopropanol, methyl ethyl ketone, and methyl isobutyl ketone.[32] Fingernail polish remover, lacquer thinners, lighter fluid, cleaning fluid, and gasoline also are used for sniffing.[32] "Spray death" may occur in asthma sufferers from pressurized aerosol bronchodilators.[33,126] Freons and related propellant (fluoroalkane) gases can no longer be considered inert.[121] Sensitization of the heart to epinephrine and fatal cardiac arrhythmia have been suggested as a cause of death.[102]

Routine toxicologic sampling in glass (not plastic) containers is recommended. If the poison was inhaled, the main bronchi should be tied and the lungs submitted separately for examination.

Sulfonamides. Best for analysis are blood, liver, and both kidneys.[130]

Interpretation of Toxicologic Reports. *Alcohol.* Ethyl alcohol is one member of the family of alcohols. In general, the toxicity increases as the number of carbon atoms in the alcohol increases. Thus, isopropyl alcohol is three times as toxic as methyl alcohol, but two thirds as toxic as isobutyl alcohol and one half as toxic as amyl alcohol. Primary alcohols are more toxic than the corresponding secondary isomers.[12]

There is no uniform method of expressing alcohol levels in body fluids. In European countries, the concentration is expressed in *promille* (grams per liter). In the United States, it has become customary to refer to concentration by percentage (grams per 100 ml), and values in these units have been written into legislation and included in the uniform vehicle codes. Unless qualified, the use of *promille* or percentage does not indicate whether the result of the analysis is weight/weight, weight/volume, or volume/volume. Another common way of expressing concentrations, mg per 100 ml, has also been used to indicate alcohol levels. It is imperative that the method of expressing concentration be clearly specified whenever the alcohol level is mentioned. The desired expression can be derived from the toxicologic report by using the following equation:

$$100 \text{ mg}/100 \text{ ml} = 1.0 \text{ } promille = 0.10\%.$$

The controversy over the "normal" body ethanol concentration remains to be resolved.[55] It is generally accepted that blood alcohol levels are negligible in the absence of ingestion of or other exposure to ethanol. "Endogenous" ethanol in human blood exists at a concentration of less than

0.15 mg/100 ml (<0.0015 *promille* or <0.00015%). Objective impairment of driving ability is observed at threshold blood alcohol levels of 35 to 40 mg/100 ml. Values less than 50 mg/100 ml are considered evidence of "not under the influence" by courts in most states. Values greater than 150 mg/100 ml are *prima facie* evidence of "under the influence"; most persons are obviously intoxicated in this range. Values of 500 to 600 mg/100 ml are associated with coma and death.[54]

If alcohol is determined in the vitreous humor, the blood alcohol concentration can be estimated by multiplying the vitreous humor alcohol concentration by 0.89.[21]

Alcohol is eliminated from the body at the rate of 10 mg/kg body weight/hr (about 10 ml of ethanol per hour for a 68-kg or 150-lb man). The rate of elimination is independent of the blood alcohol level.[54] The value of autopsy blood alcohol levels as an index of the amount of alcohol imbibed before death has been studied extensively by Plueckhahn.[94–96] His observations and conclusions may be summarized as follows:

1. Blood alcohol levels at autopsy are valid up to 48 hours after death, if certain simple principles are observed in the collection and storage of samples. High blood glucose level is the common cause of finding a falsely high blood alcohol level.

2. There is no statistically significant difference in the alcohol levels of blood samples from the intact heart chambers and the femoral vessels. Autopsy samples of blood from pooled blood in the pericardial sac or pleural cavity are unsatisfactory.

3. A significant blood alcohol level (>100 mg/100 ml) may be generated during storage of autopsy blood samples at room temperature (20 to 25 C) for 2 days, due to fermentation by enzymes, fungi, or bacteria.

4. Sodium fluoride in a concentration of 1.0% should be used as the preservative for autopsy blood samples. In concentrations less than 0.5% (recommended by most textbooks), it inhibits glycolysis but does not prevent generation of alcohol by fermentation. Mercuric chloride (recommended by some authors), at any concentration, is not a satisfactory preservative for autopsy blood samples.

5. Alcohol levels in the stomach are usually low at autopsy even when large amounts of alcohol have been consumed shortly before death. Diffusion of alcohol from the stomach to the intact heart chamber is minimal after death, even at 50 hours after postmortem instillation of 350 ml of 10% ethanol into the empty stomach.

Urine can be collected easily at autopsy and has been used extensively in some countries for estimating alcohol levels in the body. Although the kidneys do not concentrate alcohol, the urinary alcohol level is higher than the blood alcohol level because urine contains more water than blood does. In both living and dead animals under experimental conditions, the free exchange of urinary and blood alcohol through bladder mucosal capillaries tends to bring the concentrations of the alcohol in the blood and urine closer to, rather than away from, a state of equilibrium.[84]

The peak urinary alcohol level usually occurs about 20 minutes after the peak blood alcohol level. In order to allow for the variables which may occur, a regression analysis has been made on the basis of 7,653 urinary alcohol estimations and the corresponding blood alcohol concentrations.[42] It was found that, if B is the blood alcohol level and U is the urinary alcohol level, the regression can be expressed as:

$$B = 0.6582 \ U \ (\text{or the ratio } U/B = 1.52).$$

This, however, allows a 50% chance that the actual blood alcohol level is lower. The formula

$$B = 0.6582 \ U - 0.43$$

decreases this possibility to 5%, and the formula

$$B = 0.6582 \ U - 0.608$$

decreases it to 1%. In forensic laboratories in the Netherlands where analyses in a large series of cases were carried out, practical experience has suggested that the ratio, $U/B = 2$, should be used in medicolegal practice.

Strength of alcohol is measured in "proof"; absolute alcohol is 200 proof. Therefore, in the United States, alcohol content as volume percent is half the proof—for example, 100 proof whisky contains 50% alcohol by volume. The alcohol content of various beverages is shown in Table 2–6. The predicted blood alcohol level after consumption of various amounts of alcohol is shown in Table 2–7.

Glaister and Rentoul[49] and Furbank[44] have prepared tables relating blood and urinary alcohol levels to the minimal amount of whisky, wine, or beer that must have been consumed and the approximate time required for complete removal of alcohol from the body. Furbank[44] also gives correction factors to adjust the values in the tables to sex and actual body weights.

Barbiturates. According to Camps,[17] the results of toxicologic studies in acute barbiturate poisoning can be interpreted as follows: (1) if the quantity in peripheral blood is less than the quantity in liver blood and there is still drug present in the stomach, then death occurred before peak absorp-

TABLE 2–6. APPROXIMATE ALCOHOL CONTENT IN VARIOUS BEVERAGES*

Beverage	Ethanol Content (%, v/v)
Whisky and gin	40
Brandy	45.5–48.5
Sherry and port wines	16–20
Liqueurs	34–59
Rum	50–69.5
Beers	2–6
Light wines	10–15

* From Glaister J, Rentoul E: Medical Jurisprudence and Toxicology. Twelfth edition. Edinburgh, E. & S. Livingstone, Ltd., 1966.

TABLE 2–7.   PREDICTED BLOOD ALCOHOL
LEVELS*

Drinks (No.)†	Predicted Blood Alcohol Level (mg/100 ml)
1	10–30
2	30–50
3	50–80
4	80–100
5	100–130
6	130–160
8	160–200
10	190–230
12	250–320

* Within 1 hr after consumption of diluted alcohol (approximately 15%) on an empty stomach, assuming body weight of 140 to 180 pounds (63.6 to 81.7 kg).[70]

† One ounce (about 30 ml) of whisky or 12 oz (about 355 ml) of beer.

tion and probably was rapid; (2) if peripheral blood quantity is higher than liver quantity and there is only a small stomach residue, then peak absorption probably had already occurred and death was delayed; (3) if the peripheral blood quantity is higher than the liver quantity or the amount in the liver blood is low while there still remains a large quantity in the stomach, then absorption ceased before death; (4) if the peripheral blood shows a higher quantity of one drug than another (if more than one drug is present) and there is a mixture of drugs in the stomach, it is probable that a second ingestion took place; (5) the amount of alcohol in urine, stomach contents, and peripheral blood may be of assistance in deciding whether the person was intoxicated prior to taking the drug, and whether alcohol may have contributed to the fatal outcome; (6) the presence of other drugs also may be of significance.

Other Substances. In toxicologic reports, the concentration of a poison usually is reported in milligrams or micrograms per 100 gm or per 100 ml of tissue or body fluid, respectively. Chloride content of blood, as determined in cases of drowning, usually is reported as sodium chloride. For the gastric or intestinal contents, the total amount of poison found also is reported. Carbon monoxide content should be reported with reference to the hemoglobin concentration.[120] If organ blood had been extracted with water, the results are reported as percent carboxyhemoglobin saturation. In anesthesia and drug-associated deaths, the toxicologic reports are to confirm whether the incriminated substances were present and whether their concentrations were higher than the normally expected levels. If proper requests have been made to the toxicologist, the analysis also will rule out potential errors in the administration of the drug, mix-up of drugs, drug contaminants, or agents which might have affected the drug action.

The interpretation of the reported data may be extremely difficult, and comparison with earlier reported cases or animal experiments may be necessary. If the toxic substances had been determined in several tissues and body fluids, this may help to establish the mode of administration[39] and the time elapsed after intoxication. Tolerance in drug addicts, idiosyncrasies, coexisting diseases, and many other circumstances may affect the interpretation in some cases.

REFERENCES

1. Abelson PH: Death from heroin (editorial). Science *168*:1289, 1970
2. Adriani J: The Pharmacology of Anesthetic Drugs: A Syllabus for Students and Clinicians. Fourth edition. Springfield, Illinois, Charles C Thomas, Publisher, 1960
3. Baker SP, Spitz WU: Age effects and autopsy evidence of disease in fatally injured drivers. JAMA *214*:1079–1088, 1970
4. Bass M: Sudden sniffing death. JAMA *212*:2075–2079, 1970
5. Beeman J: Notes on the identification of seminal stains by means of the Florence reaction. Arch Pathol *34*:932–933, 1942
6. Bornstein: Cited by Wecht CH, Collom WD[129]
7. Bowden K: The use of x-ray examination in medico-legal autopsies. Med J Aust *2*:923–925, 1956
8. Breitenecker R: Shotgun wound patterns. Am J Clin Pathol *52*:258–269, 1969
9. Brinkhous KM: Accident Pathology. (Proceedings of an International Conference, Washington DC, June 6–8, 1968.) Washington DC, US Government Printing Office
10. Brudzynski C: Investigation of anesthetic deaths. Ann West Med Surg *6*:511–514, 1952
11. Camps FE: Gradwohl's Legal Medicine. Second edition. Baltimore, Williams & Wilkins Company, 1968, pp 123–154
12. Camps FE: Gradwohl's Legal Medicine. Second edition. Baltimore, Williams & Wilkins Company, 1968, pp 345–351
13. Camps FE: Gradwohl's Legal Medicine. Second edition. Baltimore, Williams & Wilkins Company, 1968, pp 612–615
14. Camps FE: Immersion in fluids. *In* Recent Advances in Forensic Pathology. London, J. & A. Churchill, Ltd., 1969, pp 70–79
15. Camps FE: Abortion and its complications. *In* Recent Advances in Forensic Pathology. London, J. & A. Churchill, Ltd., 1969, pp 88–100
16. Camps FE: Injuries sustained by children from violence. *In* Recent Advances in Forensic Pathology. London, J. & A. Churchill, Ltd., 1969, pp 129–136
17. Camps FE: The post-mortem findings in acute barbiturate poisoning and their interpretation. *In* Acute Barbiturate Poisoning. Edited by H Matthew. Amsterdam, Excerpta Medica, 1971, pp 351–355
18. Cherubin CE: The medical sequelae of narcotic addiction. Ann Intern Med *67*:23–33, 1967
19. Citron BP, Halpern M, McCarron M, Lundberg GD, McCormick R, Pincus IJ, Tatter D, Haverback BJ: Necrotizing angiitis associated with drug abuse. N Engl J Med *283*:1003–1011, 1970
20. Clarke EGC: Isolation and Identification of Drugs in Pharmaceuticals, Body Fluids and Post-mortem Material. London, The Pharmaceutical Press, 1969
21. Coe JI, Sherman RE: Comparative study of postmortem vitreous humor and blood alcohol. J Forensic Sci *15*:185–190, 1970
22. Curran WJ: The status of forensic pathology in the United States. N Engl J Med *283*:1033–1034, 1970
23. Curran WJ: Medicolegal investigational systems: new demands in the 1970's. N Engl J Med *284*:30–31, 1971
24. Curry A: Poison Detection in Human Organs. Second edition. Springfield, Illinois, Charles C Thomas, Publisher, 1969
25. DeGross J: Emergency treatment of drug abuse and poison ingestion. Resident Staff Physician *16*:43–51, 1970
26. De Saram GSW, Webster G, Kathirgamatamby N: Post-mortem temperature and the time of death. J Criminal Law, Criminol Police Sci *46*:562–577, 1955

27. Duguid H, Simpson RG, Stowers JM: Accidental hypothermia. Lancet 2:1213–1219, 1961

28. Dutra FR: Identification of person and determination of cause of death from skeletal remains. Arch Pathol 38:339–349, 1944

29. Eckert WG: On death and organ transplantation. INFORM (The International Reference Organization in Forensic Medicine.) 1(No. 2):3–6 (Apr.) 1969

30. Eckert WG: The forensic sciences and the drug problem. Part I. The narcotic drugs. IN-FORM (The International Reference Organization in Forensic Medicine.) 2(No. 4):3–7 (Oct.) 1970

31. Eckert WG: The forensic sciences and the drug problem. Part II. The hallucinogenic drugs. INFORM (The International Reference Organization in Forensic Medicine.) 3(No. 1):3–7 (Jan.) 1971

32. Eckert WG: The forensic sciences and the drug problem. Part III. The Depressants and stimulants. INFORM (The International Reference Organization in Forensic Medicine.) 3(No. 2):3–7 (Apr.) 1971

33. Editorial: Increasing deaths from asthma. Br Med J 1:329–330, 1968

34. Evans WED: The Chemistry of Death. Springfield, Illinois, Charles C Thomas, Publisher, 1963

35. Fatteh A: Estimation of time of death by chemical changes. Med Leg Bull 163:1–6, 1966

36. Faulkner WR, King JW, Damm HC: Handbook of Clinical Laboratory Data. Second edition. Cleveland, Ohio, The Chemical Rubber Co., 1968

37. Ferrer JM, Parsa MH: Fatal air embolism via subclavian vein (letter to the editor). N Engl J Med 282:688, 1970

38. Fiddes FS, Patten TD: Cited in Mant AK[76]

39. Finck PA: Postmortem distribution studies of cyanide: report of three cases. Med Ann DC 38:357–358, 1969

40. Freimuth HC: Toxicology in medicolegal investigations. In Legal Medicine Annual 1969. Edited by CH Wecht. New York, Appleton-Century-Crofts, Inc., 1969, pp 185–196

41. Friedman EA, Greenberg JB, Merrill JP, Dammin GJ: Consequences of ethylene glycol poisoning: report of four cases and review of the literature. Am J Med 32:891–902, 1962

42. Froentjes W: Third International Conference on Alcohol and Road Traffic. London, British Medical Association, 1963, p 179

43. Fuller RH: The clinical pathology of human near-drowning. Proc R Soc Med 56:33–38, 1963

44. Furbank RA: Conversion data, normal values, nomograms and other standards. In Modern Trends in Forensic Medicine. Vol 2. Edited by K Simpson. London, Butterworth & Co. (Publishers) Ltd., 1967, pp 344–364

45. Furuhata T, Katsuichi Y: Forensic Odontology. Springfield, Illinois, Charles C Thomas, Publisher, 1967

46. Gerlach W: Postmortale Form- und Lageveränderungen mit besonderer Berücksichtigung der Totenstarre. Ergeb Allg Path path Anat 20:259–305, 1923

47. Gettler AO: A method for the determination of death by drowning. JAMA 77:1650–1653, 1921

48. Gillett R, Warburton FG: Barbiturate blood levels found at necropsy in proven cases of acute barbiturate poisoning. J Clin Pathol 23:435–439, 1970

49. Glaister J, Rentoul E: Medical Jurisprudence and Toxicology. Twelfth edition. Edinburgh, E. & S. Livingstone, Ltd., 1966

50. Gonzales TA, Vance M, Helpern M, Umberger CJ: Legal Medicine: Pathology and Toxicology. Second edition. New York, Appleton-Century-Crofts, Inc., 1954

51. Gregory GA, Tooley WH: Gas embolism in hyaline-membrane disease. N Engl J Med 282:1141–1142, 1970

52. Gustafson G: Rôle de l'odontologie légale dans l'enquête criminelle et l'identification. Ann Med Leg 39:5–25, 1959

53. Haggerty RJ: Toxic hazards: deaths from permanent antifreeze ingestion. N Engl J Med 261:1296–1297, 1959

54. Harger RN: Ethyl alcohol. In Toxicology: Mechanisms and Analytical Methods. Vol II. Edited by CP Stewart, A Stolman. New York, Academic Press, 1961, pp 85–151

55. Harger RN, Forney RB: Aliphatic alcohols. In Progress in Chemical Toxicology. Vol 2. Edited by A Stolman. New York, Academic Press, 1967, pp 1–61

56. Hayman CR: Sexual assaults on women and girls (editorial). Ann Intern Med 72:277–278, 1970

57. Helpern M, Rho YM: Deaths from narcotism in New York City: incidence, circumstances, and postmortem findings. NY State J Med 66:2391–2408, 1966

58. Helpern M, Strassmann G: Differentiation of fetal and adult human hemoglobin: its medicolegal importance, especially in connection with alkali test for carbon monoxide in blood. Arch Pathol 35:776–782, 1943
59. Henderson AH, Pugsley DJ: Collapse after intravenous injection of hashish. Br Med J 3:229–230, 1968
60. Hirvonen J, Tiisala R, Uotila U, Tahti H, Laiho K, Martila, A, Tenhu M: Roentgeno-logical and autopsy studies on the gas content of the lungs and gastro-intestinal tract in living and stillborn infants, and sources of error in resuscitation. Deutsch Z Ges Gerichtl Med 65:73–86, 1969
61. Irey NS: Syllabus (Part I) on Diagnostic Problems and Methods in Drug-Induced Diseases. (Registry of Tissue Reactions to Drugs. American Registry of Pathology.) Washington DC, Armed Forces Institute of Pathology, 1966
62. Jelliffe RW, Stephenson RG: A fluorometric determination of myocardial digoxin at au-topsy, with identification of digitalis leaf, digitoxin, and gitoxin. Am J Clin Pathol 51:347–357, 1969
63. Jetter WW, McLean R: Poisoning by synergistic effect of phenobarbital and ethyl alcohol: experimental study. Arch Pathol 36:112–122, 1943
64. Johnston EH, Goldbaum LR, Whelton RL: Investigation of sudden death in addicts, with emphasis on the toxicologic findings in thirty cases. Med Ann DC 38:375–380, 1969
65. Joint Committee on Aviation Pathology: An Autopsy Guide for Aircraft Accident Fatalities. Washington DC, Armed Forces Institute of Pathology, 1957
66. Kevorkian J: The fundus oculi and the determination of death. Am J Pathol 32:1253–1269, 1956
67. King AB, Pechet GS, Pechet L: Intravenous injection of crude marihuana (letter to the editor). JAMA 214:1711, 1970
68. Knocker P: Effects of experimental hypothermia on vital organs. Lancet 2:837–840, 1955
69. Kulka W: Laboratory methods and technical notes: a practical device for demonstrating air embolism. Arch Pathol 48:366–369, 1949
70. Larson CP: Alcohol: fact and fallacy. In Legal Medicine Annual 1969. Edited by CH Wecht. New York, Appleton-Century-Crofts, Inc., 1969, pp 241–268
71. Lie JT: Changes of potassium concentration in the vitreous humor after death. Am J Med Sci 254:136–143, 1967
72. Lie JT, Balazs NDH, Ungar B, Cowling DC: Anaemias associated with increased foetal haemoglobin content: a study by the acid elution technique. Med J Aust 1:43–46, 1968
73. Louria DB, Hensle T, Rose J: The major medical complications of heroin addiction. Ann Intern Med 67:1–22, 1967
74. Lovell W: Joint Committee on Aviation Pathology (Memorandum No. 5). Problems in the Post Mortem Diagnosis of Hypoxia as a Contributing Factor in Aircraft Accidents. Washington DC, Armed Forces Institute of Pathology, 1959
75. Mann TP, Elliott RIK: Neonatal cold injury due to accidental exposure to cold. Lancet 1:229–233, 1957
76. Mant AK: Recent work on post-mortem changes and timing death. In Modern Trends in Forensic Medicine. Vol 2. Edited by K Simpson. New York, Appleton-Century-Crofts, Inc., 1967, pp 147–162
77. Mant AK: The postmortem diagnosis of hypothermia. Br J Hosp Med 2:1095–1098, 1969
78. Marshall TK: Temperature methods of estimating the time of death. Med Sci Law 5:224–232, 1965
79. Modell JH: The pathophysiology and treatment of drowning. Acta Anaesthesiol Scand Suppl 29:263–279, 1968
80. Modell JH, Davis JH, Giammona ST, Moya F, Mann JB: Blood gas and electrolyte changes in human near-drowning victims. JAMA 203:337–343, 1968
81. Moritz AR: Chemical methods for the determination of death by drowning. Physiol Rev 24:70–88, 1944
82. Moritz AR: Scientific evidence in establishing the time of death. Ann West Med Surg 6:302–304, 1952
83. Moritz AR: Classical mistakes in forensic pathology. Am J Clin Pathol 26:1383–1397, 1956
84. Moritz AR, Jetter WW: Antemortem and postmortem diffusion of alcohol through the mucosa of the bladder. Arch Pathol 33:939–948, 1942
85. Moritz AR, Lund H: Special evidentiary objectives of the medico-legal autopsy. J Tech Methods 23:71–85, 1943

86. Moritz AR, Morris CR: Handbook of Legal Medicine. Third edition. St. Louis, C. V. Mosby Company, 1970

87. Mueller WF: Pathology of temporal bone hemorrhage in drowning. J Forensic Sci *14*:327–336, 1969

88. Needham RWJ, Oakland MH, Fryer DI: Joint Committee of Aviation Pathology (Memorandum No. 4). Significance of Tissue Carbon Monoxide Values: Evaluation of the Method of Wilks Van Fossan and Clark. Washington DC, Armed Forces Institute of Pathology, 1959

89. Neiß A: Röntgenidentifikation. Stuttgart, Georg Thieme Verlag, 1968

90. Niles NR: Hemorrhage in middle-ear and mastoid in drowning. Am J Clin Pathol *40*:281–283, 1963

91. Nordmann M: Erfahrungen bei Exhumierungen. Zentralbl Allg Pathol *73*:81–86, 1939

92. Papper EM, Kitz RJ: Uptake and Distribution of Anesthetic Agents. New York, McGraw-Hill Book Company, Inc., 1963

93. Petty CS: Firearms injury research: the role of the practicing pathologist. Am J Clin Pathol *52*:277–288, 1969

94. Plueckhahn VD: The significance of blood alcohol levels at autopsy. Med J Aust *2*:118–124, 1967

95. Plueckhahn VD: Alcohol levels in autopsy heart blood. J Forensic Med *15*:12–21, 1968

96. Plueckhahn VD: The significance of alcohol and sugar determinations in autopsy blood. Med J Aust *1*:46–51, 1970

97. Pollak OJ: Semen and seminal stains: review of methods used in medicolegal investigations. Arch Pathol *35*:140–196, 1943

98. Polson CJ: The Scientific Aspects of Forensic Medicine. Edinburgh, Oliver & Boyd, 1969

99. Praetorius E, Poulsen H, Dupont H: Uric acid, xanthine and hypoxanthine in the cerebrospinal fluid. Scand J Clin Lab Invest *9*:133–137, 1957

100. Pryce DM, Ross CF: Post-mortem Appearances. Sixth edition. London, Oxford University Press, 1963, pp 31–32

101. Reay DT: Syllabus on Automobile Accidents. (Registry of Accident Pathology.) Washington DC, Armed Forces Institute of Pathology, 1970

102. Reinhardt CF, Azar A, Maxfield ME, Smith PE Jr, Mullin LS: Cardiac arrhythmias and aerosol "sniffing." Arch Environ Health *22*:265–279, 1971

103. Rieders F: Toxicologic considerations in deaths associated with anesthesia. *In* Legal Medicine Annual 1969. Edited by CH Wecht. New York, Appleton-Century-Crofts, Inc., 1969, pp 213–223

104. Rivers JF, Orr G, Lee HA: Drowning: its clinical sequelae and management. Br Med J *2*:157–161, 1970

105. Rupp JC: Sperm survival and prostatic acid phosphatase activity in victims of sexual assaults. J Forensic Sci *14*:177–183, 1969

106. Sammut JJ: The middle ear in accidental deaths. J Laryngol Otol *81*:137–142, 1967

107. Schleyer FL: Postmortale klinisch-chemische Diagnostik und Todeszeitbestimmung mit chemischen und physikalischen Methoden. Stuttgart, Georg Thieme Verlag, 1958

108. Sellier K: Schußentfernungsbestimmung. *In* Arbeitsmethoden der medizinischen und naturwissenschaftlichen Kriminalistik. Vol 7. Edited by E Weinig, S Berg. Lübeck, Max Schmidt-Romhild, Publisher, 1967

109. Shapiro HA: The diagnosis of death from delayed air embolism. J Forensic Med *12*:3–7, 1965

110. Siegel H, Helpern M, Ehrenreich T: The diagnosis of death from intravenous narcotism: with emphasis on the pathologic aspects. J Forensic Sci *11*:1–16, 1966

111. Snyder L: Homicide Investigation: Practical Information for Coroners, Police Officers, and Other Investigators. Springfield, Illinois, Charles C Thomas, Publisher, 1944

112. Spencer JAE, Green NM: Suicide by ingestion of halothane. JAMA *205*:702–703, 1968

113. Spitz WU: Essential postmortem findings in the traffic accident victim. Arch Pathol *90*:451–457, 1970

114. Spitz WU: Laboratory diagnosis of drowning. *In* Laboratory Diagnosis of Diseases Caused by Toxic Agents. Edited by FW Sunderman, FW Sunderman Jr. St. Louis, Warren H. Green, Inc., 1970, pp 551–553

115. Stevens PJ: Fatal Civil Aircraft Accidents: Their Medical and Pathological Investigation. Bristol, John Wright & Sons, Ltd., 1970

116. Sunderman WF, Sunderman WF Jr: Laboratory Diagnosis of Diseases Caused by Toxic Agents. St. Louis, Warren H. Green, Inc., 1970

117. Sunshine I: Manual of Analytical Toxicology. Cleveland, Chemical Rubber Company, 1971

118. Swann HG, Brucer M, Moore C, Vezien BL: Fresh water and sea water drowning: a study of the terminal cardiac and biochemical events. Tex Rep Biol Med 5:423–437, 1947

119. Swann HG, Spafford NR: Body salt and water changes during fresh and sea water drowning. Tex Rep Biol Med 9:356–382, 1951

120. Talbert WM Jr, Muelling RJ Jr: Carbon monoxide intoxication. *In* Legal Medicine Annual 1969. Edited by CH Wecht. New York, Appleton-Century-Crofts, Inc., 1969, pp 199–209

121. Taylor GJ IV, Harris WS: Cardiac toxicity of aerosol propellents. JAMA 214:81–85, 1970

122. Taylor JD: Post-mortem diagnosis of air embolism by radiography. Br Med J 1:890–893, 1952

123. Teare D: Post-mortem examinations on air-crash victims. Br Med J 2:707–708, 1951

124. US Department of Defense. Army Department: Autopsy Manual, Washington DC, US Government Printing Office, 1960

125. US Department of Defense. Navy Department: Manual of Aviation Pathology. US Naval Aviation Medical Center, Pensacola, Florida, 1962

126. Van Metre TE Jr: Adverse effects of inhalation of excessive amounts of nebulized isoproterenol in status asthmaticus. J Allergy 43:101–113, 1969

127. Virchow R: Post-mortem Examinations With Especial Reference to Medico-legal Practice. Fourth German edition. (English translation by TP Smith) Philadelphia, P. Blakiston, Son & Co., 1885

128. Waller JA: Drugs and highway crashes: can we separate fact from fancy? JAMA 215:1477–1482, 1971

129. Wecht CH, Collom WD: Medical evidence in alleged rape. *In* Legal Medicine Annual 1969. Edited by CH Wecht. New York, Appleton-Century-Crofts, Inc., 1969, pp 271–285

130. Wert EB: Suicide in relation to toxic agents. *In* Laboratory Diagnosis of Diseases Caused by Toxic Agents. Edited by WF Sunderman, WF Sunderman Jr. St. Louis, Warren H. Green, Inc., 1970, pp 558–571

131. Winek CL: Exposure to volatile or airborne toxicants. *In* Legal Medicine Annual 1969. Edited by CH Wecht. New York, Appleton-Century-Crofts, Inc., 1969, pp 227–238

CHAPTER 3

HEART AND
VASCULAR SYSTEM

With Jack L. Titus

HEART

Routine dissection.   Rokitansky began the routine dissection of the heart by first incising in situ the lateral wall of the left ventricle and continuing this incision into the left atrium.[37] This maneuver was repeated on the right side. The left ventricular outflow tract was incised from the aorta through the membranous part of the ventricular septum to the apex, leaving the pulmonary artery and valve intact. Rössle[58] also incised the heart in situ, but by a transverse section across the anterior half of both ventricles. The pulmonary outflow tract was opened from this cut; dissection was completed after the removal of the heart from the body. Hudson[20] also recommended that dissection of the heart be done by a primary transverse incision across the lower third of both ventricles after removal from the thoracic cavity. To hold the two halves together, the posterior wall should not be completely transected. If there are gross abnormalities of the myocardium, slicing is continued transversely. If the myocardium appears normal, dissection follows this sequence: (1) examination of the coronary arteries by crosswise sectioning at 2-mm intervals; (2) opening of the right atrium from the atrial appendage to the inferior vena cava; (3) opening of the right ventricular outflow tract, starting in the pulmonary artery; (4) opening of the lateral portion of the right ventricle from the base of the primary transverse incision in the right atrium; (5) cutting into the left atrial appendage and, from here, opening of the left atrium by an incision running posteriorly between the right and left pulmonary veins and to the atrioventricular junction; (6) opening of the left ventricular outflow tract

51

parallel with the anterior attachment of the ventricular septum; and, (7) if indicated, opening of the lateral wall of the left ventricle.

An excellent discussion, with illustrations, of various dissection techniques has been prepared by Reiner.[49] In our institution the following two methods are used for the routine dissection of the heart.

Following Direction of Flow of Blood. This is a modification[28] of Virchow's method.[70] The initial steps are: (1) incision of pericardium; (2) removal of pericardial contents and blood for microbiologic examination; (3) transection of innominate veins between two clamps; (4) ligation and transection of aortic arch branches; and (5) transection of trachea and esophagus at this level. The thoracic organs are now pulled downward, and the esophagus, descending aorta, and inferior vena cava are cut just above the diaphragm. In some instances, the esophagus is left attached to the stomach.

On the dissecting table the sequence is: (1) incision of the pulmonary artery above the valve; (2) opening of the artery to the hilus of both lungs; (3) longitudinal opening of the esophagus and removal of it from the heart-lung block; (4) opening of the trachea and main bronchi along their posterior membranous portion; (5) dissection and opening, with scissors, of the left inferior pulmonary vein across the left atrium into the right inferior pulmonary vein; and (6) opening of the left atrium from this primary incision toward the left atrial appendage. The heart is separated from the lungs, trachea, main bronchi, aortic arch and descending aorta, and pulmonary arteries. The epicardial coronary arteries are identified and cut in cross sections, leaving vascular rings 2 to 3 mm long. The right atrium is opened with scissors, beginning anteriorly at the ostium of the inferior vena cava and moving toward the ostium of the superior vena cava and on to the anterior surface of the right atrial appendage. The heart is turned and the right ventricle opened posteriorly with scissors or knife by an incision through the tricuspid valve along the ventricular septum to the apex of the right ventricle. The outflow tract of the right ventricle is opened by a cut along the anterior margin of the ventricular septum from the apex, passing through the pulmonary valve.

Through the previously opened left atrium, the left ventricle is opened, with a long, thin-bladed knife inserted through the mitral valve, along the most lateral aspect of the left ventricular wall; this incision passes between the papillary muscles of the left ventricle and divides the posterior leaflet of the mitral valve. The left ventricular outflow tract is opened from the apex of the left ventricle along the anterior aspect of the ventricular septum through the aortic valve. The wedge-shaped muscular mass (anterolateral part of the left ventricle) formed by these two incisions in the left ventricle and the larger muscular mass made up of septum and posterolateral portions of left ventricle are cut parallel with the endocardial surface.

Satisfactory specimens also are obtained when the inflow portion of the right ventricle is opened by cutting its lateral free wall, and the right ventricular outflow tract is opened by an incision along a straight line formed by the axis of the pulmonary artery. This procedure preserves the anterior papillary muscle intact.

Transverse Slicing of Myocardium. This method permits the best identification and localization of myocardial infarcts for electrocardiographic correlations.[4] It is indicated whenever severe coronary atherosclerosis is present. The ventricular portion of the heart is cut into slices about 1.5 cm thick.[59] The atria and the valvular plane of the heart are opened as described previously.

Measuring and Weighing Heart. Circumferences (or diameters) of valves and thicknesses of the ventricular myocardium are usually recorded. The circumference or diameter of valves is best measured with graded glass or wooden cones;[18] after the valvular ring has been opened, the circumference may be measured with a ruler. The thickness of the ventricular myocardium is conveniently measured about 1 cm below the pulmonary or mitral valve. Care should be taken that the thickness is measured radially to the center of the lumen. If several measurements have been carried out, the lowest value will be the correct one. Generally, only the compact portion of the myocardium is measured and the trabeculae carneae are not included. These latter measurements are of limited value unless heart weight, heart configuration, capacity of the chambers, and state of rigor mortis are also recorded. Some authors[49] have abandoned as worthless the practice of measuring the thickness of the ventricular walls.

The heart weight, together with the body weight, should be recorded in all cases.

The actual weight of the myocardium proper can be calculated from the specific gravity of the whole heart; this requires measurement of the volume of the heart tissue. The rationale for this calculation of muscular mass is based on the fact that the specific gravity of the myocardium and fat tissue is a relatively constant value.[38] The volume of the mass of the whole heart is determined by displacement of an isotonic sodium chloride solution. From this volume and the total weight, the specific gravity is calculated (sp. g. = total weight/total volume), and the relative weight of the myocardium can be determined from application of the appropriate factors listed in the Appendix as computed by Masshoff and co-workers.[38]

Dissection in Special Cases. *Valvular Heart Disease.* If *bacterial endocarditis* is present or suspected, material for microbiologic study should be removed by sterile techniques *before* other dissections are done (see page 211). In all other cases of valvular heart disease the first step is to determine the competence of the valves. This can be done reliably with water[3,18] poured into the aorta and into the pulmonary artery. If the aortic and pulmonary valves are competent, no water should run into the ventricles. The tricuspid and mitral valves can be tested by injecting water into the ventricles through the aortic and pulmonary valves. Clamps are applied to the aorta and pulmonary artery to prevent the reflux of water. If the tricuspid and mitral valves are competent, no water should run into the atria under reasonably physiologic pressures.

Pliable valves are measured as described above. In the presence of marked *fibroplastic deformities* and *calcification*, the opening (effective orifice) between the free edges of the valves is measured in two dimensions. In the presence of valvular disease, the dissection of the heart should follow the flow of blood but should be modified in such a way that the involved valves are left intact. The lines of incision into the heart chambers and into the great arteries remain the same.

Congenital Malformations of Heart and Associated Vascular Anomalies. The cadaver should be well supported at the level of the lower end of the scapulae. This facilitates proper exposure, identification, and dissection of vascular anomalies in the upper thoracic aperture and neck. Before the chest plate is removed, the innominate veins should be separated from the overlying bones by blunt dissection. Careful anatomic dissection is essential to identify anomalous systemic venous connections or abnormalities of the aortic arch system. This may be difficult and time-consuming, particularly in the presence of extensive postoperative hemorrhage or insufficient extension of the head and neck area.

In the presence of stenosis of the aortic isthmus, including coarctation of the aorta, dilated internal mammary and intercostal arteries can be demonstrated roentgenographically by injecting contrast medium into the lumen of the ascending aorta. By the same technique, the bronchial arteries will be demonstrated. For these procedures, the lower descending thoracic aorta, the carotid arteries in the neck, and the brachial arteries should be clamped or tied.

In the presence of congenital cardiovascular malformations, our routine method of dissecting the heart remains essentially unaltered. The chest organs may be removed en bloc or en masse—that is, together with the abdominal organs. The latter method is preferable if anomalous pulmonary or systemic venous connections with subdiaphragmatic veins are suspected. For example, in instances of isolated levocardia or isolated dextrocardia, the abdominal organs often are drained by the azygos vein which may join a persisting left superior vena cava, or the hepatic veins may drain into the right atrium, or total anomalous pulmonary venous connection may be found.[10,44] For better orientation we often leave the uppermost portion of the liver and the hepatic veins attached to the inferior vena cava and the right atrium. Modifications of the routine dissection of the heart are made whenever grafts, abnormal valves, or other lesions are to be left intact.

Excellent specimens can be prepared by wax infiltration of the heart. Schematic drawings of malformed hearts should include measurements, particularly of septal or valvular defects and of stenotic or insufficient valves.

Unrolling Techniques. Unrolling techniques are used to demonstrate the coronary artery tree in one plane. The disadvantage of these methods is that the hearts are so mutilated that they become unsuitable for demonstrating anything other than coronary artery disease.

Technique of Schlesinger.[61] This technique permits the heart and, separately, the ventricular septum to be laid out flat.

First incision (Fig. 3–1 *A*). The right ventricle is opened along a line beginning in the pulmonary artery, running to the right of the ventricular septum, and ending at the apex of the right ventricle.

Second incision (Fig. 3–1 *B*). The cut starts between the right and left anterior aortic cusps and extends down into the ventricular septum, dividing the pulmonary valve and separating the anterior border of the ventricular septum from the anterior ventricular wall.

Third incision (Fig. 3–1 *C*). The septum is severed from its posterior attachment.

Fourth incision (Fig. 3–1 *D*). The anterior leaflet of the mitral valve is bisected at the middle of its free border, and the incision is continued through the mitral and aortic ring into the left atrium, parallel with the left side of the atrial septum, and into the pulmonary veins.

Fifth incision (Fig. 3–1 *E*). The tricuspid valve ring is divided between the anterior and medial leaflets, continuing along a line between the right anterior and posterior aortic cusps to the right atrium, parallel with the right side of the atrial septum, into the superior vena cava (Fig. 3–1 *F*).

Technique of Rodriguez and Reiner.[55] This technique permits the heart, with its ventricular septum, to be laid out flat. The principle is illustrated in Figure 3–2.

First incision. This begins in the pulmonary artery and is continued down to the apex, similar to step 1 in Schlesinger's technique (Fig. 3–1 *A*).

Second incision. This cut starts from the ostium of the superior vena cava, separates the anterior right atrial wall from the atrial septum, and continues through the tricuspid valve, the crista supraventricularis, and, for the second time, through the pulmonary valve. The first incision also can be joined below the pulmonic ring by cutting into the ventral part of the right ventricular outflow tract. The right coronary artery is transected by the second incision. To avoid this, one can cut out a button of aortic wall about the coronary ostium and leave this attached instead of transecting the artery.

Third incision. The cut begins between the right superior and right inferior pulmonary veins and is continued through the mitral valve down to the apex of the left ventricle, alongside the posterior attachment of the ventricular septum. The posterior papillary muscle should be divided at its base.

Fourth incision. This is optional. The aortic valve is opened posteriorly by an incision which circumvents the mitral valve, separating the lateral segment of the aortic ring and the medial segment of the mitral ring from the base of the ventricular septum posteriorly.

Technique of Lumb and Hardy.[34] The technique permits the heart to be laid out flat with the ventricular septum projecting upward.

First incision. This passes through the pulmonary valve down to the apex, as before (Fig. 3–1 *A*).

Second incision. The cut divides the medial attachment of the anterior leaflet of the tricuspid valve, passes through the right coronary artery at its origin from the aorta, passes through the anterior wall of the right atrium, and extends into the superior vena cava.

Third incision. It is begun by passing the point of a pair of scissors through the ventricular septum from the right into the left ventricle, close

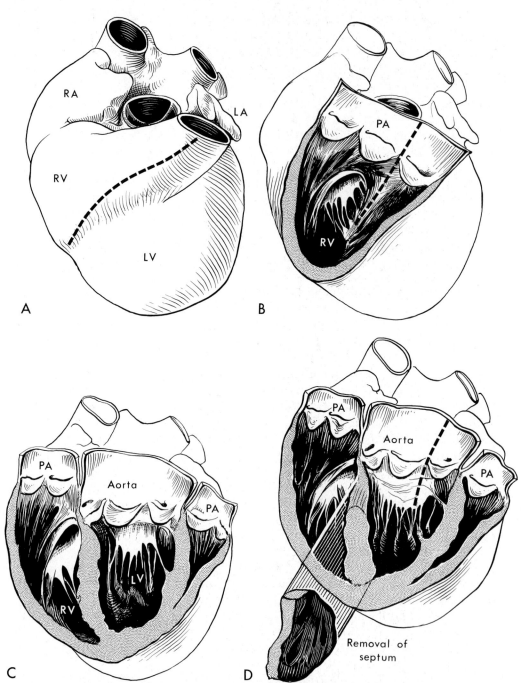

Figure 3-1.   Unrolling technique of Schlesinger. A, Broken line indicates first incision. *RA*= right atrium; *RV* = right ventricle; *LA* = left atrium; *LV* = left ventricle. B, Appearance after first incision. Broken line indicates second incision. *PA* = pulmonary artery. C, Appearance after second incision. D, Appearance after third incision. Broken line indicates fourth incision.

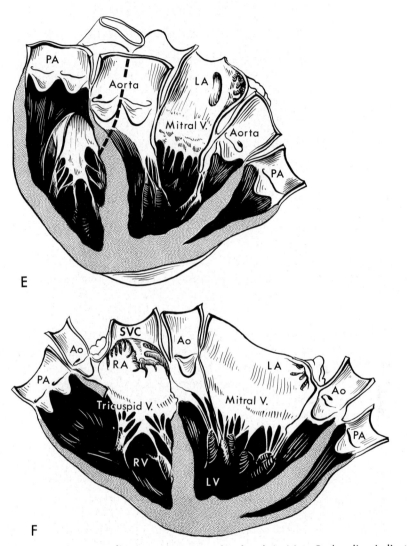

Figure 3–1 (continued). *E,* Appearance after fourth incision. Broken line indicates fifth incision. *F,* Appearance after fifth incision. SVC = superior vena cava.

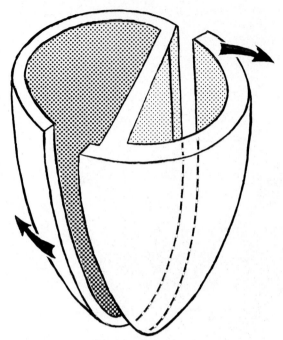

Figure 3–2. Principle of unrolling technique of Rodriguez and Reiner.[55] (Modified from Rodriguez FL, Reiner L: A new method of dissection of the heart. Arch Pathol 63:160–163, 1957.)

to the apex of the heart. From here the incision is made along the anterior margin of the ventricular septum, through the attachment of the anterior leaflet of the mitral valve, and into the aorta between the cusps.

Fourth incision. The left margin of the anterior leaflet of the mitral valve and the left atrium are cut open, ending in the left superior pulmonary vein.

Partitioning Techniques. Partitioning techniques are used to weigh the right and left ventricles separately. Removal of the coronary arteries and epicardial fat is essential. Separation of the septum into a right and a left ventricular portion generally has proved unsuccessful.

Technique of Müller.[42] The nonseptal portions of the right and left ventricles and atria, the atrial septum, and the ventricular septum are weighed separately.

Technique of Grant.[13] The heart is fixed in formalin. The atria are separated from the ventricles, and the right ventricle is dissected from the ventricular septum, leaving the septum attached to the left ventricle.

Technique of Reiner.[49] The heart first is unrolled (see technique of Rodriguez and Reiner). The chordae tendineae and the mitral and tricuspid valves are separated from the papillary muscles and the mural endocardium. Both atria, the atrioventricular ostia, and the pulmonary trunk are ablated from the ventricles. The right ventricle is separated from the ventricular septum. The atrioventricular valves and attached chordae, the aorta, and part of the pulmonary valve are removed from the atrial complex. The various portions of the heart can now be weighed.

Dissection of Atrioventricular Conduction System. Older techniques of macroscopic and microscopic examinations of the conduction system are described by Mönckeberg.[41]

Gross Dissection. The following method[66] almost always permits demonstration of the atrioventricular node, the common bundle, and the right bundle branch (Fig. 3–3). The origin of the left bundle branch (or branches) from the common bundle is sometimes noted as the dissection is carried out.

In the conventionally opened heart, the attachments of the chordae tendineae of the septal leaflet of the tricuspid valve are cut and this leaflet, sometimes with adjacent portions of the posterior and anterior leaflets, is reflected atrialward or removed. The endocardium of the right atrium above and contiguous with this leaflet—in an area bounded roughly by the coronary sinus ostium posteriorly, the fossa ovalis superiorly, and the central fibrous body anteriorly—is dissected free and reflected upward or removed. Usually, a thin band of atrial muscle running in a direction obliquely or at right angles to the tricuspid valve margin is encountered. This is carefully teased away. The atrioventricular node is then seen lying

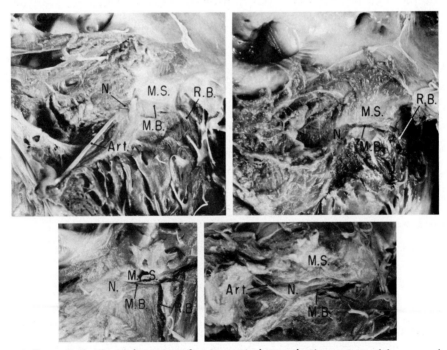

Figure 3–3. Gross dissection of atrioventricular conduction system of four normal hearts. *N.* = atrioventricular node; *M.B.* = main (common) bundle; *M.S.* = membranous septum; *R.B.* = right bundle branch; *Art.* = artery to node. (From Titus JL: The Atrioventricular Conduction System in Congenital Ventricular Septal Defect. Thesis, Graduate School, University of Minnesota, 1961.)

in the base of the atrium just above the valve margin. The central fibrous body and the adjacent membranous portion of the ventricular septum are identified. Then, either the common bundle is followed as a slender muscle fascicle extending anteriorly from the node and passing through these structures or the membranous septum is split longitudinally and the slender muscle fascicle (representing either the common bundle or the right bundle branch) is followed back through the central fibrous body to its junction with the atrioventricular node. While these methods differ only slightly, different specimens seem to be handled more easily by one method than the other.

Gross Staining of Left Bundle-Branch Radiation. Lugol's iodine solution is swept onto the septal surface of the heart, rendering blue the relatively glycogen-rich conducting fibers of the left bundle-branch radiation. The main bundle and the proximal part of the right bundle branch are not superficial enough to show with this technique. Positive results can be expected only within 90 minutes after death.

Sectioning for Histologic Study. Minor modifications of the methods of Lev and associates[29] have been used successfully by one of us[66] and appear to be the best for proper histologic examination of the atrioventricular conduction system.

An area, as outlined in Figure 3–4, is removed and two to four blocks are made of this area, depending on the size of the heart; the objective is simply to include the area under study in blocks of convenient size for handling in the tissue laboratory. The posterior limit of the blocks is approxi-

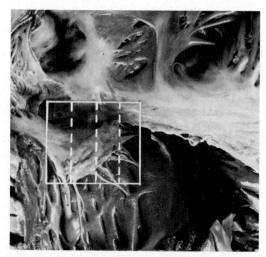

Figure 3–4. Opened tricuspid valve of normal adult heart, with right atrium above and right ventricle below. Area of gross dissection and block removed for histologic study of atrioventricular conduction system are indicated by solid rectangle. Broken lines indicate cuts made to prepare blocks of tissue for histologic sectioning. Plane of sectioning is parallel to broken lines. (From Titus JL: The Atrioventricular Conduction System in Congenital Ventricular Septal Defect. Thesis, Graduate School, University of Minnesota, 1961.)

mately level with the anterior extent of the coronary sinus ostium; the anterior limit is approximately the level of the posterior aspect of the crista supraventricularis; superiorly, approximately 1 cm of atrial septal tissue is included; inferiorly, approximately 2 cm of ventricular septal tissue is included. In thickness, the blocks include essentially all of the ventricular septum and all (or nearly all) of the atrial septum.

The plane of sectioning is parallel with the vertical plane of section used to obtain the original block (or blocks) of tissue (this is the method used in the majority of reported studies). Horizontal sections may fail to show portions of the conduction system adequately because of irregularities in the pathway of the system. For reliable and complete examination, each of the blocks should be serially sectioned in its entirety.

Dissection and Sectioning of Sinus (Sinoauricular) Node. The human sinus node is situated in the anterolateral aspect of the junction of the superior vena cava with the right atrium (the region of the crista terminalis and the most superior aspect of the right atrial appendage). It surrounds a small atrial artery and is not grossly dissectable. Identification of the sinus node may be facilitated by injection of the coronary arteries in order to fill the sinus node artery; it is the first major atrial branch of the right coronary artery in about 55% of hearts and the first major atrial branch of the left circumflex coronary artery in most, but not all, of the others.

Histologic study of cross sections of the sinus node and sinus nodal artery is carried out by removal of one or two blocks of tissue. These blocks are cut by longitudinal incisions extending from the superior vena cava into the right atrial wall (Fig. 3–5). They usually are about 3 to 4 cm long and contain approximately equal lengths of cava and atrium. Histologic sectioning is done in a plane parallel with the long axis of the block.

Postmortem Diagnosis of Early Myocardial Infarcts. *Gross Staining Techniques.* These methods are based on the absence, in ischemic myocardium, of endogenous substrates, enzymes, or coenzymes which participate in a chemical reaction whose completion is indicated by the formation, directly or indirectly, of a colored compound.

1. Nitro-BT dye test.[4,43] It is convenient to keep stock solutions of 1M Sorensen's phosphate buffer, pH 7.4, and Nitro-BT (2,2'-di-p-nitrophenyl-5,5'-diphenyl-3,3'-[3,3'-dimethoxy-4,4'-biphenylene]ditetrazolium chloride), 5 mg/ml. The incubation fluid for the test is prepared by mixing 1 volume of buffer, 1 volume of Nitro-BT, and 8 volumes of triple-distilled deionized water. This mixture is prewarmed in a water bath to 37 C.

Slices of myocardium are rinsed briefly with running cold water to remove traces of blood and tissue juices and then are placed in the incubation fluid for 30 minutes at 37 C. The slices are gently agitated and turned over in the solution. Normal myocardium turns purplish blue within a few minutes while ischemic myocardium remains unstained. Myocardial infarcts less than 6 to 8 hours old cannot be detected by this method.

After long postmortem intervals (approximately 12 hours), normal myocardium may remain unstained or poorly stained. Therefore, if there is no staining or only poor staining after 25 minutes of incubation, 1 vol-

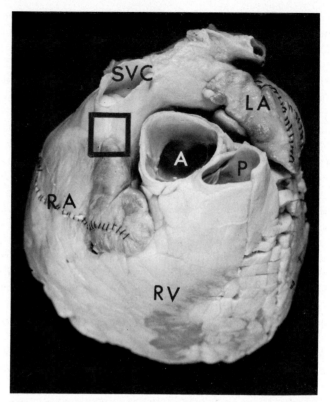

Figure 3–5. Anterior-superior view of intact heart with outline of **block for study of sinus node.** SVC = superior vena cava; RA = right atrium; RV = right ventricle; LA = left atrium; A = aorta; P = pulmonary artery.

ume of 1M sodium lactate is added to the incubation fluid; this should restore staining to normal tissue. After staining, the slices are fixed for 24 hours in neutral 10% formalin. The formazan dye is discernible on the edges of conventional histologic sections. A major disadvantage of this test is the high cost of the reagent.

2. Triphenyltetrazolium chloride (TTC) test.[26,30] The incubation fluid is TTC powder mixed with 0.2M Tris buffer, pH 8.0-8.5, to make a 1% solution. The buffer should be prewarmed in a 37 C incubator in a blackened round glass dish. Because TTC is sensitive to light, the powder or the solution should not be exposed to light for longer than required for the preparation of the incubation fluid.

Slices of myocardium, not thicker than 1 cm, are placed in the solution at 37 to 40 C in the incubator for 30 to 45 minutes. The slices are turned over once or twice during the incubation period. At the end of the incubation, the slices are placed in formol-saline in a plain glass dish.

Normal myocardium turns dark red.[26] Ischemic myocardium remains unstained, as does scar tissue (Fig. 3–6). In experimental studies,[32] positive results were obtained as early as 2 hours after coronary arterial ligation that produced infarction.

Histochemical Tests.[26] Histochemical tests on frozen sections for diphosphopyridine nucleotide diaphorase and malic dehydrogenase may be helpful. If only paraffin sections are available, the diagnosis of early myocardial infarcts on occasion can be improved by periodic acid-Schiff (PAS) stains with and without diastase treatment and with phosphotungstic acid-hematoxylin (PTAH) staining. Recently, basic fuchsin staining of paraffin sections has been shown to demonstrate ischemic myocardial fibers in the first 12 hours after the onset of ischemia.[31] The exact mechanisms of the positive reactions of ischemic fibers are uncertain but appear to be related to protein alterations.

Mitochondrial stains and fluorescent methods (acridine orange) have not been particularly useful in human autopsy material for the diagnosis of early infarction.[26]

Determination of Potassium to Sodium Ratio in Myocardium.[40,73] In normal myocardium, the ratio K^+/Na^+ is high, averaging 1.5 to 2.5. In infarcted tissue this ratio is low, approaching 1.0. The ionic ratio decreases as the age of the infarct increases for at least 24 hours; it then gradually returns to normal. Macroscopic Nitro-BT staining has been suggested as a screening test; TTC would serve equally well. In cases in which no infarct is delineated by staining, the ionic ratio should be determined in myocardium removed from standard areas.

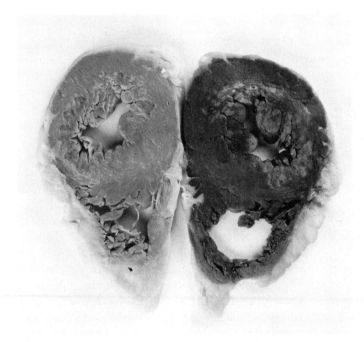

Figure 3–6. Slices of fresh myocardium from **heart with** acute (5 days) anteroseptal and posterolateral **myocardial infarction.** Mirror-image cut sections. *Left,* Slice before treatment. *Right,* Slice after treatment with TTC. Infarct is poorly defined in left slice. Clearly defined unstained areas in right slice correspond to acute infarction. (Picture courtesy of Dr. J. T. Lie.)

The analysis is performed on 1-cm cubes of myocardium (approximately 1 gm). Fat, blood clots, pericardium, and endocardium must be trimmed off the myocardium. The tissue cubes can be wrapped in aluminum foil and stored at −20 or −70 C. The trimmed myocardium is chopped into small pieces and weighed on a torsion balance. Deionized distilled water is used to wash all instruments and containers and is added to the chopped tissue to give a weight-to-volume ratio of 1:20. This mixture is homogenized for 10 minutes at room temperature in a Waring blender and then for 5 minutes in a ground-glass homogenizer. The cell debris is spun down at 1,000 rpm for 10 minutes. Analysis for sodium and potassium is carried out in a flame photometer on 1:10 and 1:50 dilutions of the supernate, respectively.

Combination of Tests. In a study[6] to delineate myocardial infarcts within 12 hours after the onset of the ischemic episode, the combination of the following four staining methods was found to be most reliable: Selye's acid fuchsin on paraffin sections, hematoxylin and eosin, acridine orange fluorescence on frozen sections, and the macroscopic Nitro-BT reaction. In the absence of the classic morphologic signs, all four staining reactions must be positive to warrant the diagnosis of early myocardial infarcts. However, it should be pointed out again that the results of such animal studies cannot always be applied to human autopsy material, as shown by the poor results in humans with acridine orange fluorescence.[26] Rather, we suggest combining conventional histologic study with the TTC test, the basic fuchsin stain on paraffin sections,[31] and possibly determination of the K^+/Na^+ ratio.

Selection of Blocks for Microscopic Study. The following sites have been suggested[14,69] for histologic examination of the formalin-fixed heart: (1) posterior border of the left atrium; (2) posterior leaflet of the mitral valve and the adjacent myocardium (1 and 2 can be combined in one block); (3) posterior papillary muscle of the left ventricle; (4) noncoronary cusp of the aortic valve and anterior leaflet of the mitral valve (one block); (5) pulmonary artery and valve; (6) right atrium and right ventricle; (7; 8) tips of the atrial appendages; and (9) coronary arteries. The precise location of most of the sections is illustrated in Figure 3–7. Section 6 (not shown) consists of 1 cm of the right atrium, the septal leaflet of the tricuspid valve, and 1 cm of the right ventricle. The incision is made about 5 cm lateral to the septal-anterior commissure. Sites and number of coronary artery sections will vary from case to case.

In the following sampling method, based on the vascular pattern of the heart,[50] the tissue blocks are selected primarily to reveal ischemic myocardial changes: (1) anterior left ventricle and adjacent ventricular septum approximately 2 cm above the anatomic apex; (2) posterolateral wall; (3) posterior basal portion of myocardium and adjacent ventricular septum, 1 to 2 cm below the atrioventricular groove; (4) (optional) anterior papillary muscle and its subjacent myocardium; (5) midposterior wall of right ventricle adjacent to the ventricular septum; (6) midanterior wall of right ventricle inferior to or including the pulmonary valve (6′); (7) posterolateral wall of the right atrium; and (8) posterior wall of the left atrium.

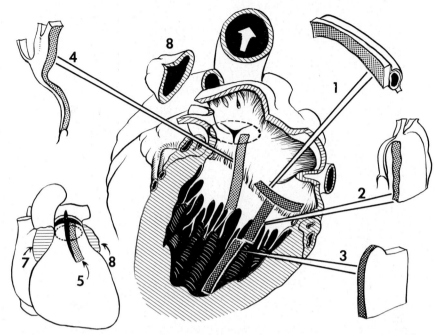

Figure 3–7. Sites for histologic examination. Numbers refer to list in text. (Redrawn and slightly modified from *Autopsy Manual,* Washington DC, Government Printing Office, July 1960, 78 pp.)

The positions of these tissue blocks are indicated in Figure 3–8.

Obviously these sampling patterns can be modified if so indicated by the gross findings. Careful dissection and inspection of the heart often will lead to a somewhat different sampling pattern, not necessarily demanding eight blocks.

In hearts without gross abnormalities, we section only one tissue block; it includes the posterior wall of the left atrium, the posterior leaflet of the mitral valve, and the adjacent myocardium.

Collection, Sterilization, and Preservation of Cadaveric Valve Homografts. In recent years, human cadaveric heart valves have been used as homografts for patients. At this time we use only aortic valves with or without the aortic arch. While the technique of removal of the homograft is fairly straightforward, the best method for preparation of the graft has not yet been established.[71] At the present time, the preferred methods are freezing-radiation and, perhaps, glutaraldehyde treatment. Some workers prefer to use nonpreserved ("fresh") grafts which are sterilized in a mixture of antibiotics in solution and stored for a few days in a nutrient medium.

Removal of Aortic Homograft With or Without Aortic Arch.[68] Grafts are selected from relatively young cadavers, usually less than 45 years of age, of either sex. The aortic valve and arch, if included, must be normal on gross morphologic examination. Grafts are obtained up to 18 hours after death. (Bacteria found in the grafts seem to be more virulent when the post-

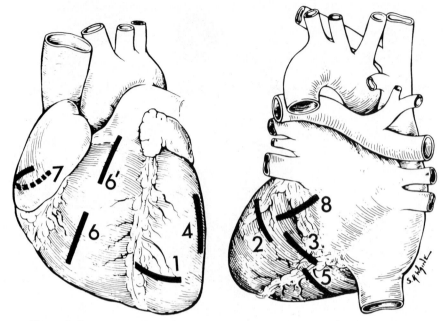

Figure 3–8. Location of tissue blocks which should be taken for **microscopic examination in ischemic heart disease.** Numbers refer to list in text. (After a suggestion by Reiner L: Selection of blocks from heart for microscopic study. Bull Pathol 9:198, 1968.)

mortem interval is long.[52]) Septicemia is not a contraindication as long as the tissues appear normal. Generally, we do not use grafts from patients who died with known "collagen disease" or who were jaundiced.

The graft obtained at autopsy includes the intact distal part of the left ventricular outflow tract, the intact aortic valve, the intact ascending thoracic aorta and aortic arch, the proximal 2 cm of the left and right coronary arteries, and the proximal 3 to 5 cm of the great arteries originating from the aortic arch. The portion of the graft proximal to the valve is composed of 3 to 5 cm of left ventricular muscle below the aortic valve and the entire anterior leaflet of the mitral valve (Fig. 3–9). The intact aortic arch is cut off from the descending thoracic aorta 1 to 3 cm distal to the origin of the left subclavian artery. Aortic valve homografts without the aortic arch are prepared by cutting off the ascending aorta about 2 cm above the aortic valve. In either case, excess muscular and fibroareolar tissues are trimmed from the external surface of the graft which is flushed with water to remove all blood. The diameter of the aortic valve is measured with a calibrated sound. The graft is then ready for further processing.

X-ray and Electron Beam Sterilization.[36,68] This is the method currently used. The graft is sealed in two or three plastic bags, one within the other. A few ordinary glass beads are placed in one of the outer bags and an appropriate identifying tag is inserted. The glass beads turn black when irradiated and thus serve to indicate that the grafts have been treated. However, they do not reflect quantitatively the dose of radiation energy.

As soon as they are sealed in plastic bags, the grafts are placed in a CO_2 freezer at -70 C. At a later time, when convenient, the grafts are sterilized with a high-energy electron beam while still frozen. After sterilization the grafts are kept at -70 C until used. No firm data are available as to the length of time that such grafts may be stored; somewhat arbitrarily, we have selected a time limit of about 6 months, although grafts stored for as long as 12 months have been used with satisfactory long-term results.

Ionizing radiation delivered to the homografts will ensure sterility if the absorbed dose is about 2.5 megarads. This dose has no apparent adverse effect on heart valves, blood vessels, bones, or nerves. This amount of radiation requires a source of high-energy photons (x-rays or gamma rays). The linear accelerator for patient therapy (6 Mev "Cliniac," Varian Associates) has provisions for extraction of the 6-Mev electron beam, and this is used for radiation of the homografts.

Since the dosage of radiation delivered is crucial to completeness of sterilization, problems of dosimetry are of major concern. The high dose rates desired restrict the choice of measurement techniques. Standardization of the dosage can be achieved by means of the thermoluminescence of lithium fluoride (LiF).[23] It was found that the reading of the rate meter

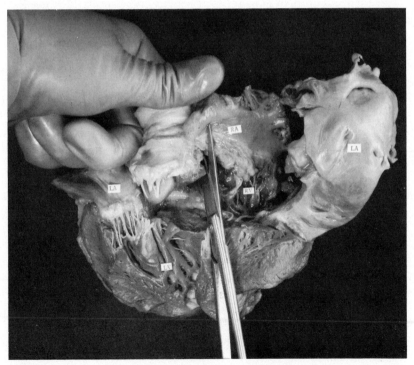

Figure 3–9. Removal of aortic valve homograft. Left index finger of prosector is in aortic valve sleeve. At fingertip, anterior leaflet of mitral valve can be seen. Wall of left atrium (LA) has been transected, and left ventricle (LV) has been separated from homograft through upper portion of ventricular septum, exposing part of right atrium (RA) and right ventricle (RV). Part of right atrium is being dissected from aortic valve sleeve.

on the control panel of the linear accelerator correlated well with the absorbed dose rate. Evaluation of the accumulated dosage of radiation was based on the change in optical density in red Perspex (Red 400) at 630 mμ.[45]

In the procedure for irradiation, a box containing the material to be irradiated, together with small pieces of Dry Ice distributed underneath and between but not above the graft, is placed in the appropriate position. A sheet of plastic, 1/16 inch (0.16 cm) thick, is placed immediately over the packaged grafts and in contact with them in order to provide buildup dose. Care must be taken to achieve adequate treatment of all portions of the packaged grafts. After half of the dose has been delivered, the electron beam is turned off, the samples are turned bottom-to-top, and the remainder of the dose is given. This improves the uniformity of dose distribution. Dosimeters of Red 400, 3/4 inch square, are placed in appropriate positions in the box before starting the irradiation to verify the dosage. At the dose of 2.5 megarads which we currently use, 25 minutes are required to complete the irradiation. Complete sterilization has been achieved by this technique.

Ethylene Oxide Sterilization.   The valvular homografts are soaked overnight in 0.2% chlorhexidine and then are trimmed, sized, and sterilized by exposure to ethylene oxide vapor for 24 hours. The grafts are freeze-dried and stored, in vacuum, in glass tubes. They are reconstituted for use by immersion in saline for 20 minutes at 37 C.[21] Most workers now agree that freeze-drying has deleterious effects on the long-term survival of nonvital cardiac valvular homografts.

Betapropiolactone Sterilization: The valves are sterilized in 1% betapropiolactone and subsequently kept at 4 C in a balanced salt solution with penicillin and streptomycin added. The sterilized valves also can be freeze-dried and reconstituted in distilled water for 30 minutes and then in isotonic saline in the operating room immediately before use. Betapropiolactone may adversely affect valvular grafts regardless of whether or not freeze-drying had been used.[63,67]

Formalin Sterilization.   Buffered formalin also has been used for both sterilization and storage of the valves.[71] The homografts are simply placed in a formalin solution which may, for instance, be buffered to about pH 5.6 at a concentration of 4%. Experiences with heterografts showed that formalin fixation was unsatisfactory in both experimental and clinical trials.[5,48]

Sterilization With Antibiotic Solutions.   In attempts to retain viability of homograft tissues, valves may be taken in a "clean" fashion at autopsy and placed in a solution containing several antibiotics for sterilization. If sterility of the graft is proved by bacteriologic cultures, it may be used after short periods of storage in nutrient medium. Care must be taken to ensure sterility; unsterile grafts stored in bacitracin and neomycin for 10 days were not effectively sterilized.[52]

Postmortem Coronary Angiography.   The main objectives of this procedure are the roentgenologic demonstration of narrowed or occluded coronary arteries and of anastomoses[54,56,64] which may have developed between the right and left coronary artery systems. The number and caliber of anastomotic vessels cannot be evaluated in any other practical way. While angiograms may clearly demonstrate vascular narrowing or occlusion, the nature of these lesions must still be determined by dissection and histologic examination. Thus, angiograms facilitate but do not replace proper dissection. The limitations of the technique and interpretation of coronary angiograms have been reviewed by Schoenmackers.[62]

In the past, various radiopaque injection media have been tried[60] such as lead phosphate in agar[61] or mixtures of lead carbonate, mercuric sulfide, and gelatin.[47] However, barium sulfate-gelatin mixtures are cheap and easy to prepare and also yield excellent results; these are now preferred by most pathologists.

Controlled-Pressure Barium-Gelatin Injection. In recent years we have routinely used this technique in all cases of suspected coronary insufficiency.[24,25]

The heart is removed with 2 to 4 cm of the major vessels attached. Postmortem clots are removed by irrigation with saline. Cannulae of suitable size are placed into the coronary ostia. Care is taken to identify an independent ostium. Ligatures are placed around the coronary arteries with an aneurysm needle and are tied as near as possible to the origins.

The cannulated heart is suspended in isotonic saline or Kaiserling I solution at about 45 C. The coronary arteries are perfused at a low pressure with isotonic saline. This is continued for several minutes, using 100 to 200 ml, until the return through the coronary sinus is free of blood.

The previously prepared barium-gelatin mixture (see below) is drawn into two 30-ml syringes. These are attached, via three-way stopcocks, to the apparatus shown in Figure 3–10, and the actual injection is begun. Care is

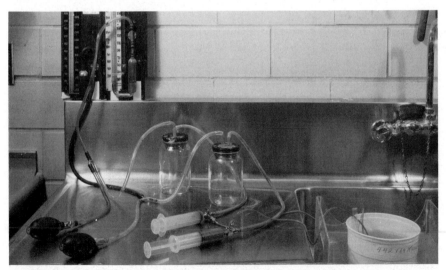

Figure 3–10. Setup for **controlled-pressure injection** of Chromopaque into coronary arteries. Each syringe contains Chromopaque of a different color and is connected to one of the coronary arteries and the pressure-regulating system. The heart is suspended in Kaiserling solution or saline in the container on the right which is in an ice-water bath. The two independent pressure-regulating systems with manometers are on the left.

taken to avoid introduction of air bubbles at any stage of the procedure. While the system is kept supplied with contrast medium by way of the syringes, the pressure is increased almost simultaneously to a maximum of 110 mm Hg. Lacerated vessels may require ligation at this stage, but these are rare in our experience.

We usually inject the right coronary artery system first. Stereoscopic roentgenograms in the anterior-posterior projection are prepared and then the uninjected coronary artery system is filled (Fig. 3–11). The heart chambers may be irrigated to remove any contrast material that enters into the lumens, although this is unusual with controlled pressures. With the coronary cannulae still in place and maintaining a pressure of 100 to 120 mm Hg, the chambers are packed with formalin-soaked cotton to their approximately normal size and shape and the specimen is immersed in cold Kaiserling I or formalin solution. The heart is cooled for 1 to 3 hours to permit the gelatin to set and is then x-rayed again.

As injection medium, Micropaque* (Damancy & Co., Ltd.), or Chromopaque* (Damancy & Co., Ltd.) if colored contrast material is desired, is satisfactory. Masses of different colors may be prepared for use in the right and left coronary artery systems if desired. The colored contrast material is composed of the following: Chromopaque, 25 ml; Micropaque, 25 gm; water, 20 ml; and gelatin, 1.5 gm. The coloring of Chromopaque is of sufficient intensity to be well preserved at this dilution. The gelatin solution is prepared in advance with a small amount of thymol added as a preservative. Prior to injection, the gelatin solution is warmed to 45 C and the Chromopaque and Micropaque are added, with care to avoid air bubbles. With the above formula, approximately 50 ml of injection medium of each color can be prepared; this amount is sufficient to fill the coronary artery

---

* Available from Picker X-Ray Corporation.

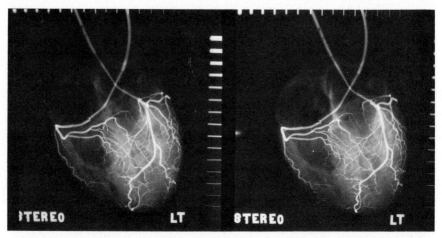

Figure 3–11. Stereoscopic views of normal **coronary angiogram** after controlled-pressure injection of both right and left coronary arteries by means of cannulae (above).

tree. At the approximately physiologic perfusion pressure of 100 mm Hg, with this contrast medium small arteries and even arterioles may be filled, but the capillary bed usually is not.

Double Contrast Technique With Visualization of Coronary Ostia.[51] Angiographic demonstration of ostial stenosis is not possible after cannulation of the coronary arteries from the aorta. It can be achieved by using a Foley catheter with a 30-ml balloon. The catheter is passed through a tightly fitting hole in a rubber stopper so that the bottom of the stopper is positioned about 2 cm above the top of the balloon. The stopper is glued to the catheter in this position. Two new openings are made in the catheter between the stopper and the balloon, taking care not to damage the small side tube in the catheter wall which is used to inflate the balloon. The catheter lumen must be closed below the new openings. A fairly large-bore needle equipped with an obturator is passed through the rubber stopper close to the catheter.

To put the catheter in place, the balloon is inflated, with air or water, below the aortic valve so that its top can be palpated on the aortic side. The rubber stopper is tied into the aorta with its base a fingerbreadth above the aortic valve. At the start of the injection, air is allowed to escape through the needle inserted in the stopper.

For this technique a medium is used which (1) retains its fluidity in the coronary arteries, (2) when poured out, a thin layer adheres to the vascular wall, and (3) has sufficient radiopacity to cast a thin shadow in the angiogram. The contrast medium should be freshly prepared for each use as follows:

Stock solution A. 2-Octanol (secondary *n*-octyl alcohol; secondary capryl alcohol), 20.0 ml, plus phenol (USP solution), 30 ml.

Stock mixture B. Bacto-gelatin, 8.7 gm, plus potassium iodide, 50 gm, plus buffer (sodium and potassium phosphate, pH 6.2), 2.3 gm.

Preparation of medium. Place 163 ml of distilled water in the Waring blender. Add 1 ml of stock solution A and mix for 30 seconds. Add 61.0 gm of stock mixture B and mix for 60 seconds. Add 100 gm of barium sulfate and mix for 2 minutes.

The medium is injected with a pressure of 80 mm Hg. Fine-grain-film roentgenograms are prepared. After conventional coronary angiography, the heart is inverted and the medium is allowed to flow out. This can be aided by slightly "milking" the coronary arteries toward their takeoff points. Air is then passed into the aorta and coronary arteries at a pressure of 50 mm Hg and, with this pressure maintained, double contrast coronary angiography is carried out. This permits visualization of the coronary artery walls by two thin lines of contrast medium.

The disadvantage of the Foley catheter apparatus is that the coronary arteries have to be injected simultaneously and so retrograde filling via collaterals cannot be evaluated. Unless ostial stenosis is too severe or ostial thrombosis is present, the advantages of this method and of the one described previously could be combined by first injecting the double contrast medium through catheters tied into the coronary arteries and then removing the catheters and preparing the heart for double contrast arteriography to permit visualization of the coronary ostia.

Simplified Barium Injection Technique Without Pressure Control or Gelatin. A simplified technique,[65] not requiring measurement of the injection pressure and without gelatin in the dye solution, has been found to demonstrate satisfactorily the collateral circulation in areas of occlusion. With the exception of the sinoatrial node artery, the vessels supplying the conduction system were also demonstrated.

The Micropaque solution is prepared by mixing equal parts (w/v) of tap water and Micropaque and adding a dash of liquid detergent for each 50 ml. Two 8-F Foley catheters with 3-ml inflatable bulbs are prepared by wrapping 1-0 silk suture material around the inflatable bulb so as to leave 1.5 ml of bulb retaining its original inflated diameter. The tips of the catheters are cut off, so that a minimum of catheter would be inserted into the coronary ostia, along with the inflatable bulb. Three-way stopcocks are tied to the ends of the catheters with silk suture material.

The heart should be obtained intact and already rinsed. It is not necessary to wash the vessels by infusion of saline. The pulmonary trunk and aorta are marked with wire sutures. The Foley catheters are filled with Micropaque solution by injection with a 12-ml syringe attached to the stopcock. A catheter is inserted into each ostium and the bulbs are inflated with a 5-ml syringe and 20-gauge needle and clamped with hemostats. A light tug on the catheters ensures their proper placement. With the catheters in place the heart is lowered into a plastic container at least 15 cm deep and filled with tap water; it is positioned so that its anterior surface is facing up. A final depth of approximately 13 cm is obtained by adding or removing water. Cotton gauze pads are used to keep the heart in position. The container is then placed on top of an 8- by 10-inch x-ray cassette under the x-ray tube and a preliminary film is taken. Next, 1 ml of Micropaque solution is injected through each of the catheters and a second film is taken. A film is taken after each succeeding 1 ml of solution is injected, until arteries 1 mm in diameter are visualized on the film, usually after 5 or 6 ml. A stereoscopic set is then taken.

In Situ Injection Without Pressure Control. The anterior chest wall can be removed or the sternum can be split lengthwise. The ascending aorta is exposed and clamped with a hemostat about 3 cm above the aortic valve. The contrast medium is injected with a large syringe and needle into the ascending aorta just above the valve. If the aortic valve is competent and the hemostat is clamped tightly enough, only the proximal ascending aorta and the coronary arteries will fill (Fig. 3–12). In situ cannulation of the coronary arteries can also be carried out but is more difficult.

Coronary Arteriograms in One Plane. The preparation of such angiograms requires mutilating dissection of the heart and is not recommended for routine use. Its major value is for specialized studies of various types. The unrolling techniques have been described earlier in this chapter. Figure 3–13 shows a coronary angiogram of a heart which had been dissected by Schlesinger's method. Preparations of this type could be adapted for a

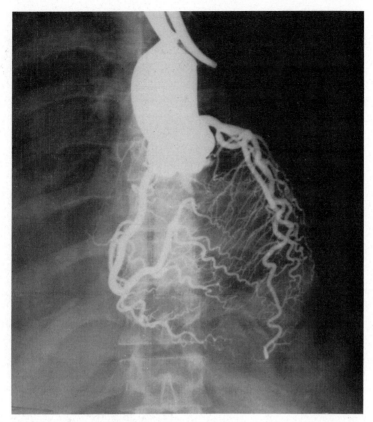

Figure 3–12. Coronary angiogram of normal heart made in situ. Sternum was split in midline and about 300 ml of barium sulfate-gelatin mixture was injected into ascending aorta, without pressure regulation, by hand with large syringe. Superior portion of ascending aorta had been clamped off.

sort of quantitative determination of coronary arterial narrowing by a radioisotope dilution technique as described by Davis.[8]

Plastic Casts of Coronary Artery Tree. Although these techniques yield fine specimens of the coronary artery tree, they are used only under exceptional conditions because the corrosion precludes proper pathologic study of the whole heart. Latex injection without corrosion may be indicated in some situations. The technique of coronary latex injection is similar to the one described for pulmonary vessels (see chapter 4). Excellent corrosion specimens of coronary arteries and veins have been prepared by Baroldi and Scomazzoni[1] using Geon latex 576 and neoprene 842 A. The coronary artery casts showed vessels as small as precapillaries.

To prepare vinyl plastic casts,[22] a glass rod is placed through the inferior and superior venae cavae where they enter the right atrium. A plastic catheter is inserted into the right atrium and secured with a purse-string suture. Purse-string sutures are applied and tied around both venae cavae with the glass rod in place. (The glass rod aids in handling the delicate spec-

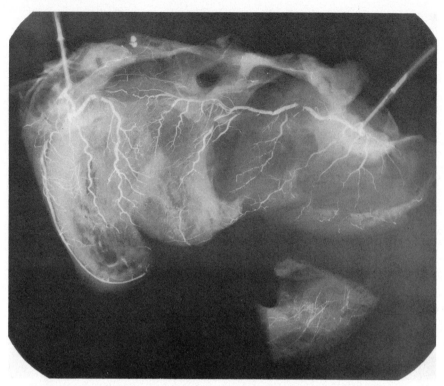

Figure 3–13. Coronary angiogram of specimen prepared by Schlesinger's unrolling technique. Severe coronary atherosclerosis is present with atheromatous occlusion of left descending and right coronary arteries. (From Smith RL Jr: An Injection Study of Intercoronary Anastomoses in the Human Heart. Thesis, Graduate School, University of Minnesota, 1941.)

imen during later steps.) A clamp is applied to the pulmonary artery about 2 cm above the valve. Glass cannulae in the right and left coronary arteries are secured by ligatures near the ostia of the vessels.

Blue liquid vinyl plastic is injected with a syringe via the catheter in the right atrium. An amount sufficient to restore the normal contours is used. Additional blue vinyl plastic is injected by needle puncture if portions of the coronary sinus or coronary veins have not been filled via the right atrium. Yellow vinyl plastic is then injected from a syringe via the cannula into the right coronary artery. Gentle pressure, and light massage at places, is used to fill the major epicardial right coronary artery branches. Red vinyl is then injected into the left coronary artery in a similar manner. All injections are made with the specimen nearly submerged in cold water. If any of the vinyl plastic leaks, it floats to the surface where it hardens and can be removed readily.

After about an hour in cold water, the injected mass is solidified. The heart is then placed in 10% formalin solution for 18 hours for fixation, after which it is placed in concentrated hydrochloric acid for 48 hours for digestion of the muscle tissue from the plastic cast of the vessels. Large hearts may require digestion for 72 hours or longer.

On removal from the hydrochloric acid, the cast is gently floated in water and carefully washed with tap water to remove debris still lodged within the cast. The preparation is then air dried (Fig. 3–14).

We have used vinyl plastics manufactured by Wards Natural Science Establishment, Inc. (Rochester, N.Y., or Monterey, Cal.). With this material we have been able to prepare excellent specimens by adjusting the injection pressure solely by hand and visual control. For other plastics, manometric control of the injection pressure is recommended—for in-

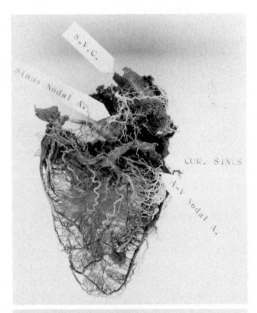

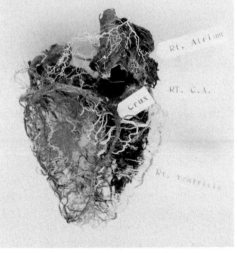

Figure 3–14. Vinyl plastic cast of coronary artery lumen, right atrium, right ventricle, and coronary sinus lumen of normal heart from 46-year-old woman. (Courtesy of Dr. A. J. Kennel.)

stance, for the mixture of Arcon 200, Polylite 8151, Polylite promoter (cobalt naphthenate), and powdered copper.[53]

Injection of Myocardial Microvasculature.   Myocardial arterioles can be studied by injecting Chromopaque (Damancy & Co., Ltd.) neutral medium with 5% added gelatin. For the injection of capillaries, the viscosity is decreased by adding saline to the medium.[11] The vessels are studied by roentgenography of transverse slices through the heart, 5 mm or less in thickness, or by the contact method, using Kodak high resolution plates.[11]

Corrosion casts of precapillaries can be prepared with Geon latex 576 and neoprene 842 A.[1]

Injection of Coronary Veins.   While the methods described above deal predominantly with the coronary arterial system, adaptation of most of these techniques to the study of the coronary veins is possible in most instances. The coronary sinus system can be filled with contrast medium from a cannula tied into its ostium; for latex-neoprene medium, an injection pressure in the coronary sinus of 50 to 80 mm Hg has been recommended.[1] The anterior cardiac venous system is best filled by injecting the contrast medium directly into the right atrium; for latex-neoprene medium, an injection pressure in the right atrium of 30 to 50 mm Hg has been recommended.[1] From the coronary sinus and the anterior cardiac veins, a more or less complete filling of the coronary venous system can be expected because of the presence of numerous venous anastomoses. Direct and exclusive demonstration of the thebesian venous system does not appear possible. Injection of plastic substances into the cardiac cavities will not permit differentiation between the true venous thebesian vessels and arterioluminal vessels.

Dry Preservation of Heart.   Dry preservation of the heart is of great didactic value[7] and in many ways superior to any other method of preparing permanent specimens for the demonstration of congenital cardiac malformations or acquired valvular heart diseases. The methods are elaborate and do not lend themselves to routine use. The hearts are dehydrated and infiltrated with substances such as paraffin and beeswax[12,72] or diglycol stearate.[27] We use a slight modification of the paraffin infiltration method of Gross and Leslie.[15]

Blood clots are removed from the isolated, unopened heart, both by squeezing the clots through the severed veins and by flushing the atria and ventricles with isotonic saline. If immediate inspection of the heart is essential, small windows may be cut into the atria and ventricles, but these always must be smaller than the outline of the windows to be made in the infiltrated specimen. Any preliminary openings preferably should be cut in such a way that they can be closed by plugs of some type; usually the quality of the specimen will suffer from these preliminary procedures. Gross and Leslie[15] used an electrically lighted nasal speculum passed through a vascular channel for inspection of the unopened heart.

Glass cannulas of appropriate sizes, with small sloping flanges, are tied into the aorta, pulmonary artery, superior vena cava, and one of the pulmonary veins. Wooden plugs of appropriate size or glass cannulas which are closed at one end are tied into the pulmonary venous orifices and into the inferior vena cava. Use of such plugs prevents puckering and collapse of the atria. The cannulas in the pulmonary artery and aorta are connected via rubber tubes and a glass Y tube. A hook under the glass Y tube suspends the heart in a container holding about 3 liters of 10% buffered formalin solution. Rubber tubes are also attached to the cannulas in the atria. The cannulas are suspended in the axis of the respective veins to prevent distortion of the atrial wall.

A large tank containing 10% buffered formalin solution is placed about 60 cm above the level of the apex of the heart (Fig. 3–15); the heart is kept floating about 3 cm above the bottom of the container. If the semilunar valves are somewhat incompetent, formalin will flow retrogradely through them into the cardiac chambers and into the atrial cannulas. If the semilunar valves are competent, the atria and ventricles are first filled with formalin through the atrial cannulas. In either situation, the rubber hoses attached to the atrial cannulas are eventually clamped off and

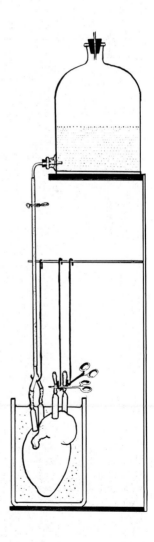

Figure 3–15. Method of suspending heart and perfusing with formalin solution. (From Gross L, Leslie E: Paraffin infiltration of hearts: a permanent method for preservation. Am Heart J 6:665–671, 1931. By permission of C. V. Mosby Company.)

the perfusion is continued through the arteries. Formalin fixation usually renders the semilunar valves somewhat incompetent. We change the formalin inside and outside the heart twice daily for 3 days.

After fixation, the cannulas are removed and the heart is dried with a towel. The plugs are left in place. The heart then is placed in 2 to 2.5 liters of 65% alcohol for 1 to 2 days, the duration depending on its size. A layer of cotton should be placed on the bottom of the container. This procedure is repeated with 80%, 90%, 95%, and absolute alcohol. The absolute alcohol has to be replaced until the alcoholometer indicates at least 98% after 24 to 48 hours.

The heart is then placed in xylol for 48 hours. The xylol is replaced after the first 24 hours. The xylol is then drained off rapidly and the heart is placed in a mixture, at 56 C in an incubator, of paraffin of melting point 53 to 55 C (95 parts by weight) and pure unbleached beeswax (5 parts by weight). After 24 hours the paraffin-wax bath is replaced and the heart is kept in the new bath for another 24 hours. Finally, the heart is removed and suspended upside down with a hook through the apex. After the paraffin-wax has been drained off, windows are cut in the atria and ventricles as described below.

See Figure 3–16 for a diagram of these steps. A knife is inserted into the inferior vena cava so that its edge is pointing toward the anterior surface of the heart. The blade is pushed through the superior wall of the right atrium until the superior vena cava is reached, cutting as close to the atrial septum as possible (Cut *A*). The knife is reinserted into the inferior vena cava with the edge pointing toward the acute margin. An incision is made in the posterolateral wall of the right atrium until the atrioventricular sulcus is reached (Cut *B*). The knife is inserted into the superior vena cava with the edge pointing toward the

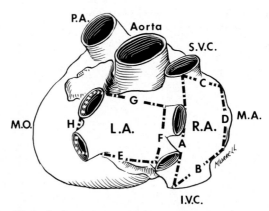

Figure 3–16. **Method of opening atria** in paraffin-infiltrated heart (see text). Cuts are shown by broken lines. *I.V.C.* = inferior vena cava; *S.V.C.* = superior vena cava; *L.A.* = left atrium; *M.A.* = acute margin; *M.O.* = obtuse margin; *P.A.* = pulmonary artery; *R.A.* = right atrium. (Modified from Gross L, Leslie E: Paraffin infiltration of hearts: a permanent method for preservation. Am Heart J 6:665–671, 1931.)

acute margin. An incision is made along an imaginary line which joins the superior vena cava with a point 5 mm posterior to the junction of the inferior border of the right atrial appendage with the atrioventricular sulcus (Cut C). The distal point of this incision is connected with the posterolateral atrial incision previously made (Cut D). In this manner the top of the right atrium is easily removed.

See Figure 3–17 for a diagram of these steps. The pulmonary artery is trimmed to within 1 cm of the level of the valve commissures. The aorta is trimmed to any level desired. The point of the knife is inserted slightly below the right atrioventricular sulcus at the junction of the latter with the acute margin. The edge of the knife points toward the pulmonary artery. The blade is pushed through the myocardium into the right ventricle, with care not to strike the delicate tricuspid valve. The blade is carried forward, following the contour of the atrioventricular sulcus, until the incision reaches to within 0.5 cm of the lower border of the pulmonary cusps (Cut A). This can be seen by looking down the pulmonary orifice. The blade is turned downward and this incision is continued parallel with the plane of the pulmonary cusps until the ventricular septum is reached (Cut B). The blade is now turned and the incision is carried to the apex of the right ventricle, keeping the knife at all times close to the ventricular septum (Cut C). This incision can be watched easily through the pulmonary orifice. The blade of the knife is inserted into the acute margin at the first point of the original right ventricular incision, and the incision is carried down toward the apex to join the last part of the incision along the ventricular septum (Cut D). While this incision is being made, one should look through the tricuspid orifice to make sure that the tricuspid valve is not injured. This window should be gently raised off the right ventricular myocardium. It will be found that the trabeculum septomarginalis or the anterior papillary muscle makes it impossible to remove this myocardial segment completely. This connection is severed by the knife at a convenient site, and the right ventricular chamber is thus opened for inspection.

See Figure 3–16 for a diagram of these steps. The blade of the knife is inserted through one of the pulmonary veins (preferably the right inferior) with the edge pointing toward the obtuse margin. An incision is made across the superior wall of the left atrium until the atrioventricular sulcus is reached (Cut E). Starting with the first point of this incision, the knife edge is turned superiorly and the posterior wall of the left atrium is cut through until a point is reached on the latter approximately opposite the superior vena cava of the right atrium (Cut F). The edge of the knife is turned toward the obtuse margin and an incision is made along a line which runs to a point approximately 5 mm posterior to the junction of the left atrial appendage with the atrioventricular sulcus (Cut G). The final incision is parallel with the line of the atrioventricular sulcus (Cut H) and connects the first and third incisions. Thus, a window in the left atrium is made which leaves enough of the inferior wall to show pathologic lesions.

See Figure 3–17 for a diagram of these steps. The last and most difficult incisions remain to be made in the left ventricle. The knife blade is inserted into the anterior wall of the left ventricle at a point approximately 1 cm below the junction of the left coronary artery with the left

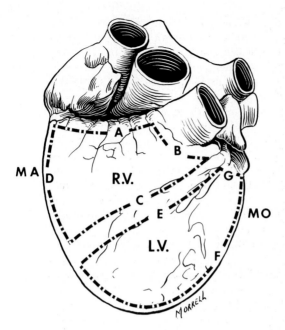

Figure 3–17. **Method of opening ventricles** in paraffin-infiltrated heart (see text). Broken lines indicate cuts. *L.V.* = left ventricle; *R.V.* = right ventricle. (Modified from Gross L, Leslie E: Paraffin infiltration of hearts: a permanent method for preservation. Am Heart J 6:665–671, 1931.)

anterior descending branch. The cutting edge should point toward the inferior border of the ventricular septum. While watching the contour of the ventricular septum and estimating the thickness of the latter as closely as possible, an incision is made parallel with the right ventricular septal incision (Cut *C*) with the object in mind of exposing as much left ventricle as possible without actually cutting into the ventricular septum (Cut *E*). The incision should be carried as far as the acute margin. The knife is inserted at a point 1 cm below the atrioventricular sulcus at the latter's junction with the obtuse margin, with the cutting edge pointing toward the apex of the heart. One should look through the mitral valve orifice to make sure that the mitral cusp is not perforated by the point of the knife. With the blade penetrating through the entire thickness of the left ventricular wall, the incision is carried down to the apex of the heart and continued around the apex until it joins the left ventricular septal incision described above (Cut *F*). A connecting incision is made between the upper ends of the ventricular septal and obtuse marginal incisions (Cut *G*). If the tissue has been cut cleanly, it will be possible to raise slightly the lower border of this left ventricular flap, but it will be impossible to remove the flap because of the stout anterolateral papillary muscle which connects the muscular window to the mitral valve. This papillary muscle is severed close to its apex by a knife, and then the left ventricular flap can be removed. Any residual clotted blood is carefully cleaned out.

If the opening of the heart is performed, as it should be, while the myocardium is slightly warm, it is simple to remove blocks for histologic study. In order to examine the coronary arteries, however, it is desirable that coronal incisions of the vessels are made during one of the dehydration stages in alcohol. Blocks can then be removed after paraffin infiltration. If it is necessary to cut additional tissue blocks at some future time, the heart should be placed in an incubator at 56 C for about 15 or 20 minutes until the paraffin softens.

The size and shape of the windows may be changed as needed. We prefer to first cut the window in the left ventricle before the heart cools and hardens. If the heart is dissected in the sequence described, it may be necessary to reincubate it during the procedure. We also have found it useful

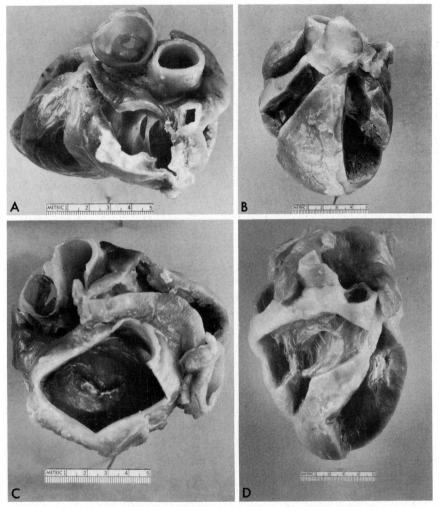

Figure 3–18. Paraffin-infiltrated hearts. *A* and *B,* From 49-year-old woman with congenital heart disease who died of paradoxic cerebral emboli. *A,* Dome-shaped pulmonary stenosis with poststenotic dilatation of pulmonary artery. Window in left atrium shows atrial septal defect. *B,* Windows in right and left ventricles reveal right ventricular hypertrophy with jet lesions in pulmonary outflow tract. *C* and *D,* From 49-year-old woman who died in congestive heart failure secondary to post-rheumatic stenosis and insufficiency of mitral valve. *C,* "Fishmouth" mitral valve in view from above through window in roof of left atrium. *D,* Windows in hypertrophied right and left ventricles reveal hypertrophic moderator band in right ventricle.

to cut small windows which then are enlarged to give the best view of the lesions of particular interest. In either case instructive specimens are obtained (Fig. 3–18). The histologic sections prepared from these hearts are of excellent quality. Previous coronary angiography does not interfere with the paraffin infiltration method.

VASCULAR SYSTEM

In this section, autopsy examination of some of the major blood vessels is considered. The vascular systems of specific organs will be discussed in the sections dealing with each organ.

Arteries. *Aorta and Other Major Arteries.* When a major abnormality of the aorta is suspected, generally en masse removal of the organs is indicated. As a rule, the descending thoracic and abdominal portions of the aorta are opened posteriorly between the origins of the right and left intercostal and lumbar arteries. In this way the main branches of the aorta remain attached and intact.

In cases of aortic aneurysm, cross sections through the fixed specimen often are most instructive. Aortic isthmus stenosis (including coarctation) is kept intact. Widened intercostal arteries can be demonstrated roentgenologically and then dissected; maceration of the ribs will facilitate their demonstration. The celiac artery system is best demonstrated by arteriography followed by dissection. Fibromuscular dysplasia of renal and other arteries should be studied by opening the vessels lengthwise.

As a rule, in the United States, major arteries of the extremities can be dissected only after embalming, so arrangements should be made with the funeral director. The femoral-popliteal vessels can be removed without an additional skin incision, as described below.

Postmortem Arteriograms of Lower Extremities. These are useful for the study of thromboses, embolic occlusions, atherosclerotic changes, and vascular anatomy of abnormal conditions such as malignant tumors. The variations in caliber of atherosclerotic vessels as seen in roentgenograms correlate well with the gross and histologic findings;[9] however, the absence of roentgenologic abnormalities does not necessarily indicate normality of the vessels.[9] One of the main difficulties in the interpretation of abnormal roentgenograms is the presence of postmortem clots. They may imitate thrombotic occlusions or they may be dislodged by the contrast medium and occlude distal vessels as an embolus.[57]

For the injection of contrast medium into the arteries of the extremities, an apparatus (Fig. 3–19) has been devised by Ross and Keele.[57] With this apparatus or with that described above for coronary angiography (Fig. 3–10), a barium sulfate preparation is injected through a cannula tied into the external iliac artery. The contrast medium is injected at a pressure which is slowly increased to 250 to 300 mm Hg and maintained for about 5 minutes. Air bubbles are avoided by making the system airtight and by compressing the tissues and vessels surrounding the cannulated artery.

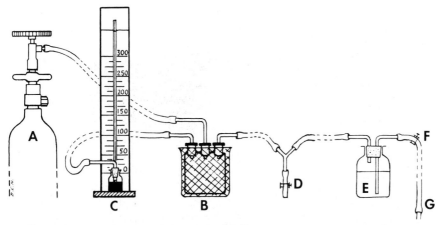

Figure 3–19. Apparatus of Ross and Keele[57] for injection of contrast medium into arteries of extremities. A = oxygen or compressed air cylinder with needle valve; B = three-necked Woulff bottle in wire basket (1-liter capacity); C = mercury manometer; D = rubber tubing with screw clamp; E = bottle with contrast medium; F = pressure tubing with screw clamp; G = injection cannula. (From Ross CF, Keele KD: Post mortem arteriography in "normal" lower limbs. Angiology 2:374–385, 1951. By permission of Angiology Research Foundation.)

Grading of Atherosclerotic Lesions. 1. Evaluation of vessels opened lengthwise, with or without staining of lesions. The method of Holman et al.[19] has been found useful and consistent in a recent international atherosclerosis project in which the specimens had to be shipped and graded by different observers.[16] The aorta, arteries of the neck, circle of Willis, and coronary arteries are dissected, opened lengthwise, placed on cardboard or cork, and fixed in 10% neutral buffered formalin solution. Fatty streaks and atheromatous plaques are stained with Sudan IV solution (Sudan IV [National Aniline No. 542], 0.5 gm; acetone, 50 ml; 70% ethyl alcohol, 50 ml) which is poured over the vessels. After a few minutes, the atheromatous plaques turn red. The time of exposure varies somewhat and the specimen has to be watched constantly to ensure the correct staining intensity. The specimen is then allowed to differentiate in 80% ethyl alcohol for about 5 minutes. The surplus alcohol-Sudan IV solution is rinsed off and the specimen is washed in tap water. The stained vessels can be kept in formalin solution.

This method has been used to identify and record the extent of fatty streaks, fibrous plaques, complicated lesions (areas of hemorrhage, necrosis, ulceration, or thrombosis, with or without calcium), and calcified lesions.[16]

2. Evaluation of vessels opened lengthwise by comparison with panel of photographs. For the grading of atherosclerosis in human coronary arteries and aortas, a committee of the American Heart Association prepared two series of color photographs of arteries which are opened lengthwise and which show atherosclerotic lesions of increasing severity.[39] Specimens are graded by matching them with the picture on the panel

which resembles most closely the prevailing degree of atherosclerosis. This method provides seven possible scores for each coronary artery and for the aorta.

3. Grading of narrowing of lumen on cross sections of arteries. We prefer this method, particularly for the routine grading of coronary atherosclerosis. Starting at their origins from the aorta, the coronary arteries are cross sectioned with a sharp, short-bladed knife at intervals of not more than 2 to 3 mm. The degree of narrowing of the lumen is estimated by assigning to the vascular segment one of four scores: grade 1, 0 to 25% narrowing; grade 2, 25 to 50% narrowing; grade 3, 50 to 75% narrowing; and grade 4, 75 to 100% narrowing (complete occlusion should be specified). Widening of the lumen or the presence of complicated lesions such as hemorrhages and thromboses is recorded separately. For routine use, the major degree of narrowing in the right, left, left anterior descending, and left circumflex coronary arteries is noted; isolated areas of narrowing are identified as "focal"—for instance, "atherosclerosis of left anterior descending coronary artery grade 2, focal 4, 0.5 cm from origin."

Veins. *In Air Embolism.* Particular care must be taken to clamp but not lacerate upper thoracic and neck veins in cases of suspected air embolism. The site of entrance of air into the venous system can be documented by identifying air bubbles in the lumens of the veins leading from it to the right heart. Gas resulting from putrefaction may simulate air embolism.

Lesions of Inferior Vena Cava System. The inferior vena cava system can be dissected and exposed in situ from the anterior aspect or posteriorly after the en masse or en bloc removal of the abdominal organs. Thromboses and intraluminal tumor growth (Fig. 3–20) are the main pathologic lesions which can be found in the inferior vena cava.

Lesions of Femoral Veins. Recent thrombi in the femoral veins sometimes can be pushed toward the pelvis and demonstrated after they protrude from the iliac veins, by "milking" the femoral veins from the knee toward the groin along the vascular bed. Because in situ dissection of the femoral-popliteal vessels often causes problems for the funeral director, a method has been developed for removing these vessels without additional skin incisions.[2] A string is tied around the femoral artery and vein just proximal to the inguinal ligament. The string is passed through an aluminum tube, internal diameter approximately 1.5 cm and length approximately 75 cm, the distal end of which is sharpened to form a cutting edge (Fig. 3–21). A constant tension of approximately 4.5 kg is placed on the vessel and the tubing is pushed down the thigh, with a twisting motion, toward the mid-distal popliteal fossa. The tension on the string is released and the vessels are cut by twisting the sharpened edge of the tube. Femoral and popliteal vessels are removed intact within the tube.

Dissection of Venous Thromboses. Thromboses can be demonstrated by opening the vein lengthwise with the clot left attached to a portion of the wall. In another approach, the window technique, the vein is left in its natural shape and a rectangular window is cut into the wall of the vein overlying a thrombus which is apparent through the thin-walled vein.

Postmortem Phlebography. The preparation of phlebograms of the infe-

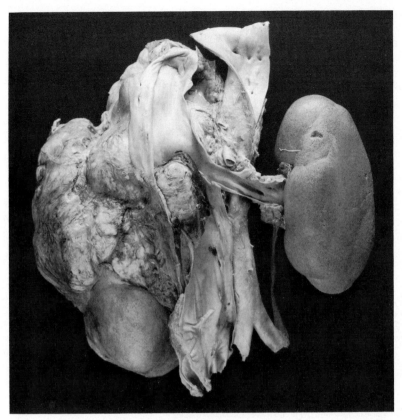

Figure 3–20. **Adenocarcinoma of right kidney** growing through right renal vein into inferior vena cava. Left renal vein and inferior vena cava are opened anteriorly.

rior vena cava system by direct injection of contrast medium into the vein with the vessel occluded by an inflatable rubber balloon will be discussed in connection with the demonstration of renal veins (chapter 5).

Thoracic veins and the inferior vena cava system also can be demonstrated by methods primarily designed for phlebography of leg veins.[35] A stasis tube is applied just proximal to the ankle to prevent incidental filling of superficial veins. An injection needle, of the Seldinger "simple" type (single-cannula Seldinger PE 90 5, No. 31683-97, AB Stille-Werner, Bondegatan 21, Stockholm 4, Sweden), is bored into the spongiosa of the calcaneus. About 300 to 400 ml of a barium sulfate solution (diluted with water to a specific gravity of approximately 1.1) is injected into each calcaneus. Better filling of the veins is achieved if, during the injection, the body is first in a prone position and then is moved to an ordinary supine position. The injection pressure varies considerably, and small veins occasionally rupture. Previously refrigerated bodies have to be kept at room temperature for at least 12 hours prior to injection to restore to normal the consistency of the fat tissue which otherwise may compress the veins.

Superficial leg vein phlebography can be achieved by injection of

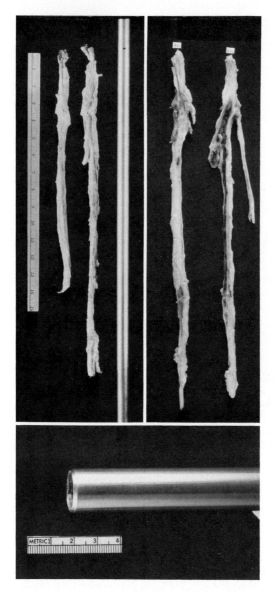

Figure 3–21. Removal of femoral-popliteal vessels. *Upper Left,* Metal tube (at right side) and extracted femoral-popliteal vessels. *Upper Right,* Bilateral venous thrombosis found in longitudinally opened femoral and popliteal veins obtained by method described in text. *Lower,* Cutting edge of tube. (From Beckering RE Jr, Titus JL: Laboratory suggestion: a method for the autopsy study of the femoral-popliteal vessels. Am J Clin Pathol 47:652–653, 1967. By permission of J. B. Lippincott Company.)

superficial veins of the foot or by using the method of deep leg vein phlebography without the stasis tube.

Phlebography generally demonstrates thrombi; it was partially unsuccessful in 7 of 65 legs with thrombosed vessels and completely negative in 2 of these cases.[35]

Lymphatic Vessels. Study of the lymphatic system at autopsy is difficult and time-consuming. Under normal circumstances, only the thoracic duct and its main tributaries can be dissected. Smaller lymphatic vessels seem to collapse and become invisible, particularly when the tissues under study are allowed to dry superficially. On the other hand, lymphatic congestion, as observed in many cases of liver cirrhosis or chronic heart failure, may render identifiable even small lymphatic vessels so that dissection and injection studies can be carried out.

Dissection of Thoracic Duct. The thoracic duct can easily be found in the fat tissue behind the descending thoracic aorta. The thoracic duct usually runs medial to the azygos vein and crosses over to the left side of the spinal column at the level of the aortic arch. Thus, the inferior portion of the thoracic duct can be exposed from either side. We prefer the left side even during the dissection of the immediate supradiaphragmatic portion of the duct. The dissection then can be continued to the cervical portion without having to change sides.

The left posterior mediastinum is exposed by lifting the left lung out of the chest cavity. The lung is then held in this position by an assistant or by mechanical fixation. In the inferior portion of the mediastinum the intercostal arteries are transected close to the aorta. The vascular stumps are clamped with hemostats and the aorta is pulled to the right in order to expose the retroaortic fat tissue. A portion of the thoracic duct is isolated with an anatomic forceps (Fig. 3–22). The remaining intercostal arteries are transected, and the thoracic duct, including its cervical portion, can be dissected. Care must be taken not to lacerate the thoracic duct at the distal (posterior) end of the aortic arch, to which the duct is closely related.

Because of variations of the thoracic duct, dissection is best combined with injection of a warm (72 C), 5% gelatin solution with 3 parts of liquid

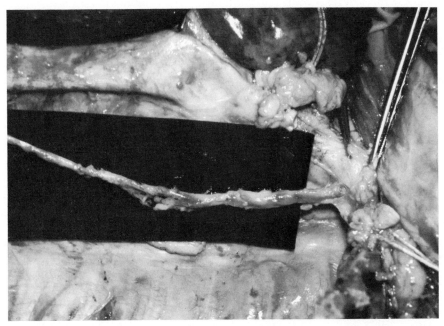

Figure 3–22. Thoracic duct in situ injected with Ethiodol and a green dye. Left lung has been lifted out of thoracic cavity and aorta has been pulled anteriorly and to the right. Duct has been dissected out of posterior mediastinal fat tissue.

phenol added to 100 parts gelatin solution. If lymphangiography is intended, barium sulfate can be added to the mixture, or Ethiodol (ethyl ester of the fatty acid of poppyseed oil, 37% iodine by weight) can be used. We found it useful to stain the medium with a few drops of green oil paint. Retrograde injection is not possible in most cases. When the abdominal portion of the thoracic duct or its lumbar trunks are to be demonstrated, the organs should be removed en masse and the tributaries of the thoracic duct should be dissected in a retrograde way from the portion exposed in the inferior mediastinum.

Some pathologists prefer to dissect the thoracic duct after the chest organs have been lifted out of the chest cavity. This technique requires separation of the mediastinum from the spinal column immediately above the periosteum of the spine. Otherwise, the duct can easily be lacerated. If injection of the duct and its tributaries is intended, this has to be carried out before the en bloc or en masse removal of the organs.

Demonstration of Peripheral Lymphatic Vessels. 1. Hydrogen peroxide method. Subserosal lymphatic vessels can be demonstrated by application of a 3% hydrogen peroxide solution to the surface of the organ or tissue. This results in spontaneous inflation of the lymphatic vessels with oxygen after a short period. The method is not always successful. Tissue clefts also may fill with oxygen.[17] The results are improved when the tissues first are aged for 12 to 24 hours and then soaked for 4 to 8 hours in a 1:10 dilution of a stock solution of 10 gallons of water, 20 lb of crystalline phenol, 5 lb of potassium nitrate, 1.5 lb of sodium arsenite, 1.5 gallons of glycerine, 1.5 gallons of ethanol, and 0.5 gallon of formalin. After this, they are immersed for several minutes in 1% hydrogen peroxide.[46]

2. Postmortem lymphangiography. This technique has not yet been used widely. Since retrograde injection rarely is successful, postmortem lymphangiography requires cannulation of a peripheral lymphatic vessel. In some cases, satisfactory lymphangiograms can be made by introducing the needle into a lymph node.

A conventional lymph injector is used, equipped with a 20-ml glass syringe with a Luer-Lok tip and a 27-gauge needle, fitted to an 18-inch plastic tube. The contrast medium is Ethiodol stained with a few drops of green oil paint, which facilitates the identification and dissection of the lymphatic vessels. The amount of contrast medium injected will vary from case to case, averaging about 6 to 10 ml of heated (72 C) contrast medium. The injection takes about 15 to 30 minutes, depending on how long free flow can be achieved. High injection pressures are needed to force the oily contrast medium through the needle. Our injector is designed to stop automatically when the pressure in the tube reaches about 630 mm Hg. If the lymphatic vessels are collapsed, this pressure will be reached relatively early during the procedure in many cases and no satisfactory lymphangiograms can be prepared. Rupture of lymphatic vessels under conditions of free flow of the contrast medium is rare.

We have had good results with this method.[33] For example, we have been able to demonstrate retrosternal and retroperitoneal lymphatic vessels by injecting pathologically dilated lymphatic vessels at the base of the falciform ligament of the liver or the hepatoduodenal ligament, respectively (Fig. 3–23).

Other injection media which can be used for postmortem lymphangiography are diluted barium sulfate mixtures (see section on coronary angiography) or silicon rubber such as Microfil (Canton Bio-Medical Products, Boulder, Colo.) which has low viscosity and shrinkage. Casts can also be prepared from Microfil which is resistant to clearing fluid. This preparation is available in various colors.

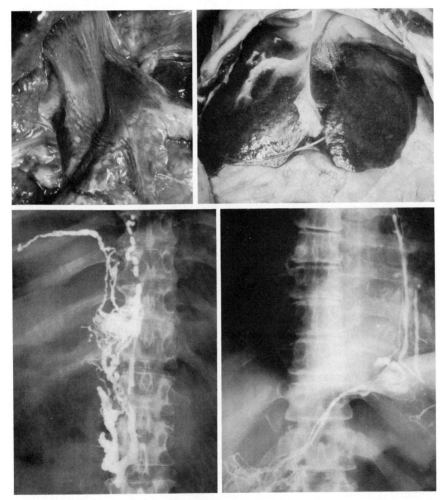

Figure 3–23. *Upper Left,* **Dilated lymphatic vessels** in hepatoduodenal ligament, before cannulation. *Upper Right,* Markedly **dilated lymphatic vessels** at convexity of liver and near base of falciform ligament. Plastic tube and needle for lymphangiography in place. *Lower Left,* **Postmortem lymphangiogram** showing dilated and varicose parapancreatic and para-aortic lymphatic vessels. The thoracic duct was dilated and tortuous. *Lower Right,* **Postmortem lymphangiogram** showing retrosternal lymphaticovenous shunt. (From Ludwig J, Linhart P, Baggenstoss AH: Hepatic lymph drainage in cirrhosis and congestive heart failure: a postmortem lymphangiographic study. Arch Pathol 86:551–562, 1968. By permission of the American Medical Association.)

REFERENCES

1. Baroldi G, Scomazzoni G: Coronary Circulation in the Normal and the Pathologic Heart. Washington DC, US Government Printing Office, 1967, p 59
2. Beckering RE Jr, Titus JL: Laboratory suggestion: a method for the autopsy study of the femoral-popliteal vessels. Am J Clin Pathol 47:652–653, 1967
3. Box CR: Post-mortem Manual: A Handbook of Morbid Anatomy and Post-mortem Technique. London, J. & A. Churchill, Ltd., 1910
4. Brody GL, Belding AW, Belding MR, Feldman SA: The identification and delineation of myocardial infarcts. Arch Pathol 84:312–317, 1967
5. Buch WS, Kosek JC, Angell WW: Deterioration of formalin-treated aortic valve heterografts. J Thorac Cardiovasc Surg 60:673–682, 1970
6. Buss H: Histochemische Frühdiagnose des experimentellen Herzinfarktes unter Berücksichtigung der Autolyse. Beitr Pathol Anat 140:257–279, 1970
7. Chapman CB: On the study of the heart. Arch Intern Med 113:318–322, 1964
8. Davis NA: A radioisotope dilution technique for the quantitative study of coronary artery disease postmortem. Lab Invest 12:1198–1203, 1963
9. Dejdar R, Roubková H, Cachovan M, Kruml J, Linhart J: Vergleich postmortaler Angiogramme mit makro- und mikroskopischen Befunden an A. femoralis und A. poplitea. Arch Kreislaufforsch 54:309–335, 1967
10. Edwards JE: Malformations of the thoracic veins. In Pathology of the Heart and Blood Vessels. Third edition. Edited by SE Gould. Springfield, Illinois, Charles C Thomas, Publisher, 1968, pp 463–478
11. Farrer-Brown G, Wartman WB: The microvasculature of the cardiac ventricles. Pathol Microbiol (Basel) 30:695–708, 1967
12. Fredericq L: Communication préalable sur quelques procédés nouveaux de préparation des pièces anatomiques sèches. Bull l'acad roy Belgique, Series 2, 41:1319–1325, 1876
13. Grant RP: Architectonics of the heart. Am Heart J 46:405–431, 1953
14. Gross L, Antopol W, Sacks B: A standardized procedure suggested for microscopic studies on the heart: with observations on rheumatic hearts. Arch Pathol 10:840–852, 1930
15. Gross L, Leslie E: Paraffin infiltration of hearts: a permanent method for preservation. Am Heart J 6:665–671, 1931
16. Guzman MA, McMahan CA, McGill HC Jr, Strong JP, Tejada C, Restrepo C, Eggen DA, Robertson WB, Solberg LB: Selected methodologic aspects of the International Atherosclerosis Project. Lab Invest 18:479–497, 1968
17. Hass H: Die Architektur der Lymphgefässe der Leberkapsel in ihren Beziehungen zur Bindegewebsstruktur und Flüssigkeitsströmung. Virchows Arch [Pathol Anat] 297:384–403, 1936
18. Hektoen L: The Technique of Post-mortem Examination. Chicago, The W. S. Keener Co., 1894
19. Holman RL, McGill HC Jr, Strong JP, Geer JC: The natural history of atherosclerosis: the early aortic lesions as seen in New Orleans in the middle of the 20th century. Am J Pathol 34:209–236, 1958
20. Hudson REB: Cardiovascular Pathology. London, Edward Arnold (Publishers), Ltd., 1965
21. Hudson REB: Pathology of the human aortic valve homograft. Br Heart J 28:291–301, 1966
22. James TN: Anatomy of the Coronary Arteries. New York, Paul B. Hoeber, Inc., 1961
23. Karzmark CJ, White J, Fowler JF: Lithium fluoride thermoluminescence dosimetry. Phys Med Biol 9:273–286, 1964
24. Kennel AJ: Coronary Atherosclerosis, Arrhythmias, and Heart Block: Pathology of the Conduction System and Its Vasculature. Thesis, Graduate School, University of Minnesota, 1970
25. Kennel AJ, Pruitt RD, McCallister BD, Titus JL: Pathologic findings in the conduction system and its vasculature in cardiac arrhythmias (abstract). Am J Cardiol 25:108, 1970
26. Knight B: The post-mortem demonstration of early myocardial infarction. Med Sci Law 5:31–34, 1965
27. Kramer FM: Dry preservation of museum specimens: a review, with introduction of simplified technique. J Tech Methods 18:42–50, 1938
28. Layman TE, Edwards JE: A method for dissection of the heart and major pulmonary vessels. Arch Pathol 82:314–320, 1966
29. Lev M, Widran J, Erickson EE: A method for the histopathologic study of the atrioventricular node, bundle, and branches. Arch Pathol 52:73–83, 1951

30. Lie JT: Personal communication
31. Lie JT, Holley KE, Kampa WR, Titus JL: New histochemical method for morphologic diagnosis of early stages of myocardial ischemia. Mayo Clin Proc 46:319–327, 1971
32. Lie JT, Pairolero PC, Holley KE, Titus JL: Unpublished data
33. Ludwig J, Linhart P, Baggenstoss AH: Hepatic lymph drainage in cirrhosis and congestive heart failure: a postmortem lymphangiographic study. Arch Pathol 86:551–562, 1968
34. Lumb G, Hardy LB: Technique for dissection and perfusion of heart. Arch Pathol 77:233–238, 1964
35. Lund F, Diener L, Ericsson JLE: Postmortem intraosseous phlebography as an aid in studies of venous thromboembolism. Angiology 20:155–176, 1969
36. Malm JR, Borman FO Jr, Harris PD, Kowalik ATW: An evaluation of aortic valve homografts sterilized by electron beam energy. J Thorac Cardiovasc Surg 54:471–477, 1967
37. Maresch R, Chiari H: Anleitung zuŕ Vornahme von Leichenöffnungen. Wien, Urban & Schwarzenberg, 1933
38. Masshoff W, Scheidt D, Reimers HF: Quantitative Bestimmung des Fett- und Myokardgewebes im Leichenherzen. Virchows Arch [Pathol Anat] 342:184–189, 1967
39. McGill HC, Brown BW, Gore I, McMillan GC, Paterson JC, Pollak OJ, Roberts JC Jr, Wissler RW: Grading human atherosclerotic lesions using a panel of photographs. Circulation 37:455–459, 1968
40. McVie JG: Postmortem detection of inapparent myocardial infarction. J Clin Pathol 23:203–209, 1970
41. Mönckeberg JG: Die Methoden zur morphologischen Untersuchung erkrankter Herzen. In Handbuch der biologischen Arbeitsmethoden. Vol VIII, part 1 (1). Edited by E Abderhalden. Berlin, Urban & Schwarzenberg, 1924, pp 635–650
42. Müller W: Die Massenverhältnisse des menschlichen Herzens. Hamburg, I. Voss, 1883
43. Nachlas MM, Shnitka TK: Macroscopic identification of early myocardial infarcts by alterations in dehydrogenase activity. Am J Pathol 42:379–405, 1963
44. Ongley PA, Titus JL, Khoury GH, Rahimtoola SH, Marshall HJ, Edwards JE: Anomalous connection of pulmonary veins to right atrium associated with anomalous inferior vena cava, situs inversus and multiple spleens: a developmental complex. Mayo Clin Proc 40:609–624, 1965
45. Orton CG: Red Perspex dosimetry. Phys Med Biol 11:551–562, 1966
46. Parke WW, Michels NA: A method for demonstrating subserous lymphatics with hydrogen peroxide. Anat Rec 146:165–171, 1963
47. Prinzmetal M, Kayland S, Margoles C, Tragerman LJ: A quantitative method for determining collateral coronary circulation: preliminary report on normal human hearts. Mt Sinai J Med NY 8:933–945, 1942
48. Rastelli GC, Titus JL: Experimental mitral valvular tissue grafts. In Biological Tissue in Heart Valve Replacement. Edited by MI Ionescu, DM Ross, GH Wooler. London, Butterworth & Co. (Publishers) Ltd., in press
49. Reiner L: Gross examination of the heart. In Pathology of the Heart and Blood Vessels. Third edition. Edited by SE Gould. Springfield, Illinois, Charles C Thomas, Publisher, 1968, pp 1111–1149
50. Reiner L: Selection of blocks from heart for microscopic study. Bull Pathol 9:198, 1968
51. Rissanen VT: Double contrast technique for postmortem coronary angiography. Lab Invest 23:517–520, 1970
52. Rittenhouse EA, Sands MP, Mohri H, Merendino AK: Sterilization of aortic valve grafts for transplantation. Arch Surg 101:1–5, 1970
53. Robbins SL, Fish SJ: A new angiographic technic providing a simultaneous permanent cast of the coronary arterial lumen. Am J Clin Pathol 42:156–163, 1964
54. Robbins SL, Solomon M, Bennett A: Demonstration of intercoronary anastomoses in human hearts with low viscosity perfusion mass. Circulation 33:733–743, 1966
55. Rodriguez FL, Reiner L: A new method of dissection of the heart. Arch Pathol 63:160–163, 1957
56. Rodriguez FL, Robbins SL: Postmortem angiographic studies on the coronary arterial circulation: intercoronary arterial anastomoses in adult human hearts. Am Heart J 70:348–364, 1965
57. Ross CF, Keele KD: Post mortem arteriography in "normal" lower limbs. Angiology 2:374–385, 1951
58. Rössle R: Technik der Obduktion mit Einschluss der Massmethoden an Leichenorganen. In Handbuch der biologischen Arbeitsmethoden. Vol VIII, part 1 (2). Edited by E Abderhalden. Berlin, Urban & Schwarzenberg, 1935, pp 1093–1246
59. Roussy G, Ameuille P: Technique des autopsies et des recherches anatomopathologiques à l'amphithéatre. Paris, O. Doin & Fils, 1910

60. Saphir O: Gross examination of the heart: injection of coronary arteries; weight and measurements of heart. *In* Pathology of the Heart. Second edition. Edited by SE Gould. Springfield, Illinois, Charles C Thomas, Publisher, 1960, pp 1043–1066
61. Schlesinger MJ: An injection plus dissection study of coronary artery occlusions and anastomoses. Am Heart J *15*:528–568, 1938
62. Schoenmackers J: Die Blutversorgung des Herzmuskels und ihre Störungen. *In* Kaufmann's Lehrbuch der speziellen pathologischen Anatomie. Vol 1, part 1, Suppl. Eleventh and twelfth edition. Edited by M Staemmler. Berlin, Walter de Gruyter & Co., 1969, pp 59–224
63. Smith JC: The pathology of human aortic valve homografts. Thorax *22*:114–138, 1967
64. Smith RL Jr: An Injection Study of Intercoronary Anastomoses in the Human Heart. Thesis, Graduate School, University of Minnesota, 1941
65. Suberman CO, Suberman RI, Dalldorf FG, Orlando FG: Radiographic visualization of coronary arteries in postmortem hearts: a simple technic. Am J Clin Pathol *53*:254–257, 1970
66. Titus JL: The Atrioventricular Conduction System in Congenital Ventricular Septal Defect. Thesis, Graduate School, University of Minnesota, 1961
67. Titus JL: Pathology of grafted heart valves. *In* Long-Term Prognosis Following Valve Replacement. Edited by JHK Vogel, Basel, S. Karger AG, 1972, pp 149–162
68. Titus JL, Feldman A, Anderson JA: Unpublished data
69. US Department of Defense. Army Department: Autopsy Manual, Washington DC, US Government Printing Office, 1960
70. Virchow R: Post-mortem Examinations With Especial Reference to Medico-legal Practice. Fourth German Edition. (English translation by TP Smith.) Philadelphia, P. Blakiston, Son & Co., 1885
71. Welch W: A comparative study of different methods of processing aortic homografts. Thorax *24*:746–749, 1969
72. Wolhard D: Eine neue Methode zur Konservierung des Herzens. Int Assoc Med Mus Bull *5*:48–49, 1915
73. Zugibe FT, Bell P Jr, Conley T, Standish ML: Determination of myocardial alterations at autopsy in the absence of gross and microscopic changes. Arch Pathol *81*:409–411, 1966

TRACHEOBRONCHIAL TREE AND LUNGS

DISSECTION AND FIXATION TECHNIQUES

Dissection of Larynx. Routinely, the larynx is opened along the posterior midline, and the lateral portions are pulled apart to expose the mucosa. In adults this maneuver may require breakage of the ossified laryngeal cartilage.

I prefer to slice the larynx into serial cross sections; this yields good histologic specimens for the demonstration of mucosal changes and also of the cricoarytenoid joint. This joint is found just beneath the level of the vocal cords, at both sides of the posterior midline of the larynx. Laryngeal joints are readily accessible at autopsy, and we now save them routinely in all cases, together with the sternoclavicular joints.

Dissection of Trachea and Main Bronchi. The trachea and main bronchi usually are opened along their posterior membranous walls. Anterior incisions in situ may be indicated in cases of aspiration and drowning. Tracheo-esophageal fistulas also are best demonstrated by anterior midline incision or complete removal of the anterior half of the trachea (Fig. 4–1).

Dissection of Fresh Lungs. *Dissection From Hilus.* The pulmonary arteries and bronchi are opened from the hilus toward the periphery of the mediastinal surface of the lung. Subsequently, the lungs are cut into several sagittal slices—that is, parallel with the mediastinal surface. This method permits study of many cross sections of bronchovascular units and gives a good overall view of the parenchyma. There are two disadvantages. First, the continuity of the organ is lost, so that it may be difficult to identify the original site of individual slices. Second, vessels and bronchi running in a more frontal plane cannot be dissected without at least partly destroying the slices. Instead of preparing sagittal sections, one can combine this method with the one in the following section.

93

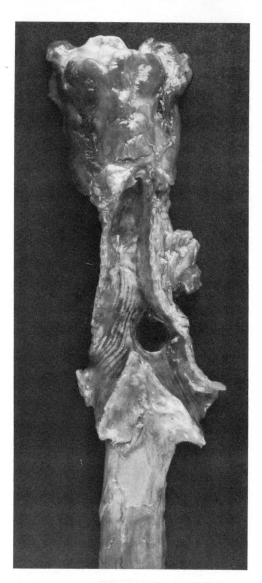

Figure 4–1. Larynx, trachea with carina, and esophagus with anterior half of trachea and adjacent main bronchi removed. Note perforation of carcinoma of esophagus into left main bronchus at carina.

Dissection From Incisions Along Lateral Surface of Lung. The hilus of the lung is held in the hand of the prosector. An incision is made from the apex to the base of the pulmonary lobes along their longest lateral axis. For the right middle lobe this axis lies almost in the horizontal plane. The incisions into the upper and lower lobes reach toward but not into the hilus and are connected by a third incision which lies at a right angle to the first and second. This third incision divides part of the wall of a main pulmonary artery, which usually shines through the pleura in the interlobular fissure close to the hilus. One blade of a pair of scissors is introduced into this opening, and the pulmonary arteries are opened radially in all directions. The cuts are continued peripherally from the vessels through the pleura so that the lung can be laid out well (Fig. 4–2). Subsequently, the bronchial tree is dissected in the same fashion (Fig. 4–3). This cannot be done without cutting through many pulmonary arteries.

This method leaves the dissected lung in continuity and permits easy reconstruction of the original position of pulmonary lesions. The disadvantage of this method is it may be difficult to leave the hilus intact unless there is a bronchopulmonary cuff.

Histologic Sampling. For routine histologic sampling, we use a stainless steel formalin container with three compartments for the right pulmonary lobes and two compartments for the left lobes. These compartments are created by removable stainless steel dividers.

Wet Fixation of Whole Lungs. Wet fixation of lungs provides excellent specimens, both by reconstituting the size of the lung at full inspiration and by providing good fixation for histologic study. The more important techniques have been reviewed by Silverton.[49]

If none of the perfusion apparatuses described below is available, lungs can be reinflated with 10% formalin solution through the main bronchus. About 2 liters of formalin solution is needed for an adult lung.

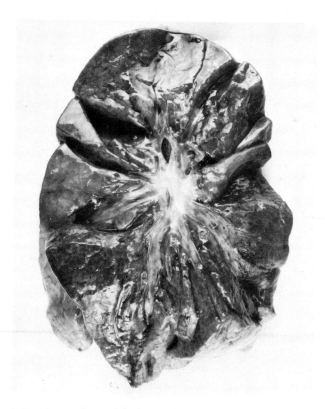

Figure 4–2. Cut surface of lung dissected from incisions along lateral surfaces of lobes. Hilus is left intact. Pulmonary artery tree has been opened lengthwise in radial fashion.

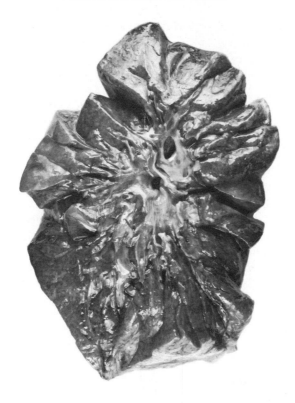

Figure 4–3. Same lung as in Figure 4–2. Bronchial tree has been opened lengthwise in radial fashion, sacrificing continuity of some overriding arteries.

The inflation can be done with a large syringe or, better still, by delivering the formalin solution from a bottle 30 to 50 cm above the specimen. Subsequently, the main bronchus is clamped and the lung is floated in a formalin bath. The disadvantage of this method is that the lung shrinks considerably.[56]

We routinely perfuse one lung and dissect the other in the fresh state to obtain material for microbiologic examination and for smears, for instance when we suspect *Pneumocystis carinii*. Pulmonary edema and embolism are best assessed on the fresh lung and, as a rule, the heavier one should be selected for this purpose.[56]

Removal and Preparation of Lungs. For most special studies on isolated lungs it is essential not to lacerate the organ during removal. We usually first produce a pneumothorax through a small parasternal incision. Subsequently, the anterior attachments of the diaphragm to the rib cage are incised so that the hand of an assistant can be introduced to hold back and protect the lung when the chest plate is removed. The remaining rib ends must be covered with towels immediately (not only can the sharp rib ends easily lacerate the visceral pleura but they also are dangerous to the pathologist and his assistant). Before the lungs are removed, adhesions must be carefully dissected as close to the parietal pleura as possible. This is particularly difficult at the posterior base of the lower lobes, where adhesions are frequently encountered. Extensive pulmonary adhesions may make it very difficult to remove the lungs intact. One may attempt to remove the lungs extrapleurally—that is, together with the parietal pleura which must be dissected from the bony and muscular parts of the chest wall.

Small rents in the pleura should be tied off before wet or steam fixation is attempted. Rents also can be sealed with wound spray ("artificial skin") and gauze reinforcement.[40]

Connection of the lung with the nozzle of the inflation or perfusion apparatus is greatly facilitated if an extrapulmonary bronchial or pulmonary artery cuff is left attached to the lung. A ring of the extrapulmonary bronchial wall should be removed for histologic examination before the glass nozzles and clamps are used. After removal of the heart, one also can inflate or perfuse both lungs simultaneously from the trachea or prepare pulmonary angiograms by injecting the main pulmonary artery. Both procedures can be carried out in situ.

Before inflation or perfusion, mucus or purulent material should be suctioned from the bronchi. If this cannot be done successfully, perfusion should be carried out through the pulmonary vessels.

Fixation Time. With perfusion methods, fixation time is about 3 days. Consolidated and fibrosed lungs may need longer. Plugging of bronchi may completely prevent proper expansion and fixation.

Formalin Perfusion Techniques (Pressure Fixation). Simple versions of the apparatus are shown in Figures 4–4 and 4–5. They consist essentially of

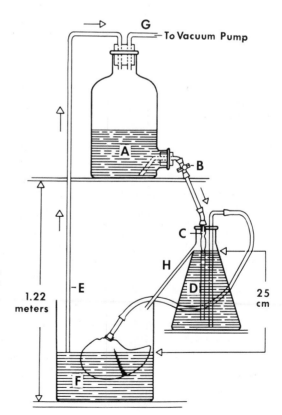

Figure 4–4. Simple version of lung perfusion apparatus of Heard with vacuum pump. Perfusion pressure of 25 cm H$_2$O (formalin) is maintained by appropriate setting of height of flask (D). See text. E: tube from container F to A; G: tube to vacuum pump; B: clip adjusted to prevent flask D from overflowing when vacuum breaks in tube E; C: one-way glass valve. (From Heard BE: A pathological study of emphysema of the lungs with chronic bronchitis. Thorax 13:136–149, 1958. By permission of the British Medical Association.)

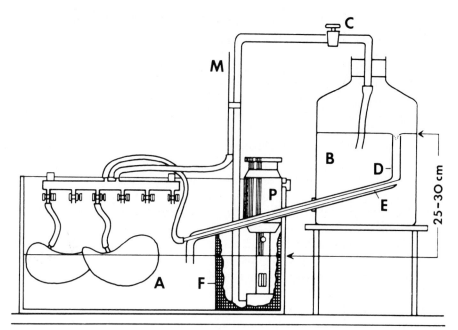

Figure 4–5. Lung perfusion (pressure fixation) apparatus of Heard. Same principle as apparatus in Figure 4–4, but using electrical centrifugal pump (P) to raise formalin to upper container (B) from which it overflows down pipe D. Manifold is supplied by tube E. Tap C controls output from pump. Filter F prevents pump from becoming clogged with debris from lower container. Manometer (M) serves to indicate that no unused taps on manifold are left open. Six lungs can be fixed simultaneously. (From Heard BE: Pathology of pulmonary emphysema: methods of study. Am Rev Resp Dis 82:792–799, 1960. By permission of the National Tuberculosis and Respiratory Disease Association.)

two containers, one the formalin bath with the specimen and the other an elevated formalin container from which the formalin flows under pressure into the lungs. The formalin is kept in circulation either by an electric vacuum pump and a glass valve to fill the upper container intermittently, or by an electric centrifugal pump to fill the upper container continuously. The desired pressure is maintained by setting the height of an overflow.

We are using modifications of this apparatus as shown in Figures 4–6, 4–7, and 4–8. The fixed specimens are of good quality (Fig. 4–9).

Because the overflow may cause excessive formalin fumes and foaming and continuous pumping wears out the motor, an apparatus was designed[21] which worked without overflow and required only occasional pumping (Fig. 4–10). The formalin solution (15%) is raised by a pump from the fixing bath to an elevated container until the control float is lifted. This moves a microswitch which operates the relay and stops the pump. When the level of formalin solution in the raised container falls a short distance, the float drops, activating a second microswitch which restarts the pump. Filters remove blood and exudate that would otherwise be injected deep into the lungs. Sedimentation in both containers also helps in this respect. The diagram does not show an overflow that is fitted near the top

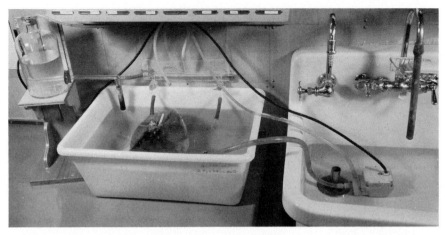

Figure 4–6. Pressure fixation of lung. Simple modification of apparatus shown in Figure 4–5. Lid of plastic formalin bath containing lung has been removed. Black electric cable leads to continuously running submersible pump. Plastic hoses connect pump with elevated formalin container and overflow and with formalin bath.

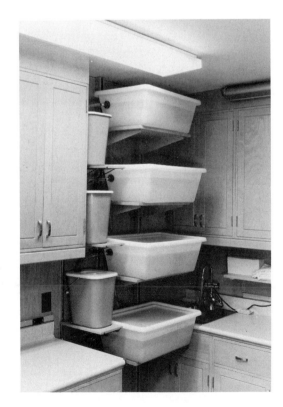

Figure 4–7. Pressure fixation of lung. Modification of apparatus shown in Figure 4–6, permitting simultaneous fixation of 12 or more lungs. Two sets of shelves with formalin reservoirs and plastic containers with lungs can slide up and down on rails fixed to wall. In position shown here, uppermost formalin bath cannot be used. Pump in sink (at right) supplies entire system.

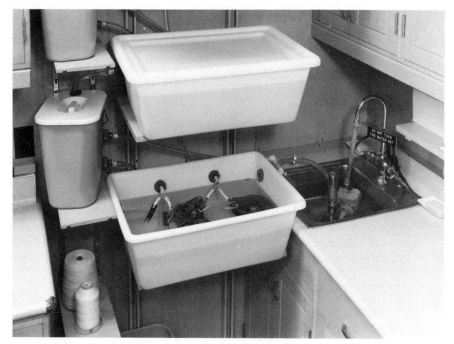

Figure 4–8. **View of lowermost formalin bath in Figure 4–7** with lid removed. Two lungs are attached to one Y connection; other Y connection is unused and is clamped. Submersible pump is in sink at right. At left is elevated formalin container and overflow.

of the upper container and drains into the lower container; this is a safety measure in case the float fails to switch off the pump. The pressure in the manifold is checked with an open-end manometer. The filter F^2 has to be cleaned frequently. The whole apparatus is drained and cleaned twice a year.

Pressure-Free Perfusion Fixation (Hartung). In this method[15] the fixative is not forced into the bronchial system by pressure but rather is aspirated from a separate container. The lung can be fixed at any desired state of expansion.[17] The isolated lung is kept submerged by a padded wire mesh in a container, 45 by 30 by 25 cm, filled with formalin solution (Fig. 4–11). The level of the wire mesh can be adjusted. A tube is tied into the main bronchus of the lung, run through the lid of the formalin container, and connected with another container at the same level. The container with the specimen is freed of air by forcing in formalin solution through a second tube which perforates the lid and connects to the extrapulmonary fluid space in the main container. The air escapes through an air trap on top of the lid. After all the air has escaped, this air trap is closed. The lung will now adjust to any volume changes in the main container. Removal of formalin solution will cause expansion of the lung and vice versa. When the lung expands, formalin solution will flow through the tube into the main bronchus, but the pressure will remain atmospheric.

Expansion to about two thirds of the inspiration volume is considered optimal and requires removal of about 0.6 to 1.5 liters in adults, 0.4 to 0.8 liter in 10-year olds, and 0.2 liter in 4-year olds.

Gaseous Fixation. Fixation with vaporous media can be achieved with formaldehyde gas or with formalin steam. Use of formaldehyde gas provides dry lungs. If air is blown through these lungs, desiccation or mummification occurs, as with the method of Blumenthal and Boren.[5] Since desiccation is not usually desired, afterfixation is recommended for both techniques.

Preparation of Lungs. The procedures of removing the lungs are similar to the ones described in the previous section. For gaseous fixation it is even more important not to lacerate the pleura. Pleural rents should be sealed. The average fixation time is 3 days. With the method of Weibel and Vidone[54] (see below) fixation sufficient for cutting histologic blocks is achieved after only 2 hours. Afterfixation of the tissue with Zenker's fluid is recommended by these authors. If 40% formaldehyde solution is used, this secondary fixation seems to be unnecessary.[48]

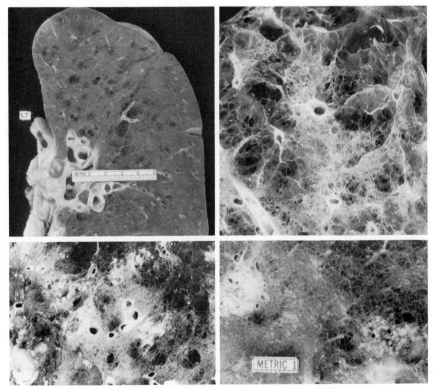

Figure 4–9. Lung specimens after pressure fixation with modified system (see text). *Upper Left,* Mild centriacinar emphysema in 65-year-old man. *Upper Right,* Severe destructive panacinar emphysema in 74-year-old man. Barium-gelatin injection of pulmonary arteries. *Lower Left,* Close-up of destructive centriacinar and irregular emphysema, purulent bronchitis and bronchiolitis, and bronchopneumonia in 52-year-old man. *Lower Right,* Close-up of mild panacinar and irregular emphysema and metastasis of anaplastic bronchogenic squamous cell carcinoma in 81-year-old man.

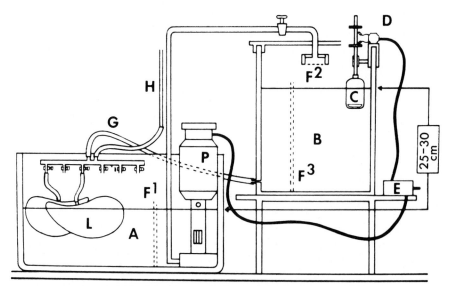

Figure 4–10. Modified apparatus for lung perfusion (pressure fixation). Aqueous formalin is supplied continuously from raised container (*B*), replenished by electric pump (*P*) acting intermittently and controlled by float (*C*) and switch (*E*). F^1, F^2, and F^3 are filters. (From Heard BE, Esterly JR, Wootliff JS: A modified apparatus for fixing lungs to study the pathology of emphysema. Am Rev Resp Dis 95:311–312, 1967. By permission of the National Tuberculosis and Respiratory Disease Association.)

Formaldehyde Gas: Method of Cureton and Trapnell.[6] A rubber stopper is tied into the main bronchus and is perforated by a needle through which the lung is inflated with formaldehyde gas at a pressure not exceeding 40 to 50 mm Hg (Fig. 4–12). The formaldehyde gas is produced by filling half of a large carboy with 40% formaldehyde solution and bubbling air through the solution. The formaldehyde vapor above the fluid is used to inflate the lungs. Occasionally, mucus or other bronchial obstructions have to be removed. After roentgenograms have been taken, the whole lung is floated for at least 2 to 3 days in 20% formalin solution and covered with a cloth soaked in the same fixative. Subsequently, the whole fixed lung or slices can be roentgenographed again.

Formalin Steam: Method of Weibel and Vidone.[54] This method makes use of a more sophisticated apparatus which permits control of the state of inflation. In the following description, the letters refer to the labels in Figure 4–13.

The lung is mounted in a clear plastic (Lucite) box (*N*) so that the bronchus is open to the exterior (at *C*). Several holes in the walls of the box permit various manipulations such as vascular injections. One hole is fitted with a manometer (*F*); another hole (*E*) is fitted with a connection to a pump (*J*) for removing air from the box (the air so removed is passed through water in a flask [*G*] to trap formalin fumes). The negative pressure in the box is regulated by means of a screw clamp on a side arm (*H*). The cover (*O*) is held firmly to the box by the negative pres-

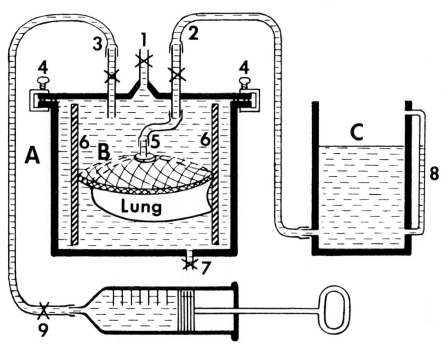

Figure 4–11. Pressure-free lung fixation by volume complement method. A = Air-tight container with lid fixed by screw clamps (4), air trap and stopcock (1), and tubes leading to lung (2), to container (3), and to drain (7), all with stopcocks. B = Concave wire mesh which keeps lung submerged; opening in wire mesh for tube tied into main bronchus (5). Four rods (6) guide and stabilize wire mesh. C = Container with fixative connected to tube leading to main bronchus and fitted with fluid level indicator (8). D = Syringe (300 to 500 ml), with stopcock (9) for regulating fluid volume in container. See text for method. (From Hartung W: Gefrier-Großschnitte von ganzen Organen, speziell der Lunge. Zentralbl Allg Pathol 100:408–413, 1960. By permission of Gustav Fischer Verlag.)

Figure 4–12. Apparatus of Cureton and Trapnell[6] **for gaseous fixation of whole lung.** 1 = Carboy of concentrated form-aldehyde solution; 2 = aneroid pressure gauge; 3 = rubber syringe. (From Cureton RJR, Trapnell DH: Post-mortem radiography and gaseous fixation of the lung. Thorax 16:138–143, 1961. By permission of the British Medical Association.)

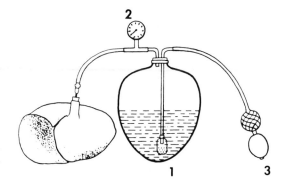

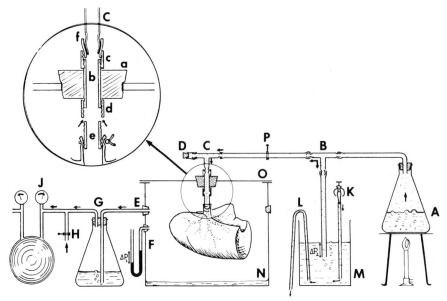

Figure 4–13.   Apparatus of Weibel and Vidone[54] **for formalin steam fixation** of whole lung. This permits fixation in controlled state of inflation. See text for explanation. (From Weibel ER, Vidone RA: Fixation of the lung by formalin steam in a controlled state of air inflation. Am Rev Resp Dis 84:856–861, 1961. By permission of the National Tuberculosis and Respiratory Disease Association.)

sure. By adjustment of the negative pressure in the box ("pleural" pressure) the lung can be inflated to any desired extent. Also the lung can be made to "breathe" by changing the pressure.

Formalin steam is generated in a 3-liter flask (A) containing approximately 1,500 ml of a mixture of 2 parts of 37% formaldehyde solution and 1 part of water. The steam is led through a T tube (B) whose side arm is immersed in water (M) to a depth of 5 to 10 cm to act as an escape valve and keep the pressure constant. The formaldehyde vapor which escapes through the side arm is absorbed by the water which is changed continuously by inflow (K) of fresh water and drainage through a siphon (L).

The steam is passed into the bronchial tree through a T tube (C) which is fitted to a connector system (see *inset*). By use of the side arm (D) and clamp (P), the lung can be inflated with room air before the treatment with formalin steam is started.

The connecting arrangement (C), constructed according to the recommendations of Moolten[37] and Liebow et al,[29] consists of two short lengths of threaded metal pipe (b,e) and two corresponding sleeves (c,d). One length of pipe (b) is fitted tightly into a rubber stopper (a); to the ends of this pipe the sleeves (c,d) are tightly screwed. The other length of pipe (e) is used to cannulate the trachea or bronchus; its other end screws into the lower sleeve (d). The conical end (f) of the glass T tube (C) is fitted with a piece of rubber tubing which is inserted tightly into the opening of the sleeve (c).

If blood vessels are to be injected, they should be cannulated after the bronchus is tied to the pipe but before the lung is placed in the box. Otherwise, the major branches should be ligated to prevent exsanguination, if possible, in situ before transection of the vessels. After the free end of the pipe (*e*) is screwed into the sleeve (*d*) but before the lung is lowered into the box, the pleural surface is coated lightly, with a cotton swab, with glycerin diluted with water to prevent excessive drying of the surface.

When the apparatus is assembled, clamp (*P*) is closed and the side arm (*D*) is opened. The clamp at *H* is opened and closed to vary the negative pressure in the box; this inflates the lung with room air and is continued until the whole lung is well inflated. Inflation of the lung should be carried out gradually until almost the maximum is reached—at this point a change in pressure causes only a slight change in volume. Then the pressure is decreased slightly and the inflation corresponding to 75% of maximal inflation is maintained constant.

With clamp *P* still closed, heat is applied to flask *A*. A marking pencil is used to trace the contour of the expanded lung onto the front panel of the box, so that the degree of shrinkage due to fixation can be determined.

When sufficient steam pressure builds up, clamp *P* is opened slowly and side arm *D* is closed gradually with a rubber stopper. One must be careful not to let the lung collapse at this time. Because much of the first steam may condense in the lung, *D* must be open enough to keep the lung inflated until the steam pressure builds up sufficiently. This state will be indicated by a stream of bubbles coming out of the escape valve (*B*). Varying the heat controls the steam production.

When steam production is sufficient to maintain the inflated state, the treatment is continued for $1\frac{1}{2}$ to 2 hours; at this time the surface of the lung should appear uniformly gray-brown. To end the procedure, the heat at the steam generator is turned off, clamp *P* is closed rapidly, and side arm *D* is opened immediately. It is very important that the airways should be opened to the atmosphere immediately after the steam line is closed. Otherwise, condensation of the vapors inside the lung would permit the lung to collapse and, since it is fixed, it could not be inflated again. Collapse will be prevented if the external pressure is never allowed to exceed the internal pressure. As the vapor in the steam generator cools, water from *M* will flow through *B* into *A* and thus dilute the strong formaldehyde solution.

After the lung has cooled, it is held by the pipe (*e*), disconnected from the T tube, and immersed in Zenker's fluid in a large bucket. A layer of cotton saturated with the same fluid is placed over the floating lung. All handling must be with care to avoid crushing the lung.

During overnight soaking, the Zenker fluid infiltrates and hardens a layer approximately 3 to 4 cm deep. The lung now can be handled easily and is cut into slices 1 to 2 cm thick. These slices are wrapped together loosely with gauze and soaked in Zenker's fluid for 12 hours. The lung tissue then is stiff enough to withstand manipulation, such as slicing and embedding, without collapsing.

Advantages and Disadvantages of Wet and Gaseous Fixation Methods. The main advantages and disadvantages of these techniques are compared in Table 4–1. The reader will have to weigh for himself the arguments of

TABLE 4–1.   COMPARISON OF GASEOUS AND WET FIXATION METHODS

Method	Advantages	Disadvantages
Gaseous fixation	More accurate volume measurements; lungs can be fixed in any desired dimension[24] Roentgenograms of slices are not obscured by collection of fixation fluids Alveolar ducts can be identified more easily[19]	Fixation may be incomplete, particularly in cases of chronic bronchitis, pulmonary fibrosis, or other types of pulmonary consolidation[41] "Artifact emphysema," probably due to autolysis[44]
Wet fixation	Complete fixation in most situations with preservation of good cytologic details	State of expansion is poorly controlled except by method of Hartung Intrapulmonary injection of formalin solution tends to overinflate lungs, particularly in emphysema and old age Formalin washes mucus down bronchial tree[9] Roentgenograms of fixed slices are obscured by fixation fluid

the various authors. For quantitative studies in emphysema requiring exact volume control, Dunnill[8] advocated the gaseous fixation technique of Weibel and Vidone. However, volume control appears to be even superior with the wet fixation method of Hartung. Overinflation, which is produced by the other wet fixation methods, could be prevented by fixing the lungs within the thoracic cavity. The lungs would then be fixed in a position closer to expiration. This in turn is compensated for to some extent by rigor mortis which causes some inspiratory movement of the chest.[11] Unfortunately, in situ formalin fixation[30] is too time-consuming for routine autopsies. The in situ fixation which is achieved by embalming is always insufficient for the requirements of pathologists. Freezing methods[30] are accompanied by many difficulties and rarely can be recommended. These are beyond the scope of this discussion.

For routine use and for qualitative study of emphysema, we prefer the wet fixation technique with a perfusion pressure of 25 to 30 cm H_2O. This provides good histologic detail and excellent museum specimens (Fig. 4–9).

Dry Preservation of Lungs.   Kramer[27] has reviewed obsolete mummification methods. A few more recent papers have described air-drying techniques.[5,38,52] We occasionally have mummified lungs; this provides durable specimens which are economical and excellent for teaching purposes. There is little loss of volume (Fig. 4–14) but complete loss of color and normal consistency. Histologic sections of such lungs are far from good but still are much better than one would expect—for instance, bronchopneumonia can still be diagnosed.

The intact lung is formalin-fixed by one of the previously mentioned methods. The lung is then thoroughly perfused and washed with tap water for about 1 day in order to prevent subsequent precipitation of formalin crystals. A hose from the laboratory air outlet is connected with the main

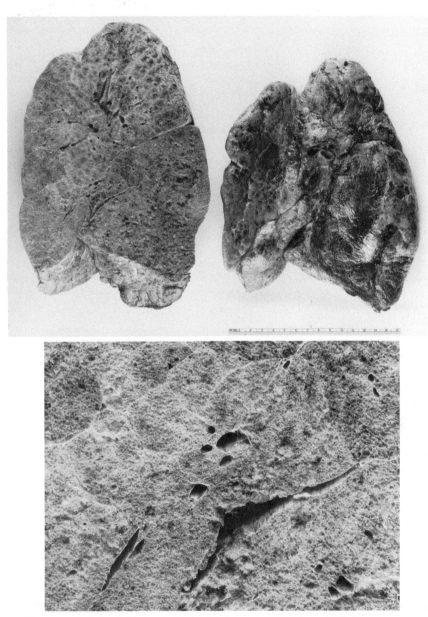

Figure 4–14. *Upper,* Right lung with minimal centrilobular emphysema in upper lobe. This lung was air dried (mummified) after perfusion fixation with formalin solution. *Lower,* Close-up of area in lower center of cut surface shown at right in *Upper.*

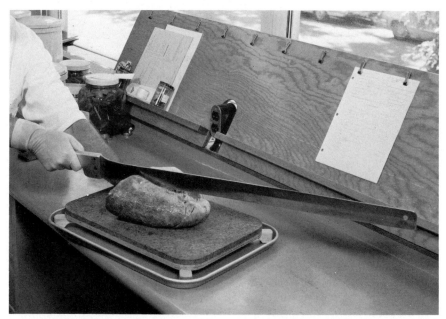

Figure 4–15. **Slicing of lung** fixed by perfusion method of Heard. If lung is cut with uninterrupted pulling motion and special long-bladed knife, there will be no knife marks on cut surface. Cork cutting board rests on metal tray which collects draining formalin solution.

bronchus, and the air pressure is adjusted so that the specimen maintains approximately its normal size.

Formaldehyde vapor fixation can be combined with the subsequent air-drying process[5] by simply bubbling the air through a flask containing formalin. The fixation time is 3 to 5 days. Alcohol fume fixation can be used if color preservation is desired. After fixation with alcohol or form-aldehyde vapor, air alone is passed into the lungs through the same system.

With all of these techniques, air-drying requires about 1 week. The lung becomes rigid and dry but not fragile. Large, thick slices can be stained by various techniques.[5] Thus, the lungs can be studied in three dimensions.

Infiltration methods for pulmonary tissues, such as infiltration with paraffin or diglycol stearate,[27] are similar to those used for dry preservation of the heart (see chapter 3). I have found that, for museum specimens, wet preparations are superior, both economically and esthetically.

Slicing of Fixed Lungs.   I use a special knife and slicing board (Fig. 4–15). The cork slicing board is mounted in a metal tray where the draining formalin solution collects. The knife has a 78-cm-long blade which permits the whole lung to be cut with an uninterrupted pulling mo-tion. This ensures a smooth and even cut surface without knife marks. This knife also works well to prepare even slices of livers or large spleens. The lung usually is cut in the frontal or sagittal plane in slices about 1.5 cm thick. For frontal sectioning, the lung is placed so that the hilus is uppermost. I usually make the first cut immediately adjacent to the hilus (Fig. 4–9 *upper left*). If the cut section is to be along the axis of a bronchus, the knife is guided along metal probes or glass rods previously inserted into the major airways.

Thin slices can be prepared by freezing the fixed lung and cutting the block with a meat slicer or a band saw. For still thinner slices, wax infiltration is required (see below).

IMPREGNATION AND STORAGE OF LUNG SLICES

Barium Sulfate Impregnation. Barium sulfate impregnation renders pulmonary tissue opaque. This makes it considerably easier to quantitate lung changes such as in pulmonary emphysema. After impregnation with barium sulfate the lung slices sink in water and can easily be photographed and studied with the naked eye or with a dissecting microscope (Fig. 4–16).

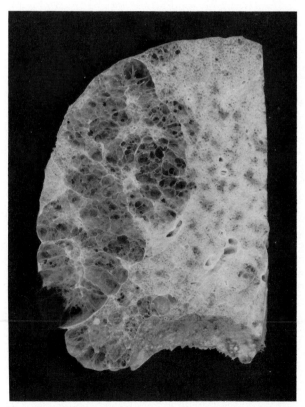

Figure 4–16. Slice of lung fixed by perfusion method of Heard, impregnated with barium sulfate, and photographed under water, showing focal panacinar emphysema.

Method of Heard.[20]   A slice of fixed lung is placed in a solution of 75 gm of barium nitrate dissolved in 1 liter of warm water. The lung tissue is slightly squeezed so that the solution penetrates the tissue. After about 1 minute, the slice is taken out of this solution and excess fluid is squeezed out.

Next, the tissue is submerged in a solution of 100 gm of sodium sulfate dissolved in 1 liter of warm water. The lung tissue is again slightly squeezed and then taken out of the solution, drained, and returned to the barium nitrate bath. This procedure is repeated several times until all air bubbles have been squeezed out and the barium sulfate precipitate has rendered the lung tissue opaque and grayish white. Gas bubbles are considerably less bothersome when the lung had previously been inflated with carbon dioxide.

Storage.   Fresh lungs can be stored in a refrigerator for a few days at temperatures just above the freezing point. Fresh lungs also can be kept deep frozen for months and remain satisfactory for histologic studies or vascular injection. However, complete thawing is essential. The lungs should be transferred to a refrigerator at 0 C for 3 days, then left at room temperature overnight, and finally placed in an incubator at 40 C for 1 hour.[40] I cannot recommend this as a routine procedure.

Fixed lungs are best sliced and stored flat in heat-sealed plastic bags filled with 5 to 20% formalin solution. Several slices can be stored in a stack without distorting the lung tissue.

MOUNTED GROSS SECTIONS

Paper-Mounted Sections.   *Technique of Gough.*   The following is the original technique of Gough with some recent modifications.[12] Eleven days are required to complete the sections.[55] The completed preparations can be stiffened with cellophane.[12] Gough kept unstained sections for 20 years without noting any change. Sections stained with hematoxylin and aniline dyes tend to fade in light while Perls' stain for iron remains unchanged.

The intact lungs are perfused, under pressure, through the bronchi with a solution consisting of formalin (40% formaldehyde solution), 500 ml; sodium acetate, 200 gm; and water, 5,000 ml. Slices of fixed lung, 2 cm thick, are washed in running water for 3 days. Care must be taken to keep the containers free of microorganisms, including algae, which can digest the gelatin in which the slices are to be embedded.

The embedding solution, which contains a disinfectant, has the following components: gelatin, 300 gm; ethylene glycol monoethyl ether, 40 ml; capryl alcohol, 5 ml; glycerin, 100 ml; water, 1,250 ml; dichlorophene (Panacide), 3 drops. The lung slices are placed in this solution which is preheated to about 60 C and subjected to a partial vacuum to remove the air from the tissue and to cause the gelatin to penetrate. The gelatin solution with the specimen is left in an incubator at 35 C for 48 hours. The gelatin then is allowed to set, and the gelatin block is placed on a warm microtome holder with some weight on top. The gelatin block is now kept in a deep freezer at −25 C overnight. The sections are cut at 400 μ with the MSE "large section" microtome (Measuring and Scientific Equipment, Ltd., 14-29 Spenser Street, London, S. W. 1) and put in the 10% formalin-acetate solution used for perfusion (see above). After 1 to 2 days in this solution, the gelatin is hardened again and can be washed for 1 to 2 hours.

For the paper mounting, a second gelatin solution is used which has the following composition: gelatin (80–100 bloom), 75 gm; glycerin, 70 ml; Cellosolve, 40 ml; water, 850 ml; dichlorophene, 3 drops. The 400-μ lung slice is taken from the water bath, surplus gelatin is cut off, and the tissue is placed on a piece of plexiglass onto which some of this gelatin solution has been poured. More of the second gelatin solution is poured over this preparation which then is covered by a sheet of Whatman No. 1 filter paper. Surplus solution and air bubbles are removed, the preparation is dried, and, finally, the paper with the tissue slice is lifted from the plexiglass.

Modification for Rapid Preparations. The original method of paper-mounted sections of Gough requires 11 days. The modification of Whimster[55] is based on shorter fixation, washing, and embedding procedures. The gelatin used is somewhat less viscous. The preparation of the sections requires 1 to 2 days. The 24-hour method yields good sections, but the results of the 48-hour method are superior.

Film-Strip Mounting. A 70-mm film-strip mounting system for large serial sections of animal lungs has recently been described[57] and appears to be applicable for research work on human lungs. Cost is said to be low.

QUANTITATIVE ESTIMATION
OF PULMONARY CHANGES

Volume Determination. The trachea is clamped before the chest is opened. After the chest plate has been removed, hilar bronchi and vessels are also clamped. The lungs then are removed and weighed and their volume is measured by water displacement. Care must be taken that the bronchi or any rents in the pleura are closed airtight. Large bullae should be injected with gelatin prior to submersion.[4]

Grid Methods for Wet Specimens or Paper-Mounted Sections. For all these methods, appropriate fixation is essential, preferably by formalin gas or by the wet fixation method of Hartung.

The simplest type of grid is subdivided into squares. The grid is placed on a slice of lung tissue and those squares in which the lung tissue is affected by whatever pathologic process is being studied are counted.[42] Such grids also are used for stratified random sampling.

The Ryder grid[45] consists of 10 triangular segments. Emphysema is scored 0, 1, 2, or 3 ("none," "mild," "moderate," or "severe") in each of the segments in a grid overlying paper-mounted sections. Standards are used for scoring the segments. The scores for the 10 segments are added and the total score is expressed as a percentage of the total possible score of 30. The use of a panel of standards, although arbitrary and intuitive, has been found to be the quickest and most accurate method of grading from paper-mounted sections.[51]

For the measurement of bronchi and bronchioli, a system with concentric circles has been used incorporated into a 12.5× ocular of a Leitz microscope projector.[4]

More commonly used are grids with points. The statistical basis of point-counting techniques has been discussed in detail by Weibel.[53] It has been applied to the study of bronchitis by Hale et al[14] and Dunnill et al[10] and to the study of emphysema by Dunnill[8] and by Weibel.[53] Emphysema is evaluated with a transparent cellophane grid with points 1 cm apart at the apices of equilateral triangles. This cellophane grid is placed on the lung slice and each point is ascribed to one of the three components: (1) non-parenchyma (bronchi and blood vessels larger than 2 mm in diameter), (2) normal parenchyma, and (3) abnormal air spaces. A total of 2,000 to 3,000 points is assessed.

Blocks for histologic study are selected by stratified random sampling for which a grid with 1-cm squares is used. Histologic slides are assessed by the same principles as in macroscopic preparations. The mean shrinkage coefficient usually is calculated from randomized samples. With this technique, volume proportions and surface area are estimated.

Thurlbeck[50] used a dissecting microscope for the point-count assessment. Excluding "non-parenchyma," he expressed emphysema as a percentage of total lung parenchyma.

Planimetric Study From Photomicrographic Transparencies. This method was used by Anderson and Foraker[1] to measure cross sections of the terminal bronchioli, parenchymal air spaces, and vasculature in normal and emphysematous lungs. The measurements were carried out on photomicrographic transparencies by using tracing paper with a compensating planimeter. The measurements were first made in square centimeters and then reduced to square microns on the microscopic slide.

Light Absorption Methods. *Diazo Print Technique.*[47] Frozen sections 400 to 500 μ thick are prepared; this thickness seems to be crucial for this method. A modified Gough-Wentworth technique is used. The frozen sections are placed on a sheet of clear plastic and blotted with filter paper. The dry undersurface of the plastic sheet is placed on the sensitized surface of diazo paper. This preparation is put between two glass plates and exposed to 150-watt photographic floodlights. The bulb should be more than 30 cm from the section. A 30-second exposure provides a well-differentiated image. Optimal exposure is of critical importance. The exposed paper is developed in a chamber or hood with ammonia fumes. The diazo copies can then be used for planimetric studies.

Photometric Measurement of Tungsten-Filament Light Absorption.[31] Sections 0.6 to 0.8 cm thick of formalin-steam-fixed lungs are placed on a scanner frame support and the absorption of tungsten-filament light is measured by placing the light and the light-sensitive tube on opposite sides of the specimen. The light falling on the photo tube is measured by a densitometer. A computer counter is used to record the densitometer output. The light absorption method is said[31] to give an adequate measure of lung destruction.

Measurement of Sound Transmission and Beta Radiation Absorption. There is no satisfactory correlation between absorption of sound or transmission of beta radiation and lung destruction when evaluated by modifications of the previously described method for measuring tungsten-filament light absorption.[31]

Microradiographic Techniques. The absorption of roentgen rays by air-dried lungs is measured.[38] Slices 0.5 mm thick are roentgenographed in a vacuum chamber, using 2.5 kv in a modification of the Philips microradiographic unit. Tissue slices more than 2 mm thick are roentgenographed with a General Electric grain unit using 10 to 30 kv. For thicker slices and the whole lung, Eastman Type M Industrial x-ray film is used.

POSTMORTEM PULMONARY ANGIOGRAPHY AND BRONCHOGRAPHY

Satisfactory injection can be achieved only with inflated lungs. Therefore, careful removal of the lungs and sealing of accidental lacerations of the pleura are essential.

Pulmonary Arteriography. *In Situ or Isolated Adult Lungs.* Barium-gelatin mixtures are the preferred media. A suitable preparation has been described in chapter 3. The viscosity of the gelatin preparations depends on many factors, so that the optimal concentration of gelatin will vary and has to be tested.

The pulmonary arteries can be injected in situ, using the technique described in chapter 3 for in situ coronary angiography. A 13-gauge needle is introduced into the pulmonary artery just above the pulmonary valve. This technique is particularly useful when tumors, adhesions, or other pathologic lesions prevent the removal of intact lungs.

For pulmonary arteriography on isolated lungs (Fig. 4–17), one glass cannula is tied into the pulmonary artery and one into the main bronchus. The lung is inflated through the bronchus with air or carbon dioxide at a pressure of 20 mm Hg. The barium-gelatin medium is warmed to about 60 C and injected into the inflated lung at a pressure of about 70 to 80 mm Hg (other authors use higher pressures[41]). Differences in required injection pressure result from differences in viscosity of the medium, temperature, types of syringes, and other factors. With our method, the smallest vessels filled have an internal diameter of about 60 μ. For an average-sized lung, about 150 ml of medium is needed. The injection takes 5 to 10 minutes. When the vascular tree is filled, the pressure increases suddenly, so that this end point cannot easily be missed. The lung should be kept warm during the injection so that the gelatin does not set too quickly.

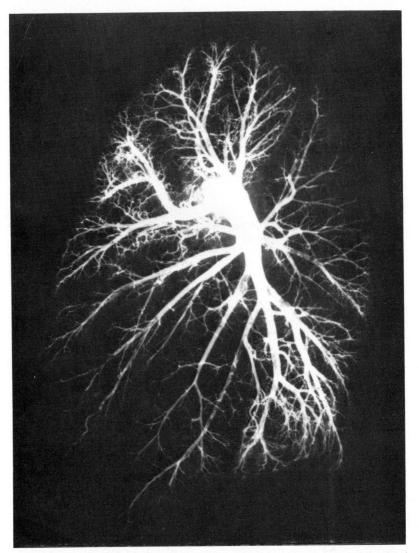

Figure 4–17. Arteriogram of left lung; lung inflated with carbon dioxide and pulmonary artery injected with barium sulfate-gelatin mixture. Note marked rarefication of vascular tree in this emphysematous lung.

Isolated Infant Lungs.[26] The pulmonary artery and its branches, including the arterioles, are filled with contrast medium under standardized conditions. The injection is pulsatile while the lungs are rhythmically ventilated by negative insufflation pressure. Both injection and ventilation pressures are in "physiologic" ranges.

The pressure source of the perfusion apparatus is a pump (Filamatic Vial Filler, Model AB, 50 ml, National Instrument Co., Baltimore, Md.) with variable stroke volume and providing unidirectional flow. The cyclic pressure is transmitted to a container in which the contrast medium is kept continuously agitated to avoid sedimentation of the barium sulfate. The contrast medium is usually injected at a pressure of 80/50 mm Hg at room temperature.

The contrast medium is 7.5% barium sulfate (Micropaque) suspended in 6% Rheomacrodex to make a concentration of approximately 340 mmoles/liter. The pH of this suspension is 4.8.

The lung is suspended in a vacuum chamber and the trachea is connected to an air inlet (Fig. 4–18). The pulmonary artery or vein is connected to the catheter which delivers the contrast medium. By moving the airtight plexiglass cylinder upward, a negative pressure is created around the lung; the lung can be made to "breathe" by moving

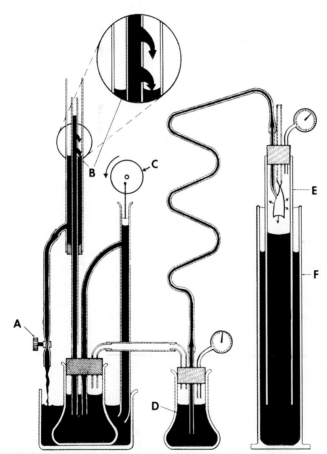

Figure 4–18. Apparatus for pulmonary arteriography and microangiography of infant lungs. Lung is suspended in airtight cylinder (**E**). Respiratory pressure changes are reproduced by moving cylinder up and down in water-filled jacket (**F**). Contrast medium (**D**) is injected under cyclic pressure generated by pump (**C**). Pressure and amplitude are controlled by height of water column (**B**) which can be adjusted by changing outflow resistance (**A**) and stroke amplitude of pump (**C**). (From Ivemark BI, Wallgren G: The pulmonary vascular pattern in idiopathic respiratory distress: a micro-angiographic study. Acta Pathol Microbiol Scand 76:203–214, 1969. By permission of Munksgaard.)

the tube up and down. The pressure in the vacuum chamber is usually made to oscillate between −15 and +10 mm Hg which in all cases causes pronounced cyclic volume changes of the lungs with visible aeration of all alveoli lining the surface. The respiratory rate is kept at 15/min and the injection time is standardized to 30 minutes.

After cannulation of the trachea, lobar bronchi can be ligated if aeration is to be limited to only one lobe. The contrast medium is injected into the main pulmonary artery after ligation of the ductus arteriosus.

After the injection the trachea is clamped and the aerated specimen is disconnected from the cannula and submerged in neutral formalin solution. After fixation for 2 to 3 days, slices 2 to 4 mm thick are roentgenographed. Ordinary x-ray film can be used. Stereomicroangiography is carried out on paraffin-embedded 1,000-μ blocks. Histologic sections are prepared from the same blocks.

In the technique of Davies and Reid,[7] a mixture of gelatin and Micropaque is injected at 60 C under a pressure of 74 mm Hg. Arteries down to a diameter of 15 to 25 μ are filled. Prior to injection the lungs are placed into an incubator at 37 C for 1 hour to ensure even injection. It should be noted, however, that this warming procedure will interfere with fine cellular detail.

Pulmonary Venography.   The injection technique is basically similar to that for pulmonary arteriography. The apparatus shown in Figure 4–18 also can be used for venography. In situ filling can be achieved by injecting contrast medium into the left atrium through a catheter in the mitral valve or by clamping the aorta and injecting the contrast medium into the left atrium. After the heart chambers are filled, the contrast medium will flow in a retrograde fashion into the pulmonary veins. Postmortem blood clots may cause filling defects. The same technique may be used on isolated heart-lung blocks. Pulmonary venography on an isolated lung is facilitated if a part of the left atrium has been left attached so that glass cannulas can be tied into the veins. The recommended injection pressure is 20 mm Hg.[4]

Bronchial Arteriography.   For injection through the aorta in situ,[29] the axillary arteries, thyrocervical trunks, internal mammary arteries, vertebral arteries, and common carotid arteries are ligated. The axillary arteries are tied distal to the costocervical trunks so that the upper intercostal vessels, from which bronchial arteries may take off, are also injected. The aorta is washed out, and the supravalvular portion of it is tied. The aorta is then injected from above the celiac axis. A mixture of 80% barium sulfate (Micropaque) and 3% gelatin will give satisfactory results.[36] A useful non-pulsatile injection pressure is 150 mm Hg in adults and 80 to 120 mm Hg in infants. The injection time may be more than 30 minutes.[43] The injection can be terminated when the minute subpleural vessels begin to fill in the periphery of the lungs.[36]

On isolated lungs, the bronchial arteries can be cannulated at the posterior-superior aspect of the main bronchus.[36] A 30-gauge polyethylene catheter is tied into the isolated bronchial artery (or arteries). The lung is then inflated with carbon dioxide or air, and the contrast medium (see previous section) is injected through the catheter. The injection pressure is 150 mm Hg. The end point of the injection has been discussed in the previous section. After bronchopulmonary anastomoses have opened, bronchial arteriograms may also show segments of pulmonary arteries (Fig. 4–19).

Injection of Pulmonary Capillaries. The injection of pulmonary capillaries can be achieved easily with media of low viscosity. Because of overlapping, pulmonary capillaries can be studied only in fairly thin sections.

Figure 4–20 shows schematically the apparatus used by Reid and Heard[39] to inject pulmonary capillaries. The injection mixture consists of 400 ml of Pelican waterproof drawing ink and 45 gm of gelatin in 100 ml of hot water. The lung is kept in the refrigerator until the gelatin has set and then it is perfused with formalin solution through the bronchial tree. The capillaries are studied on $200\text{-}\mu$-thick frozen sections.

Bronchography. *Barium-Gelatin Injection.* Attempts to prepare bronchograms with barium-gelatin mixtures often result in overfilling. This can be avoided to some extent by increasing the viscosity of the medium and by repeated roentgenographic control of the filling procedure.

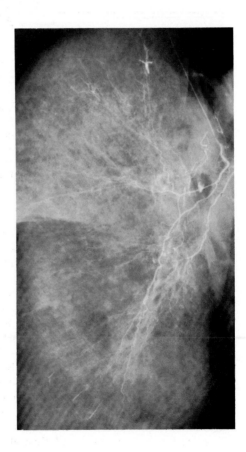

Figure 4–19. Bronchial arteriogram of right lung. Two bronchial artery branches were directly cannulated with plastic tubes. Some of injected barium sulfate-gelatin mixture entered pulmonary artery via broncho-pulmonary anastomosis near apex.

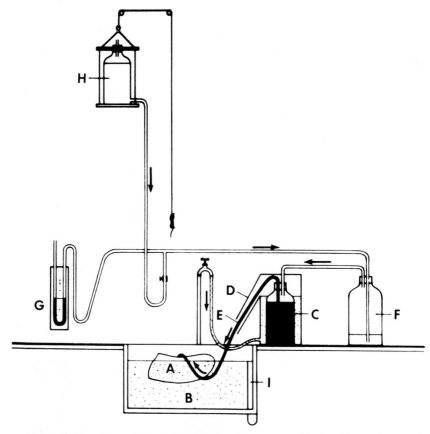

Figure 4–20. Apparatus used to inject pulmonary capillaries. Mixture in container (*C*) is heated by hot running water from tap. Pressure for injection is supplied by air from container (*F*) displaced by water from elevated container (*H*) at pressure of 60 mm Hg on manometer (*G*). Hot water flowing down channel (*D*) warms tubing (*E*) and lung (*A*) floating in sink (*B*). (From Reid A, Heard BE: Preliminary studies of human pulmonary capillaries by India ink injection. Med Thorac 19:215–219, 1962. By permission of S. Karger AG.)

Lead Particle Coating.   Excellent bronchograms can be prepared with airborne lead particles which coat the air passages and render them radiopaque without occluding their lumen.[28]

The unfixed lung is suspended in a transparent negative-pressure box (Fig. 4–21). Cannulae of various sizes must be available because the main bronchi may vary considerably in diameter. The greater extrapulmonary length of the left main bronchus makes the left lung the easier to handle. Both the apparatus and the lung must be airtight. Results are not entirely satisfactory when there is a tear in the lung, even though it is repaired. A negative pressure of about 20 cm H_2O is used to expand the lung, but as high as -40 cm H_2O has been used without harm. Generally, the higher pressures are used only to overcome the surface tension between opposed alveolar walls when expansion first is attempted. The lung is expanded and then allowed to retract, the cycle being repeated 15 to 20 times. During the expansion, which simulates the inspiratory phase of respiration, 2 to 3 ml of lead dust is insufflated into the bronchial cannula. Much of the insufflated dust is rejected by the lung at each deflation. Between successive expansions it is important, particularly with emphysematous lungs, that adequate time be allowed to permit full collapse of the lung. At the end of the procedure, the cannula is closed with a rubber stopper to keep the lung expanded.

To insufflate the lead powder, one uses a small hand-insufflator such as is commonly used for dusting wounds. Use of a pressurized air supply instead of the rubber hand bulb is more effective in making the lead dust airborne, but this has the disadvantage, early in the procedure, of creating a heavy load of dust which clogs the moist bronchial pathway and prevents the finest particles from penetrating to the periphery. Use of a continuous supply of air under pressure from a pump or cylinder is reserved for cases in which, because of tears in the lung or blockage of the air passages by mucus, the hand insufflator is not effective. In these cases, it is not necessary to use a negative-pressure container to expand the lung.

A fine-grain film (Crystallex, a Kodak industrial x-ray film) and a small anode (0.3 mm focus) are used to provide clarity of detail in the roentgenogram. These films can be enlarged 5 to 10 magnifications without loss of detail. The usual exposure has been 30 ma, 50 kv at 0.8 second.

After the roentgenograms are made, fixation is achieved by filling the lung with 10% formalin solution (neutral or slightly alkaline with sodium bicarbonate) run into the main bronchus at low pressure; it is not necessary to clamp the bronchus subsequently. The bicarbonate is added to prevent the slight solubilization of lead that occurs in soft water; it is not needed with hard water. After fixation for 1 week, the lung is cut sagittally. The lead coating, clearly visible on the bronchi and in the lung tissue, adheres to the surfaces during the stages of histologic

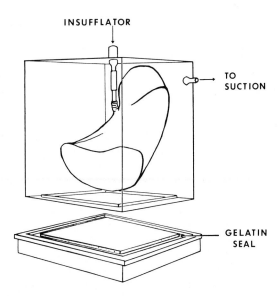

Figure 4–21. Transparent negative-pressure expansion box for postmortem bronchography with airborne lead particles. (From Leopold JG, Gough J: Postmortem bronchography in the study of bronchitis and emphysema. Thorax 18:172–177, 1963. By permission of the British Medical Association.)

INSUFFLATOR

TO SUCTION

GELATIN SEAL

preparation, and this helps in the correlation of histologic features with features seen on the bronchogram. As an additional aid, roentgenograms of slices of the lung can be made. The lead does not interfere with any of the commonly used staining methods and does not smear. The preparation of paper-mounted sections has been recommended for the study of these lungs.[28]

Cinefluorobronchograms. Cinefluorobronchograms have been used for the study of expiratory collapse.[32]

The unfixed lung is ventilated in an artificial thorax, with lung volume always greater than forced residual capacity, at a frequency of 15 breaths/min (2-second inspiration, 2-second expiration). The respirator is set to provide an inspiratory pressure of -20 cm H_2O and an expiratory pressure of $+10$ cm H_2O; these are approximately the performance pressures of the in vivo 1-second forced expiratory volume. By using an atomizer and compressed air at a flow rate of 5 to 7 liters/min, about 2 ml of dry Micropaque powder is blown into the main bronchus. Fluoroscopic observation permits control of the amount of radiopaque material used; it should be just enough to provide good visualization of the airways down to those 2 to 3 mm in diameter. The bronchogram is made with a 35-mm cinefluorography camera at 60 frames/sec. A recording device is used to supply a permanent record of flow, volume, and box pressure. Morphologic studies can be carried out after wet perfusion fixation. The inventors of postmortem cinefluorobronchography used 1.8% (isosmotic) neutral buffered glutaraldehyde solution. The lungs were perfused through the main bronchus at a pressure of 20 to 25 cm H_2O for 5 to 7 days.

PREPARATION OF PULMONARY VASCULAR AND BRONCHIAL CASTS

Polyvinyl Chloride Corrosion. This method may yield excellent instructive casts. Tissues for histologic study must be secured after plastic injection and before the lung tissue is destroyed by the corrosion. A great variety of plastics can be purchased, and the factory specifications must be followed. The following technique was described by Liebow et al.[29]

A solution of polyvinyl chloride (Vinylite) in acetone (28% by weight) is used; for the injection of small vessels or other fine structures, the solution is further diluted. Silica gel or diatomaceous earth is used as a filler when shrinkage of the plastic is a problem. Complete casts are prepared by injecting dilute plastic first, followed by concentrated plastic with a filler substance for the coarse portion of the cast. The plastic is mixed with green, red, or black pigments which are able to withstand the subsequent use of concentrated hydrochloric acid and which do not diffuse into the adjacent tissues. Radiopacity is achieved by adding lead chromate. The bronchial arteries are injected in situ through the aorta with a pressure of 250 to 500 mm Hg. The pulmonary arteries are injected through a cannula tied in the main stem of the pulmonary artery, just above the valve; the pulmonary veins are injected through a cannula inserted into the left atrium through the mitral valve.

In order to inject the lungs in the expanded state, a Pyrex glass vacuum jar is used with the trachea communicating with the outside air (Fig. 4–21). The plastic is injected through the previously cannulated pulmonary arteries and veins while the lungs are expanded in the vacuum chamber at a negative pressure of about 10 mm Hg. The vessels are filled to capacity with plastic of increasing viscosity. Plastic is also forced into the respiratory tree. The plastic hardens in 24 to 48 hours.

The casts are prepared by dissolving the pulmonary tissue for 24 to 48 hours in concentrated hydrochloric acid (or a 40% solution of potassium hydroxide).[33] Subsequently, the casts are washed and dried.

Wood's Metal Corrosion. Wood's metal is a low-melting alloy of lead, tin, bismuth, and cadmium. Casts of the bronchi can be prepared with this alloy by pouring it, molten, into the trachea before the chest is opened.[33] Subsequently, the specimen is corroded with 40% potassium hydroxide or antiformin (see chapter 7, page 202).

Latex Injection. Latex injection permits the study of the injected structures in relation to the surrounding tissues.[35] No corrosion is required.

Water-soluble colored latex (General Latex and Chemical Corporation, Cambridge, Mass.) is injected into the pulmonary vessels and airways at an injection pressure of 100 to 260 mm Hg. Solidification of the latex and tissue fixation are achieved by injecting 10% formalin solution with a small amount of dilute acetic acid into the tracheobronchial tree. The lung is then submerged for 1 to 2 days into a tank also filled with acidified formalin solution.

After fixation the lungs can be quick-frozen, sectioned with a bacon slicer into slices 3 to 4 mm thick, and studied under the dissecting microscope.

MEASUREMENT OF PULMONARY BLOOD VOLUME AND DISTRIBUTION, VASCULAR VOLUME, AND AIR CONTENT

These topics have been described in detail by Backmann.[3]

Air Content. The lung lobes are homogenized and the volume of the homogenized lung tissue is subtracted from the total lung volume (see page 111).

Total Pulmonary Blood Content. Lung homogenates are washed repeatedly with a solution of 0.2 gm of potassium ferricyanide and 0.2 gm of potassium cyanide in 1,000 ml of distilled water. The blood is hemolyzed by this procedure, and cyanhemoglobin forms which can be measured photometrically. For the calculation of blood volume, hemoglobin concentration is measured by the same method in a mixture of 5 ml of blood from the subclavian veins and 5 ml from the femoral veins. This is done to compensate for the hypostatic sedimentation of the blood after death.

Appropriate control studies have shown that the hemoglobin content of the different vascular compartments varies only by 3 to 5%. Repeated hemoglobin measurements from lung homogenates and venous blood mixtures show variations of about 1%.

Bronchial Vascular Blood Volume. The normal blood volume in intrabronchial vessels represents about 1% of the total intrapulmonary blood volume. For most studies this can be neglected.

Capillary Blood Volume. *Direct Measurement.* The capillary blood volume is measured by filling the capillaries completely under physiologic conditions and then emptying the capillary bed under increasing alveolar pressure. The lung is suspended in an air-free, water-filled glass tank with the bronchus and vessels pointing downward and connected to the outside with plastic tubes (Fig. 4–22). The lungs are expanded, without increasing the intrabronchial pressure, by draining water from the tank while the tube connected with the bronchus is left open. The vessels are filled with a 6:5 mixture of carbon tetrachloride and paraffin oil (dynamic viscosity, 5 centipoise). The pulmonary system is perfused first at an arterial pressure of 30 cm H_2O, a venous pressure of 0, and an expansion pressure of −10 cm H_2O. Subsequently, the arterial pressure is increased to 50 to 70 cm H_2O for 3 to 5 minutes. The venous pressure is now increased and the arterial pressure decreased until an equilibrium between arterial and venous sides

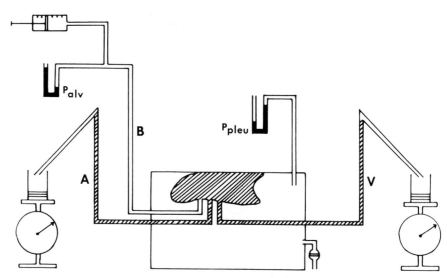

Figure 4–22. Apparatus for measurement of capillary blood volume in human lung at autopsy. Isolated lung is expanded in vacuum (artificial thorax). A = Plastic tube to pulmonary artery; V = plastic tube to pulmonary vein; P_{alv} = manometer for tube (B) to main bronchus (indicating positive pressure); P_{pleu} = manometer for container with suspended lung (indicating negative pressure). Containers on scales measure volume of oil overflowing from pulmonary arteries and veins, respectively. (From Backmann R: Blutvolumen, Gefäßbett und Blutverteilung in der Lunge. Part 79, Stuttgart, Gustav Fischer Verlag, 1969. By permission.)

is achieved at a pressure of 10 to 12 cm H_2O (after 1 to $1\frac{1}{2}$ hours). At this time the static pressure in the capillaries is assumed to be 10 to 12 cm H_2O. The intra-alveolar pressure is now increased over the intracapillary pressure, using a record syringe connected to the bronchus tube. The fluid in the capillary bed is thus transferred into the venous and arterial compartments, from which equivalent amounts of fluid flow into containers through the connecting tubes. The weight increase of the containers represents the amount of perfusion fluid in the capillary bed.

Calculation From Other Measurements.   The pulmonary capillary volume can be calculated from the difference between the total blood volume and the combined volume in the pulmonary arteries and veins.

Pulmonary Arterial Blood Volume.   First, the total pulmonary blood volume is measured. Then the blood is removed from the small pulmonary vessels by repeated increases of the intrabronchial pressure as described for capillary blood volume. The pulmonary arteries are filled, through a plastic tube, with iodized oil (Lipiodol ultrafluid, with an iodine content of 0.48 gm/ml and a viscosity of 65 centipoise at 15 C). The oil is first injected at a pressure of 50 cm H_2O and then adjusted to 16 to 17 cm H_2O. Repeated increases in pressure will fill the pulmonary arteries up to a diameter of 60 to 70 μ. One can monitor the filling process with frequent roentgenograms. The intrapulmonary volume of contrast oil at 16 to 17 cm H_2O represents the volume of the pulmonary arteries.

Pulmonary Venous Blood Volume.   After the pulmonary arterial blood volume has been determined, the pressure in the pulmonary arterial system is decreased to 0. Iodized oil is then injected into the pulmonary veins at an initial pressure of 30 cm H_2O. The procedure is similar to the one used for the pulmonary arteries. The volume of oil in the pulmonary veins is measured at a pressure of 5 to 6 cm H_2O.

POSTMORTEM PULMONARY FUNCTION STUDIES

The pioneer work in this field was carried out by Hartung.[16-18] Figure 4–23 shows equipment which this author used for dynamic measurement of the respiratory cycle in isolated lungs. Tissue elasticity and surface tension were measured on volume-pressure diagrams of lungs filled with air and subsequently with saline. Total capacity, functional residual capacity, static and dynamic compliances, tidal volume, and other pulmonary functions also were studied. The mechanics of thoracic-lung systems were tested by ventilating through a cannula tied into a bronchus. Perfusion tests with a mixture of carbon tetrachloride and paraffin oil (6:5) were performed in an attempt to reproduce pulmonary hemodynamics. Some of the postmortem pulmonary function tests showed results identical with clinical function tests; others were not altogether comparable.

The site of airway obstruction in emphysema, bronchiectasis, or bronchiolitis has been determined by wedging a small catheter into small airways of excised human lungs.[25] The catheter was placed in airways of

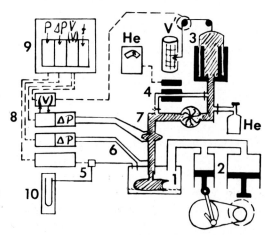

Figure 4–23. Equipment for dynamic measurement of ventilatory cycle of isolated lung. *1* = Respirator box; *2* = breathing pump *(left)* and manipulator for functional residual capacity *(right)*; *3* = spirograph; *4* = diaferometer for helium mixing technique; *5* = pressure recorder (Statham); *6* = connections for measurement of transpulmonary pressure; *7* = flow meter (pneumotachygraph) which may be replaced by volume recorder from spirograph; *8* = pressure amplifiers and transducer group; *9* = direct-writing recorder with three channels and time signal; *10* = manometer. *Hatched area,* breathing system. Flow gauge pump has not been drawn. (From Hartung W: Postmortem correlates of pulmonary function. *In* The Lung. Edited by AA Liebow, DE Smith. Baltimore, Williams & Wilkins Company, 1968, pp. 298–310. By permission.)

about 2 mm in diameter and extended through the bronchial wall, parenchyma, and pleural surface. This technique permitted comparison of airway resistance central to and peripheral to the catheter tip.

Some pulmonary function tests can be carried out on refrigerated lungs. The pressure-volume curves of refrigerated lungs remain constant for days.[13]

PARTICLE IDENTIFICATION

Histologic Analysis. Many types of particles can be identified histologically if they are within the resolution limits of the light microscope.[34] Inorganic particles can be isolated and concentrated for morphologic study by holding an unstained, uncovered paraffin section over a flame until the organic tissue has been incinerated.

For the demonstration of asbestos bodies, a frequent requirement, the following technique[2] can be used. An incision, about 1 cm deep, is made in the base of the lung, and the cut surface is scraped with a knife. The exuding fluid is smeared on standard microscopic slides. The slides are dried, fixed in alcohol, and mounted unstained in DPX under a 20- by 50-mm cover slip. Asbestos bodies show refractility, a pale central fiber, smooth or segmented yellowish encrustation, and clubbed or rounded ends.

Electron Microscopic Analysis. This is the method of choice for particles smaller than 1 μ.[34] A simple replication technique has been described by Henderson.[22] The electron micrograph of the replica of the particle is compared with a set of standard micrographs of different types of mineral particles.[23]

Chemical Analysis. In some cases, chemical analysis of ashed lungs can be used for particle identification. However, incineration may bring about chemical changes.[23] Incineration can be carried out on gross tissues or on histologic sections; the latter usually are used for morphologic analysis.

Complicated Techniques. Complicated physical and chemical techniques,[34] such as x-ray diffraction, are available in certain commercial laboratories which provide expert analysis of particles. Tissues can be sent to these laboratories, such as Walter C. McCrone Associates, Inc., Chicago, Illinois 60616.

PULMONARY SURFACTANT

Pulmonary surfactant is measured in foam or liquid lung extracts. The various methods have been described by Scarpelli.[46]

REFERENCES

1. Anderson AE Jr, Foraker AG: Relative dimensions of bronchioles and parenchymal spaces in lungs from normal subjects and emphysematous patients. Am J Med 32:218–226, 1962
2. Ashcroft T: Asbestos bodies in routine necropsies on Tyneside: a pathological and social study. Br Med J 1:614–618, 1968
3. Backmann R: Blutvolumen, Gefäßbett und Blutverteilung in der Lunge. Part 79. Stuttgart, Gustav Fischer Verlag, 1969
4. Bignon J, Khoury F, Even P, Andre J, Brouet G: Morphometric study in chronic obstructive bronchopulmonary disease: pathologic, clinical, and physiologic correlations. Am Rev Resp Dis 99:669–695, 1969
5. Blumenthal BJ, Boren HG: Lung structure in three dimensions after inflation and fume fixation. Am Rev Tuberc 79:764–772, 1959
6. Cureton RJR, Trapnell DH: Post-mortem radiography and gaseous fixation of the lung. Thorax 16:138–143, 1961
7. Davies G, Reid L: Growth of the alveoli and pulmonary arteries in childhood. Thorax 25:669–681, 1970
8. Dunnill MS: Quantitative methods in the study of pulmonary pathology. Thorax 17:320–328, 1962
9. Dunnill MS: Discussion. *In* Form and Function in the Human Lung. Edited by G Cumming, LB Hunt. Baltimore, Williams & Wilkins Company, 1968, p 184
10. Dunnill MS, Massarella GR, Anderson JA: A comparison of the quantitative anatomy of the bronchi in normal subjects, in status asthmaticus, in chronic bronchitis, and in emphysema. Thorax 24:176–179, 1969
11. Gerlach W: Postmortale Form- und Lageveränderungen mit besonderer Berücksichtigung der Totenstarre. Ergeb Allg Path path Anat 20:259–305, 1923
12. Gough J: Twenty years' experience of the technic of paper mounted sections. *In* The Lung. Edited by AA Liebow, DE Smith. Baltimore, Williams & Wilkins Company, 1968, pp 311–316
13. Gruenwald P: Normal and abnormal expansion of the lungs of newborn infants obtained at autopsy. II. Opening pressure, maximal volume, and stability of expansion. Lab Invest 12:563–576, 1963

14. Hale FC, Olsen RC, Mickey MR Jr: The measurement of bronchial wall components. Am Rev Resp Dis *98*:978–987, 1968

15. Hartung W: Gefrier-großschnitte von ganzen Organen, speziell der Lunge. Zentralbl Allg Pathol *100*:408–413, 1960

16. Hartung W: Histomechanik der Ventilationsstörungen. Verh Dtsch Ges Pathol *44*:46–59, 1960

17. Hartung W: Untersuchungsmethoden an Lungen und Thorax zur postmortalen Analyse der Atmungsfunktion. Ergeb Allg Path path Anat *43*:121–160, 1963

18. Hartung W: Postmortem correlates of pulmonary function. *In* The Lung. Edited by AA Liebow, DE Smith. Baltimore, Williams & Wilkins Company, 1968, pp 298–310

19. Hasleton PS: Discussion. *In* Form and Function in the Human Lung. Edited by G Cumming, LB Hunt. Baltimore, Williams & Wilkins Company, 1968, p. 183

20. Heard BE: Pathology of pulmonary emphysema: methods of study. Am Rev Resp Dis *82*:792–799, 1960

21. Heard BE, Esterly JR, Wootliff JS: A modified apparatus for fixing lungs to study the pathology of emphysema. Am Rev Resp Dis *95*:311–312, 1967

22. Henderson WJ: A simple replication technique for the study of biological tissues by electron microscopy. J Microsc *89*:369–372, 1969

23. Henderson WJ, Gough J, Harse J: Identification of mineral particles in pneumoconiotic lungs. J Clin Pathol *23*:104–109, 1970

24. Heppleston AG: Lung architecture in emphysema. *In* Form and Function in the Human Lung. Edited by G Cumming, LB Hunt. Baltimore, Williams & Wilkins Company, 1968, pp 6–19

25. Hogg JC, Macklem PT, Thurlbeck WM: Site and nature of airway obstruction in chronic obstructive lung disease. N Engl J Med *278*:1355–1360, 1968

26. Ivemark BI, Wallgren G: The pulmonary vascular pattern in idiopathic respiratory distress: a micro-angiographic study. Acta Pathol Microbiol Scand *76*:203–214, 1969

27. Kramer FM: Dry preservation of museum specimens: a review, with introduction of simplified technique. J Tech Methods *18*:42–50, 1938

28. Leopold JG, Gough J: Postmortem bronchography in the study of bronchitis and emphysema. Thorax *18*:172–177, 1963

29. Liebow AA, Hales MR, Lindskog GE, Bloomer WE: Plastic demonstrations of pulmonary pathology. J Tech Methods *27*:116–129, 1947

30. Loeschcke H: Methoden zur morphologischen Untersuchung der Lunge. *In* Handbuch der biologischen Arbeitsmethoden. Vol VIII, part 1 (1). Edited by E Abderhalden. Berlin, Urban & Schwarzenberg, 1924, pp 575–598

31. Longfield AN, Hentel W: Lung destruction measured by energy transmission through fume fixed lungs. Dis Chest *50*:225–231, 1966

32. Maisel JC, Silvers WG, Mitchell RS, Petty TL: Bronchial atrophy and dynamic expiratory collapse. Am Rev Resp Dis *98*:988–997, 1968

33. Marchand P, Gilroy JC, Wilson VH: An anatomical study of the bronchial vascular system and its variations in disease. Thorax *5*:207–221, 1950

34. McCrone WC, Draftz RG, Delly JG: The Particle Atlas: A Photomicrographic Reference for the Microscopical Identification of Particulate Substances. Ann Arbor, Michigan, Ann Arbor Science Publishers, Inc., 1967

35. McLaughlin RF, Tyler WS, Canada RO: A study of the subgross pulmonary anatomy in various mammals. Am J Anat *108*:149–165, 1961

36. Milne ENC: Circulation of primary and metastatic pulmonary neoplasms: a postmortem microarteriographic study. Am J Roentgenol Radium Ther Nucl Med *100*:603–619, 1967

37. Moolten SE: A simple apparatus for fixation of lungs in the inflated state. Arch Pathol *20*:77–80, 1935

38. Oderr CP, Pizzolato P, Ziskind J: Microradiographic techniques for study for emphysema. Am Rev Resp Dis *80*:104–113, 1959

39. Reid A, Heard BE: Preliminary studies of human pulmonary capillaries by India ink injection. Med Thorac *19*:215–219, 1962

40. Reid L: The Pathology of Emphysema. Chicago, Year Book Medical Publishers, Inc., 1967

41. Reid L: Discussion. *In* Form and Function in the Human Lung. Edited by G Cumming, LB Hunt. Baltimore, Williams & Wilkins Company, 1968, p 183

42. Reid L, Millard FJC: Correlation between radiological diagnosis and structural lung changes in emphysema. Clin Radiol *15*:307–311, 1964

43. Robertson B: Postnatal formation and obliteration of arterial anastomoses in the human lung: a microangiographic and histologic study. Pediatrics *43*:971–979, 1969

44. Ryan SF: Artifact emphysema. Am Rev Resp Dis *99*:801–803, 1969
45. Ryder RC, Thurlbeck WM, Gough J: A study of inter observer variation in the assessment of the amount of pulmonary emphysema in paper-mounted whole lung sections. Am Rev Resp Dis *99*:354–364, 1969
46. Scarpelli EM: The Surfactant System of the Lung. Philadelphia, Lea & Febiger, 1968
47. Sherwin RP, Wyatt SL: Diazo replication of thick sections of whole lung in the evaluation of emphysema. Am Rev Resp Dis *91*:768–772, 1965
48. Silverton RE: A comparison of formaldehyde fixation methods used in the study of pulmonary emphysema. J Med Lab Technol *21*:187–217, 1964
49. Silverton RE: Gross fixation methods used in the study of pulmonary emphysema. Thorax *20*:289–297, 1965
50. Thurlbeck WM: Internal surface area and other measurements in emphysema. Thorax *22*:483–496, 1967
51. Thurlbeck WM, Dunnill MS, Hartung W, Heard BE, Heppleston AG, Ryder RC: A comparison of three methods of measuring emphysema. Hum Pathol *1*:215–226, 1970
52. Tobin CE: Methods of preparing and studying human lungs expanded and dried with compressed air. Anat Rec *114*:453–465, 1952
53. Weibel ER: Morphometry of the Human Lung. New York, Academic Press, 1963
54. Weibel ER, Vidone RA: Fixation of the lung by formalin steam in a controlled state of air inflation. Am Rev Resp Dis *84*:856–861, 1961
55. Whimster EF: Rapid giant paper sections of lungs. Thorax *24*:737–741, 1969
56. Whimster EF: Techniques for the examination of excised lungs. Hum Pathol *1*:305–314, 1970
57. Wilson JW, Pickett JP: Serial sections of lung: the use of a 70-millimeter film-strip technique for large tissue sections. Am Rev Resp Dis *102*:268–273, 1970

CHAPTER 5

ESOPHAGUS AND ABDOMINAL VISCERA

ESOPHAGUS

For the demonstration of tracheo-esophageal fistulas or infiltrating tumors, the esophagus should be left attached to the mediastinal organs. Tracheo-esophageal fistulas are demonstrated by opening the esophagus along its posterior wall and opening the trachea anteriorly (Fig. 4–1). Infiltrating tumors are best demonstrated by cutting properly oriented sections through the previously fixed mediastinal organs. Intraluminal tumors or strictures are well displayed on fixed specimens (Fig. 5–1).

Demonstration of Esophageal Varices. *Injection of Varices.* A needle is attached to an air hose, and the air pressure is adjusted so that the air streaming out of the tip of the needle is barely perceptible. The lower portion of the esophagus and the attached gastric fundus are turned inside out. The tip of the needle is then introduced into the stretched mucosa, and one of the collapsed veins is punctured. The esophageal mucosal veins immediately become inflated and prominent. The needle must be held steady while the air supply is shut off. Barium sulfate-gelatin mixture or some other contrast medium can now be injected through the same needle. Points of hemorrhage are easily demonstrated by this method (Fig. 5-2).

Clearing Techniques. 1. Method of Chomet.[8] The esophagus is placed, without folding, in 10% formalin solution or in Kaiserling solution I.[21] After fixation for 24 hours, the mucosal layer—that is, the mucosa together with the submucosa—is stripped from the muscularis very carefully so as not to tear the specimen. While separating the submucosa from the muscularis, it is important to stay close to the muscularis, to leave the submucosal layer intact. The mucosal layer is completely submerged in absolute alcohol. Three changes of alcohol are necessary, with $\frac{1}{2}$ hour between changes. The specimen is kept flat at all times. The specimen is dried and then completely submerged in a tray of benzene (the tray is kept covered).

129

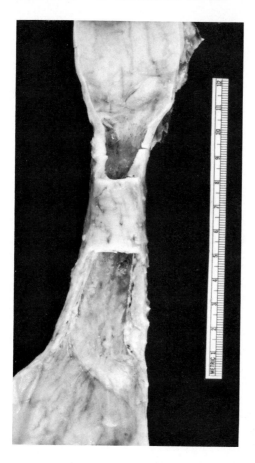

Figure 5–1. Lower esophagus and cardia; specimen prefixed in formalin solution. Midportion of stenotic segment has been left intact.

The average clearing time originally was stated to be 15 minutes, but often 30 to 60 minutes is required.[7] Inadequate clearing may give false gross impressions, and so does postmortem collapse of veins. The specimen is dried again and transferred to an opal glass tray (dental instrument tray) filled with benzene and containing a ruler made of an inert substance. The specimen must be completely submerged during photography. The tray is covered with a sheet of glass. For photography, three lights are necessary. One light is placed under the tray for transillumination (all other areas around the tray are masked with black cardboard); the other two are placed at equal distances, pointing toward the top of the specimen. After the photographs are taken, the specimen is returned to the fixing solution.

    2. Preparation of permanent museum specimens.[7] The esophagus and the cardia are tied off before the specimen is removed from the body. This prevents loss of blood from the varices before fixation. The initial fixation and stripping procedure is the same as in 1 above. After this, the mucosa is put into 70%, 90%, and absolute alcohol, in this order, with 1 hour between changes. The specimen then is dried and submerged in a tray of benzene. The benzene tray should be kept tightly covered and in a well-ventilated hood. If the benzene solution becomes cloudy, the

esophagus should be taken through two additional changes of absolute alcohol. The clearing process requires 30 to 60 minutes. A thin layer of Permount (Fisher Scientific Company, Chemical Manufacturing Division, Fair Lawn, N.J.) is poured into the inverted top of a Petri dish (150 by 20 mm). The specimen is removed from the benzene solution and, still drenched with benzene, is placed in the Petri dish. The entire specimen must be covered with Permount (Fig. 5-3 *a*). The bottom of the Petri dish is placed on the specimen, with care taken to force out all of the air bubbles from under the preparation (Fig. 5-3 *b*). "C" clamps are applied to maintain the pressure until the Permount has hardened (Fig. 5-3 *c*), and the entire assembly is placed in a 37 C incubator (the assembly is placed on an inverted beaker or jar so that the clamps do not touch the bottom of the incubator). After 24 hours of incubation Permount is added with a micropipette to force out any additional air bubbles. The incubation is continued for 5 to 7 days; if any more air pockets are noted, they are filled with Permount. After the specimen has hardened, the top of another Petri dish is placed on the rim of the inverted first dish (Fig. 5-3 *d*), and the two dishes are sealed together with transparent tape.

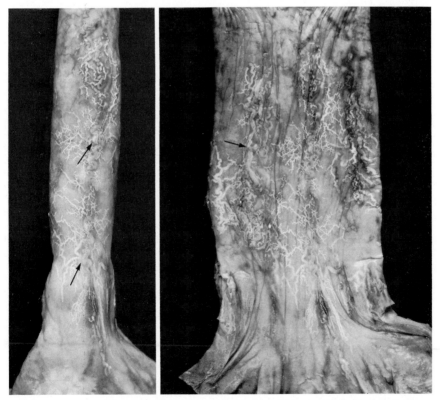

Figure 5–2. Esophageal varices, injected with barium sulfate-gelatin mixture. Varices stand out and are white (*arrows*). *Left,* Esophagus unopened but turned inside out. Air insufflation and injection are carried out at this stage (see text). *Right,* Mucosal aspect of opened esophagus. Dark staining in background is due to autolysis.

We have prepared satisfactory specimens with this method (Fig. 5–4). We found it useful to place the bottom of the Petri dish eccentrically so as to leave as much space as possible at one side where Permount can be added easily. Instead of a C clamp, 4 pounds of lead weights are placed in the middle of the dish. We incubate the specimens for 10 days at 37 C and add Permount if needed. Subsequently, the dish is placed on a warm radiator guard or otherwise exposed to a flow of warm air. The amount of weight is gradually decreased until the specimen can be sealed.

If a flow of warm air is available, the incubation in the oven can be omitted. Normal Petri dishes have somewhat uneven bottoms and lids, and dishes with better optical and mechanical properties would be preferable.

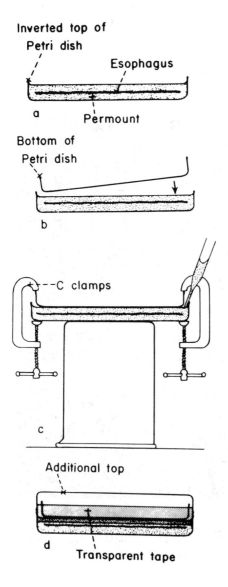

Figure 5–3. Preparation of **permanent museum specimens of esophageal varices.** *a*, Cleared specimen (see text) is placed in inverted top of Petri dish. *b*, Bottom of Petri dish is pressed against specimen. *c*, C clamps are applied to Petri dish. *d*, Top of another Petri dish is inverted on first dish. (From Chomet B, Gach BM: Demonstration of esophageal varices in museum specimens. Am J Clin Pathol 51:793–794, 1969. By permission of J. B. Lippincott Company.)

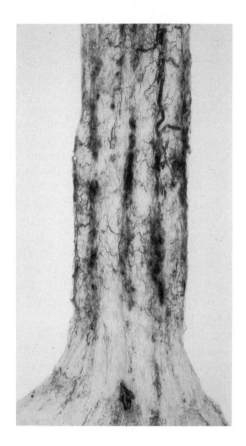

Figure 5–4. Permanent museum specimen of esophageal varices. Mucosal layer has been stripped, and specimen has been cleared in benzene by modified technique of Chomet and Gach[7] (see text, method 2).

The method also can be used for demonstrating enlarged vascular channels in the diaphragm, particularly in patients with cirrhosis.[7]

Demonstration of Lower Esophageal Rings. Lower esophageal rings (Schatzki rings) can be palpated or objectively demonstrated by roentgenography.[14] The lower half of the esophagus is removed with the upper half of the stomach and an attached ring of diaphragm. The stomach is clamped across the corpus. The preparation is then filled and slightly distended with a mixture of barium sulfate and 10% formalin solution. Roentgenograms should be prepared as soon as possible after death. Subsequently, the specimen should be fixed in the distended state. We suspend it in a formalin tank until it is to be cut.

This method also can be used for other types of strictures and stenoses of the esophagus.

STOMACH

The stomach routinely is opened along the greater curvature. Penetrating ulcers or infiltrating tumors are best displayed by fixing and sectioning the stomach together with the pancreas, a portion of the liver, or whatever the infiltrated tissue might be. Tumors with predominantly intraluminal growth and the associated obstruction can be displayed after formalin fixation of the unopened specimen and subsequent dissection. The stomach is inflated with formalin while it is submerged in a formalin bath. We use the same perfusion apparatus as for pressure fixation of the lungs (see chapter 4).

Staining for Intestinal Metaplasia.   Gross stomach specimens may be stained to demonstrate areas of alkaline phosphatase activity.[34] The reaction is positive only in the presence of intestinal metaplasia which may be associated with peptic ulcers and carcinomas. The technique gives satisfactory results on freshly resected surgical specimens. Only in rare instances will comparable autopsy material be available.

Angiography. *Gastric Arteries.* Postmortem arteriography of the stomach can be performed after removal of the organs supplied by the celiac axis. The splenic and hepatic arteries are tied as far distally as possible. A barium preparation is injected through the celiac artery. After injection, the stomach is isolated, opened along the middle of the anterior surface parallel with the longitudinal axis of the organ, spread out on an x-ray plate, and roentgenographed.[40]

Gastric Capillaries. These can be injected with India ink via the gastroepiploic artery. An adjacent portion of the gastric wall is injected while more distant portions are clamped off. For the study of mucosal capillaries, the mucosa is stripped off the muscularis, cleaned in saline, and placed on a microscope slide. Strong illumination is used while the specimen is kept moist.[40]

INTESTINAL TRACT

In the presence of tumors or other pathologic lesions involving the duodenum, papilla of Vater, head of the pancreas, or hepatoduodenal ligament, the duodenum should be opened in situ. Precise orientation may become impossible after removal of these organs. This is particularly important in postoperative autopsies.

Routinely, the intestinal tract is opened with an enterotome. This is greatly facilitated when the mesentery has been cut close to the wall of the small intestine. The specimen usually is opened in a sink under running water. Unless special precautions are taken (see below), the intestinal epithelium will be flushed off during this procedure.

Use of a stationary probe-enterotome[32] may facilitate the opening of the small bowel. Our stationary enterotome is fixed to a faucet and consists of a steel rod with a plastic and metal cone and a replaceable shielded Bard-Parker no. 11 blade (Fig. 5–5). The cone is inserted into the lumen of the small bowel which then can be slit open rapidly by the prosector pulling the organ toward him.

A tumor with predominantly intraluminal growth and its associated obstruction can be displayed after formalin fixation of the unopened speci-

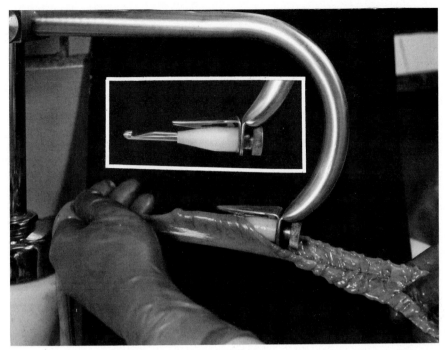

Figure 5–5. Stationary probe-enterotome (see text). *Inset,* Mounting of shielded blade.

men and subsequent dissection. The apparatus used is the same as that for lung perfusion. The glass tube at the hose from the elevated formalin vessel is simply hooked to one end of the hollow viscus; the other end is clamped or tied off. The whole preparation is suspended in a formalin bath.

For proper histologic orientation, long strips of gastric or intestinal wall can be cut parallel with the long axis of the organ, fixed, and embedded in a spiral fashion — for instance, with the proximal end in the center. Isolated histologic specimens of gastrointestinal tract should always be fixed on cardboard or corkboard.

Preservation of Small Intestinal Mucosa. The small bowel is tied at the duodenojejunal junction and at the terminal ileum close to the cecum. A T-shaped cannula is inserted into the most superficial presenting loop of the small intestine. Concentrated formalin (40% formaldehyde) solution is instilled through the cannula until the small bowel is distended and a pressure of 40 cm H_2O is reached. During this procedure it is essential to handle the small intestine only at sites where this is absolutely unavoidable. The formalin-filled bowel should be left untouched for as long as possible. The bowel is soaked for another 24 hours in 10% formalin solution. This method[39] yields satisfactory histologic sections of the mucosa if fixation is begun up to 6 hours after death.

Instillation into the small bowel of mercuric chloride in saline also may counteract autolytic changes.

Preparation of Specimens for Study Under Dissecting Microscope. Postmortem autolysis causes the loss of the intestinal epithelium. Thus, the dissecting microscope shows villi which appear thinner than the ones seen on biopsy specimens. The openings of the crypts become more prominent. In spite of these differences, the extent and character of abnormal mucosal patterns can easily be evaluated with a dissecting microscope.

In this method,[18] 1.3-cm squares of intestinal wall are gently rinsed in saline until they are free from surface contamination such as mucus or food particles. The specimens are then pinned on cardboard and fixed in buffered 10% formalin solution. After at least 24 hours of fixation, the specimens are put into one change of 70% alcohol and two changes of 95% alcohol for 2 hours each. The specimens are stained with 5% alcoholic eosin for 4 minutes and subsequently treated with two changes of absolute alcohol for 2 hours each. The fixed, stained, and dehydrated intestinal wall is placed in xylol. The preparation is now ready for examination.

The specimen also can be stained with a hematoxylin-alum solution.[11] The square blocks of formalin-fixed intestine are kept overnight in a mixture of 20 to 40 drops of Mayer's hematoxylin and 50 ml of water. Then the specimens are dehydrated and cleared as above.

Intestinal mucosal patterns also can be evaluated on unstained specimens.

Gross Staining Methods. Staining of the intestinal mucosa with alcoholic eosin[18] or hematoxylin[11] is used for study under the dissecting microscope.

The demonstration of mesenteric fat infiltration by tumor can be facilitated by staining for fat.[10] The specimen is fixed in formalin solution, and an appropriate slice is soaked for 1 day in 50% alcohol, followed by staining for 1 or 2 days in a saturated solution of Sudan III in 70% alcohol. After the fat has become deep orange red the specimen is returned to 50% alcohol solution until all nonfatty tissues return to their normal color.

Dry Preservation. Air drying[19,37] or paraffin infiltration yields interesting permanent museum specimens (Fig. 5–6). The air-dried bowel is light brown, very thin-walled, and friable. The vascular pattern is easily discernible. The methods can be combined with injection of colored plastics or other media.

No formalin fixation is necessary during this procedure. The unopened portion of the bowel is rinsed with saline. The specimen should be free of all excess fat and tissues. Glass tubes are tied into both ends, and one tube is connected to a tank of compressed air. The glass tube at the other end is fitted with a rubber tube and clamp. While air is blown through the bowel under low pressure, the clamp is slowly closed until the bowel distends slightly. This prevents shriveling and compensates for the shrinkage which occurs during the subsequent drying. The drying process takes 1 to 3 days, depending on the size of the specimen and its fat content. The drying can be accelerated by placing the bowel in front of a fan or on a frame of 1-inch wire mesh which is elevated 40 to 50 cm over a large electric hot plate. It may be necessary to readjust the air pressure from time to

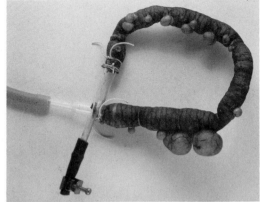

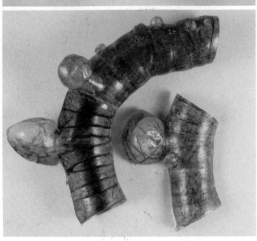

Figure 5-6. *Upper,* Air drying of unfixed jejunum. Glass tube to the left is connected to air outlet. Rubber hose at end of glass tube facing down is partly clamped to keep unfixed specimen inflated. *Lower,* Air-dried portion of jejunum coated with shellac. Vessels show up distinctly in wall of jejunum and in diverticula.

time. After the preparation is dried and cooled, it is sprayed with three coats of shellac.

Mesenteric Angiography. In the method of Reiner et al,[29,30] a solution of mercuric chloride in saline is instilled into the lumen of the intestinal tract in order to counteract autolytic changes. The abdominal viscera are removed en bloc. The celiac, superior mesenteric, and inferior mesenteric arteries are cannulated and injected with a barium sulfate-gelatin mixture with some formalin added. The final injection pressure is 200 mm Hg. The most important step for adequate stereoscopic roentgenography is the partitioning of the abdominal viscera. Three specimens are prepared (Fig. 5–7). The celiac artery specimen includes all upper abdominal organs with the root of the superior mesenteric artery and the first jejunal artery. The duodenum is rotated upward. The liver and spleen are removed from the specimen after the splenic artery and the arteria hepatica propria are tied. The superior mesenteric artery specimen consists of intestine from the first jejunal loop to the midportion of the transverse colon. The inferior mesenteric artery specimen includes the distal part of the transverse colon and

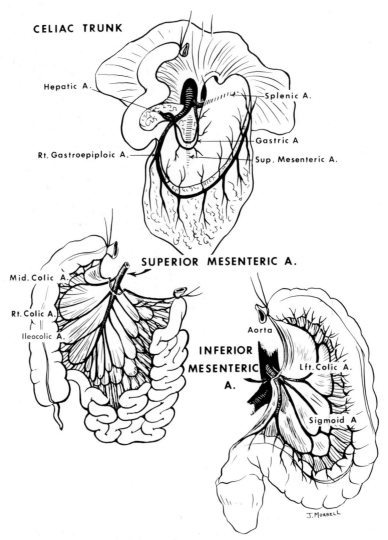

Figure 5–7. Partitioned abdominal viscera for celiac and mesenteric arteriography. *Celiac trunk specimen.* Note rotation and upward sweep of duodenum. Root of superior mesenteric artery remains with celiac artery but is hidden behind pancreas. *Superior mesenteric artery specimen.* This includes intestine from middle of first jejunal loop to middle of transverse colon. *Inferior mesenteric artery specimen.* This extends from middle transverse colon to anus; pelvic viscera (uterus and bladder) are attached. (Redrawn from Reiner L: Mesenteric vascular occlusion studied by postmortem injection of the mesenteric arterial circulation. *In* Pathologic Annual: 1966. Vol. 1. Edited by S Sommers. New York, Appleton-Century-Crofts, Inc., 1966, pp. 193–220.)

the remainder of the large intestine, including the anus and the pelvic viscera.

Telangiectases in the stomach and intestinal tract can be demonstrated by the clearing method described for esophageal varices.[7] However, the intestinal submucosa is much more dense than the esophageal submucosa, which makes stripping from the muscularis more difficult.

Other methods include injection of latex and India ink to study the microvasculature of the gastrointestinal tract.[24] The specimens are cleared with methyl salicylate or a mixture of tricresyl phosphate (one part) and tributyl phosphate (three parts).

LIVER AND HEPATODUODENAL LIGAMENT

Before removal of the liver, the hepatoduodenal ligament should be dissected. First, the common bile duct is incised and opened toward the hilus and the ampulla of Vater. The lowermost portion of the common bile duct runs retroduodenally. The duodenum must be pulled in the anterior direction and somewhat to the left if the common bile duct is to be exposed in its full length without cutting into the wall of the duodenum. Again, the best specimens can be prepared after formalin fixation (Fig. 5–8). In fetuses and newborns, dissection of the common bile duct may be difficult, and its patency is easier to check by opening the duodenum and observing whether bile can be milked out through the papilla. This is a useful test, particularly when biliary atresia is suspected.

The hepatic artery lies to the left of the common bile duct and can easily be dissected from the anterior aspect of the hepatoduodenal ligament. The portal vein is found at the posterior aspect of the ligament. In the presence of portal vein thrombosis or tumor growth in portal veins or after portacaval shunt, dissection from the posterior aspect of the hepatoduodenal ligament gives the most instructive results (Fig. 5–9). In these instances en bloc or en masse removal is recommended.

Slicing. It is almost impossible to slice livers with normal-sized knives without leaving knife marks on the cut surface. Smooth cut sections of cirrhotic livers are even more difficult to prepare. We use a knife with a 78-cm blade (Fig. 4–15) which in most instances permits slicing of the whole organ with an uninterrupted pulling motion.

Usually the liver is sliced in the frontal plane, each slice being about 2 cm thick. The hilar structures may remain attached to one of the central slices. Demonstration of hepatic atrophy on such slices can be accomplished by photographing the slice within the silhouette of the normal-sized liver of a body weight-matched control case (Fig. 5–10).

Sometimes it is necessary to expose, on one cut section, a large parenchymatous surface or to leave the hilar structures intact. In these instances, a horizontal section through the liver is the method of choice.

Fixation. Complete fixation of the intact liver by perfusion is very difficult to achieve. In many instances, portions of the liver remain unfixed.

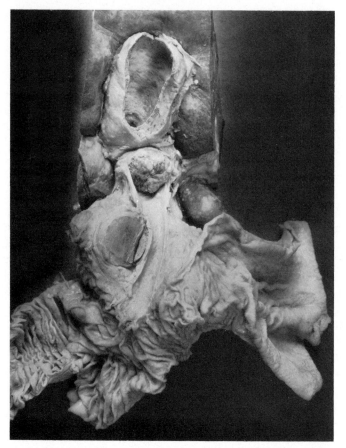

Figure 5–8. Portion of **liver, common bile duct, gall bladder, and duodenum,** showing intraluminal, exophytic adenocarcinoma of common bile duct, hepatoduodenal lymph node metastasis, and chronic cholecystitis and cholelithiasis (gallstones are removed). Specimen had been fixed in formalin solution prior to dissection.

Furthermore, the organ becomes rock hard and difficult to slice. Large slices, 3 to 4 mm thick, fix readily but usually with considerable distortion. For the preparation of large histologic sections the slices of hepatic tissue have to be kept flat during fixation—for example, by use of an appropriate capsule. A less recommendable method is to take the section from the fixed surface of a large tissue block.

Gross Staining for Iron. This method is used particularly in cases of hemochromatosis. Hemosiderin storage in other organs (pancreas, myocardium) also can be demonstrated by this technique.

A slice of liver is placed for several minutes in a 1 to 5% aqueous solution of potassium ferrocyanide and then is transferred to 2% hydrochloric acid. One can also use a solution of equal parts of 10% HCl and 5% aqueous potassium ferrocyanide.[28] The specimen is then washed for 12 hours in running water. In the presence of abundant hemosiderin, the

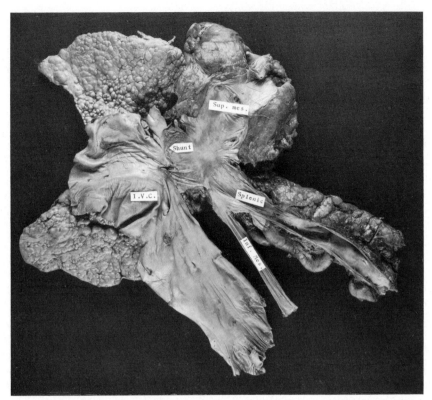

Figure 5–9. **Portacaval shunt** had been created 4 years previously and remained patent and functioning until patient died in hepatic coma. Veins have been dissected from their posterior aspect. *I.V.C.* = inferior vena cava; *Sup. mes.* = superior mesenteric vein; *Splenic* = splenic vein; *Inf. Mes.* = inferior mesenteric vein.

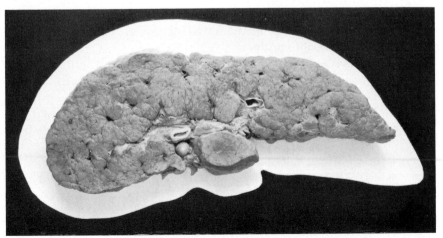

Figure 5–10. Demonstration of **hepatic atrophy in cirrhosis.** Frontal slice of atrophic liver is photographed within silhouette of corresponding slice of normal-sized control liver.

tissue will rapidly turn dark blue. Mount in 5% formalin-saline. In hemochromatosis specimens, the color tends to diffuse out.[28]

Hepatic Angiography.   The liver should be removed together with the diaphragm, the hepatoduodenal ligament, and a long segment of inferior vena cava. The vessels are cannulated and blood and blood clots are flushed out with water.

Microscopic Demonstration of Two Vascular Compartments.   India ink and a carmine-gelatin mass (see below) are injected slowly and simultaneously into two vascular compartments.[25] Following injection, the cannulas are removed and the vessels are ligated. After 1 to 2 hours, multiple incisions are made into the liver which is then fixed for 3 days in 10% formalin solution. Frozen sections, 50 to 100 μ thick, are cut from uniformly injected areas. The sections are dehydrated in 70%, 95%, and absolute alcohol (30 minutes for each change), cleared in cedarwood oil for 10 to 15 minutes, rinsed in xylol, and mounted in DPX. Paraffin sections can be prepared from the same blocks. Not all blocks will be satisfactory.

To prepare the carmine-gelatin mass,[26] gelatin is dissolved in warm water and then carmine, first rubbed up with a little water, is added slowly with continual agitation. The mixture is then heated to boiling and concentrated ammonia is added drop by drop to dissolve the carmine. The color of the solution will change to dark red. The solution is then neutralized by adding 50% acetic acid drop by drop. When the smell gradually changes from ammoniacal to sour, the color reverts to bright red. A little excess acid is added and the mixture is examined under the microscope; the carmine should be present as a granular precipitate (the carmine should be in an insoluble form; otherwise it would diffuse out of the vessels).

Injection of Radiopaque Contrast Media.   Excellent arteriograms, portal venograms, and cholangiograms can be prepared with Ethiodol and barium sulfate-gelatin mixtures (see chapter 3). Distortion or occlusion of vessels and dilatation or narrowing of intrahepatic bile ducts (Fig. 5–11) are best studied by combined stereoroentgenography of the whole liver and of slices and by histologic examination. Barium sulfate crystals can be identified microscopically. The contrast medium often will lift the epithelium off the basement membrane of the intrahepatic bile ducts. However, this hardly affects the quality of the cholangiograms.

An approach to hepatic venography is described later in this chapter.

Preparation of Corrosion Casts of Hepatic Vessels and Bile Ducts.   *Vinylite Corrosion.*   Colored Vinylite, 10% in acetone, and kieselguhr, 60 gm/liter, are used;[25] the kieselguhr prevents shrinkage. The vessels are first perfused with saline and then with acetone. The injection requires high pressure. For the hepatic arteries, 8% Vinylite is used. When no more fluid can be introduced, a final filling of the larger vessels is achieved by injecting concentrated (20%) Vinylite solution. Each vascular compartment is injected separately, the artery first. After 1 hour, blocks can be removed for histologic examination. After 2 days the specimen is macerated in concentrated HCl for 3 to 5 days. The cast is then rinsed in water, dried, and defatted in ligroin.

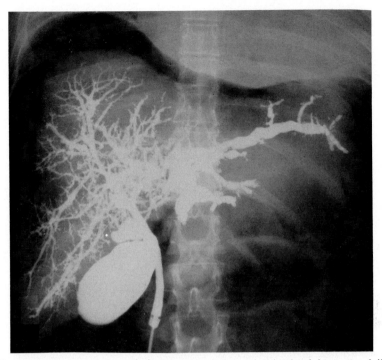

Figure 5–11. Postmortem cholangiogram, prepared with Ethiodol injection followed by barium-gelatin mixture. Note plastic tube tied into distal common bile duct. Marked dilatation and distortion of major bile ducts, particularly of left lobe of liver, are apparent. Many middle-sized ducts end abruptly. Filling of small interlobular ducts is absent in left lobe and diminished in right. Histologic examination revealed primary biliary cirrhosis with destruction of peripheral ducts. Central duct dilatation is probably due to inspissation of bile. (From Legge DA, Carlson HC, Ludwig J: Cholangiographic findings in diseases of the liver: a postmortem study. Am J Roentgenol Radium Ther Nucl Med 113:34–40, 1971. By permission of Charles C Thomas, Publisher.)

We have prepared instructive casts (Fig. 5–12) using an essentially similar technique.[22]

Latex Injection. The hepatic vessels are washed with 1.3% saline or saline and sodium bicarbonate.[2,36] Neoprene latex is injected into the portal and hepatic veins at a pressure of 40 to 100 mm Hg, into the hepatic artery at 120 to 400 mm Hg, and into the bile ducts at 40 to 60 mm Hg. The injection pressure can be obtained with a sphygmomanometer.[38] The vessels are injected simultaneously, and the injection time is 5 to 10 minutes. The liver is then fixed for 2 to 5 days in acidic formalin solution and incubated at 37 C in concentrated HCl until the corrosion is completed. The cast is then washed and dried.

Preparation of Wax Models. The following method[17] has been used to reconstruct vascular relationships in a cirrhotic liver, but it also is adaptable to other conditions.

A paraffin block of cirrhotic liver is selected. Two notching grooves are

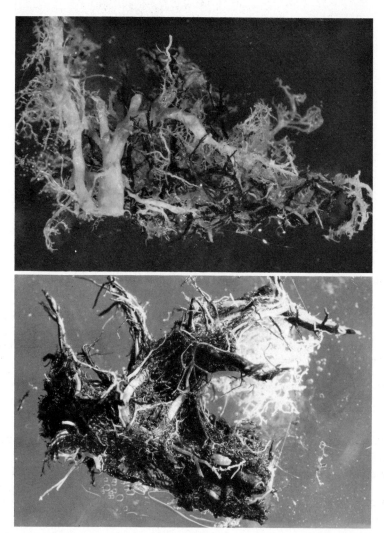

Figure 5–12. Portions of **vinyl acetate cast of cirrhotic liver.** ($\times$3.) *Upper,* Note distortion of all vascular elements. Abnormal contour of hepatic vein (white) is especially evident. *Lower,* Baskets of vessels in septa between regenerative nodules. (From Mann JD, Wakim KG, Baggenstoss AH: Alterations in the vasculature of the diseased liver. Gastroenterology 25:540–546, 1953. By permission of Williams & Wilkins Company.)

cut into the sides of the tissue block as points of reference. Serial 15-μ sections are prepared (a good knife has to be used to prevent shifting of tissue elements). Every tenth section is projected onto a white sheet of paper. The desired size of the model is determined at this point. The regenerative nodules and blood vessels are outlined on the paper sheets. Glass plates are placed on top of the paper and the projected outlines are inked onto the glass, the veins in blue and the regenerative nodules in brown. A three-dimensional figure is produced by placing the glass plates on top of each other and sealing them in blocks with a diluted solution of mounting medium (Fig. 5–13).

Wax models are prepared by using the sheets of paper with the projected outlines to trace the perimeters of the nodules on a sheet of wax. The nodules are made by placing alternate sections of red wax one on another. The authors of the method used sheets of wax which were more than two times the thickness of the tissue in a single section represented on a sheet of paper. Therefore, in this instance, only every second sheet of paper was used. The wax sections are fused with a jet flame from an alcohol lamp. The separate wax nodules are placed in proper position on a glass plate, using the glass model as a guide (Fig. 5–14). The veins are modeled from blue wax. Size, course, and relationship to the nodules are determined from the glass plates.

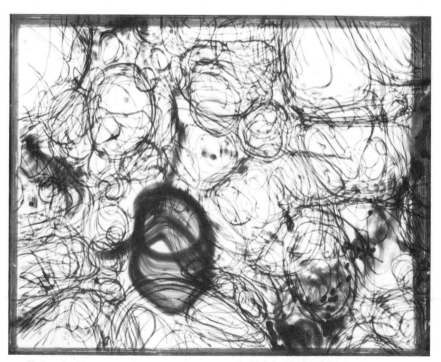

Figure 5–13. Three-dimensional **reconstruction of paraffin block of cirrhotic liver.** Regenerative nodules and accompanying veins are outlined with ink on glass plates, each plate representing a different level (see also Figure 5–14).

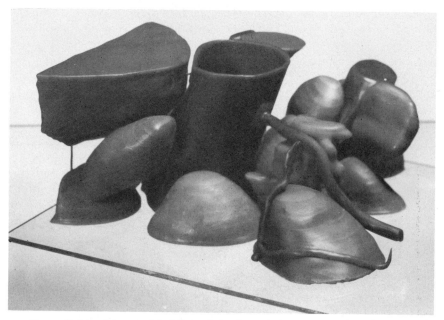

Figure 5–14. Wax model of liver cirrhosis made by reconstruction of regenerative nodules and accompanying veins, prepared from glass plates shown in Figure 5–13. Actual height of model, 8.25 cm, representing a tissue block 5.7 mm in height. (From Kelty RH, Baggenstoss AH, Butt HR: The relation of the regenerated liver nodule to the vascular bed in cirrhosis. Gastroenterology 15:285–295, 1950. By permission of Williams & Wilkins Company.)

GALLBLADDER

To avoid spilling of bile and discoloration of organs, the gallbladder usually is removed from its bed intact and opened in a fine-meshed strainer over a collecting vessel. If liver and gallbladder are to be fixed in a block, as in Figure 5–8, it is advisable to first remove the bile from the unopened gallbladder with a syringe. Before the tissue block is submerged in the formalin bath, the gallbladder and the extrahepatic bile ducts are partially opened and stuffed with formalin-soaked cotton in order to preserve the normal shape of the structures. The cystic duct is very difficult to dissect because of its numerous folds.

The intense staining of bile makes it difficult to prepare lasting museum specimens from gallbladders. Special fixation techniques are required (see chapter 9). The preparation of gallstones for museum specimens[23] requires a thin but wide-bladed jeweler's saw or a fine scroll saw. The stones may be hardened for 24 hours in concentrated formalin solution before cutting. Small and friable stones are frozen before cutting. The round half of the stone is leveled off slightly to give a flat base for mounting. A small hole is drilled through the stone and two similar holes are drilled through the plate glass foundation. A thread passed through these holes will securely anchor the stone to its base, and the unit is mounted in

10% formalin solution. Techniques to prevent green discoloration by biliverdin are described in chapter 9. Another method is to seal the dry calculi hermetically in thick-walled glass tubes; the tubes then are placed upside down in plaster of Paris.[6]

Plastic models have been used to study the hyperplastic mucosa of the gallbladder.[12]

PANCREAS

The parenchyma usually is best exposed by an incision in the frontal plane. Parallel sagittal sections are preferred when the pancreatic duct is dilated. When only one routine section of pancreatic tissue is to be studied, the tail of the pancreas is usually selected because of the abundance of islets in this region.

Lipomatosis of the pancreas can be well demonstrated by staining a slice of the organ with Sudan III (see page 136).

Fat tissue necroses also can be stained. The tissue is fixed in 10% formalin solution and subsequently placed in a concentrated copper acetate solution. After 1 day in the incubator or several days at room temperature, the fat tissue necroses turn blue-green.[4]

Injection of the mesenteric and celiac artery system (page 137) permits good roentgenographic visualization of the pancreatic arterial system.

The retrograde injection of radiopaque medium from the papilla of Vater provides excellent roentgenograms of the pancreatic duct system. Cystic dilatations, stenoses, tumors, and concrements can be identified by this technique.[1]

SPLEEN

Frontal or horizontal sections are prepared, by the same principles used for sectioning the liver. Formalin perfusion of the intact organ through the splenic vessels has proved unsatisfactory unless the blood has been previously removed (page 148). Some areas tend to remain unfixed. If formalin fixation is intended, care must be taken that the slices are very thin. Fixative does not penetrate well into the splenic pulp.

Injection from the celiac artery (page 137) or direct injection from the hilus of the spleen may be used for splenic angiography.

For histologic demonstration of the splenic reticulum,[33] slices of spleen can be macerated in 20% nitric acid or in 1 to 3% potassium hydroxide. The reticulum fibers of the spleen are more resistant to chemical maceration or digestion with trypsin than are the collagen fibers, and alcohol- or mercuric chloride-fixed material has been recommended for this technique.

The splenic reticulum also can be studied by washing the blood out of the pulp. This also facilitates fixation of the whole organ. The spleen is first perfused through the splenic artery or vein with 0.9% saline, using an injection pressure of about 100 mm Hg. After 1 hour, all blood will be removed and the splenic pulp will appear white. The perfusion is now continued with 10% formalin solution. In some instances it may be useful to fix the organ at more than its normal volume by tying the efferent vessels.

URINARY AND GENITAL SYSTEM

Kidneys and Ureters.   Renal vessels usually are opened lengthwise from the aorta or inferior vena cava to the hilus. I routinely incise the kidneys in situ. The fibrous and adipose capsule is stripped, using the unsevered renal vessels as an anchor. This prevents the organs from slipping out of one's hand after they have been removed from the retroperitoneal fat tissue. The kidneys are then incised from their convexity toward the hilus, exposing the renal pelvis. During this procedure the organ can be held in a firm grip by applying some tension to the renal vessels.

The ureters are opened lengthwise, starting from the renal pelvis and, if necessary, cutting through some undissected parenchyma at the lower pole of the kidneys.

The renal vessels and ureters can now be severed, or the kidneys can be removed together with the aorta, inferior vena cava, and pelvic organs.

Blocks for histologic examination should include renal cortex, medulla with a papilla, and a portion of the renal pelvis.

Microdissection for Isolation of Nephrons and Collecting Tubules.   In this method,[27] tissue blocks 3 to 10 mm thick, which include cortex, medulla, and a portion of the renal pelvis or whole kidneys of embryos and small fetuses, are placed in concentrated HCl at room temperature until they reach an optimal degree of maceration. This varies from 3 to 36 hours depending on the room temperature, the size of the specimen, and the amount of connective tissue. When the desired point is reached, the acid is poured off and the tissues are carefully rinsed three to four times with distilled water and left in the same container. The water becomes very dilute acid and will preserve the tissue for 1 to 2 weeks without producing further maceration if kept under refrigeration.

The dissection is carried out in a Petri dish under distilled water. Very fine needles and a binocular dissecting microscope are needed. The general topography of the nephrons and collecting tubules is first noted, and the tissue then is gently teased into smaller and smaller pieces. With experience, individual collecting tubules with all their attached nephrons can be dissected free of other tissues. Photographs should be made with the tissues still in the containers in which they were dissected in order to avoid distortion or separation of tubules.

During the preparation for microdissection, shrinkage and subsequent expansion and color changes of the tissue will occur. Excessive maceration causes the tissue to become fragile; glomeruli become detached, and other artifacts are so readily produced that it may be impossible to distinguish them from pathologic changes. Only with experience can one tell whether the tissue has been properly prepared for dissection.

Isolation of Glomeruli. Relatively pure preparations of glomeruli, free of Bowman's capsule, may be required for the preparation of antigens or other purposes. A rapid method[13] yielding glomeruli in less than 20 minutes is based on the use of sieves of different sizes.

Normal kidneys are obtained at autopsy and immediately perfused with ice-cold isotonic saline through the renal artery until they become pale brown. They are then bisected, and each half is cut into triangular fragments along the pyramids. The medulla is removed with an iris scissors and discarded. The cortex is cut into small fragments (about 2 mm³) with a razor blade and gently forced through a 80-mesh stainless steel sieve. The material remaining on the top of the sieve is discarded. The cortical mesh on the bottom surface of the wire cloth is collected with an angular spatula and suspended in 50 ml of ice-cold isotonic saline; this material contains glomeruli, small tubular fragments, and cellular debris.

After thorough mixing, the suspension is poured onto a 120-mesh wire cloth which is placed 10 cm above a 200-mesh sieve. Each sieve is washed with 200 ml of ice-cold saline. The material on top of the 120-mesh sieve contains small tubular fragments, while all glomeruli are retained on the 200-mesh cloth. The glomeruli are suspended in saline and transferred into 12-ml conical centrifuge tubes with a Pasteur pipette; each sample is diluted to 10 ml and centrifuged at $1,060 \times g$ for 3 minutes. The supernate is discarded and the glomerular pellet is buttered through a clean 200-mesh sieve resting on a 50-ml beaker placed in an ice bath. The sieve is washed with 10 ml of ice-cold saline. The suspension in the beaker contains uniformly decapsulated glomeruli with minimal glomerular disintegration.

These glomeruli are washed twice with saline and three times with ice-cold distilled water. They are collected by centrifugation at $1,060 \times g$ for 2 minutes and lyophilized. The glomerular pellet obtained from one kidney weighs 10 ± 3.0 mg.

Perfusion Fixation. A cannula is tied into the renal artery and 0.9% saline is perfused through the kidneys.[35] The perfusion time is 20 minutes at a pressure of 100 mm Hg. Subsequently, the perfusion is continued for 2 hours with 7% formalin-saline. This step seems to increase the washing out of blood clots in the renal veins.

Angiography and Urography. 1. In situ arteriograms.[15] The aorta is cross clamped proximal to the celiac axis and near the aortic bifurcation. A polyethylene catheter is inserted into the aorta via the severed superior mesenteric artery and secured by a ligature. The celiac and inferior mesenteric arteries are ligated. Thirty to 50 ml of 50% sodium acetrizoate (Urokon) is rapidly injected through the catheter, and a roentgenogram of the aorta, renal arteries, and kidneys is obtained (Fig. 5–15). Barium sulfate-gelatin mixtures also produce excellent renal arteriograms.

2. Arteriograms after en bloc removal.[3] The entire abdominal aorta is removed with the attached renal arteries, kidneys, and perirenal fat. The

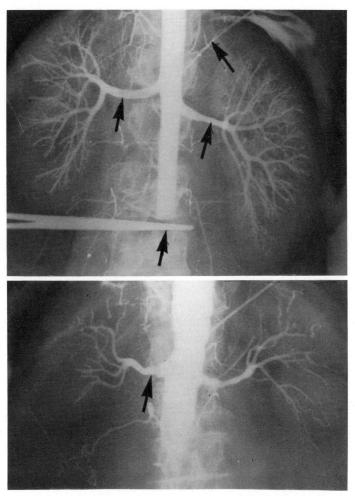

Figure 5–15. **In situ renal arteriograms.** *Upper,* Polyethylene catheter in superior mesenteric artery. Main renal arteries had minimal histologic evidence of atherosclerosis (*arrows*). Cross clamping of aorta is evident at base of film (*arrow*). *Lower,* Evidence of narrowing in both renal arteries but more pronounced in right renal artery (*arrow*). Histologically, stenosis was graded as severe. (From Holley KE, Hunt JC, Brown AL Jr, Kincaid OW, Sheps SG: Renal artery stenosis: a clinical-pathologic study in normotensive and hypertensive patients. Am J Med *37*:14–22, 1964. By permission of Reuben H. Donnelley Corporation.)

nonrenal artery branches and both ends of the abdominal aorta are tied, except for the celiac artery which is cannulated for injection of the radiopaque material.

3. Venography. The techniques are essentially similar to the ones used for arteriography. We have prepared in situ venograms by injection of contrast medium into a segment of the inferior vena cava which was sealed off by inflatable cuffs (Fig. 5–16). The tube with the cuffs can be introduced

from the iliac or femoral veins without handling of the inferior vena cava system. By moving the cuffs a little higher, excellent hepatic venograms can be prepared.

4. Urography. Retrograde urograms are easy to prepare with any of the conventional contrast media. The ureter is cannulated either from the urinary bladder or through the wall of the distal ureter.

Preparation of Plastic Casts. Plastic casts can be used for the demonstration of the renal vasculature, the pelvic system, and cysts or other abnormal cavities. The methods[3,16,31] are similar to those described for the coronary arteries (chapter 3). For injection of the plastic mixture of Arcon and Polylite,[3] a pressure of 100 mm Hg is recommended, controlled with a standard Schlesinger manometric apparatus. The injection time is 3 to 4 minutes.

Preparation of Renal Tissue for Immunofluorescent Microscopy. Immunofluorescent microscopy is of great diagnostic value in suspected immune complex diseases, such as poststreptococcal glomerulonephritis, and in anti-glomerular-basement-membrane antibody (anti-GBM) diseases, such as glomerulonephritis with pulmonary hemorrhages (Goodpasture's syndrome). Immune complex diseases are characterized by irregular (granular) fluorescence (Fig. 5–17 *A*), whereas anti-GBM diseases show regular (linear) fluorescence (Fig. 5–17 *B*). Methodologic details have been

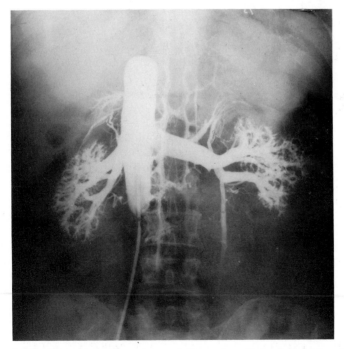

Figure 5–16. Normal renal venogram. Rubber tube with two inflatable cuffs was introduced to seal off inferior vena cava above and below renal veins. Barium sulfate-gelatin mixture was injected through midportion of tube. There is also filling of lumbar, prevertebral, adrenal, and left testicular veins.

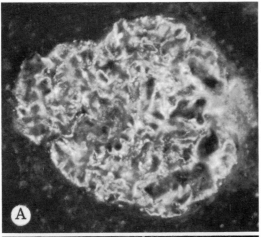

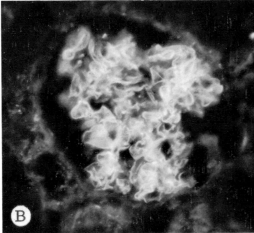

Figure 5–17. Autopsy material prepared for **immunofluorescence microscopy.** A, Diffuse granular immunofluorescence of glomerular basement membrane in lupus erythematosus. B, Linear immunofluorescence of glomerular basement membrane in rapidly progressive glomerulonephritis.

discussed by Coons.[9] The technique which we use has been applied successfully to both renal biopsies and suitably procured autopsy material.

1. Remove renal tissue as soon as possible after death.

2. Snap-freeze small pieces of kidney (6 by 3 by 2 mm) and store in methylbutanol at −70 C.

3. Cut tissue on cryostat at 4-micron thickness; fix by placing slides in incubator at 37 C for 1 hour just prior to staining (extra tissue sections not used immediately may be stored at −40 C in a covered container).

4. Remove slides from incubator and wash in phosphate buffer (pH 7.2) for 5 minutes at room temperature with one change of buffer and constant agitation of slides in the buffer.

5. Remove excess moisture from the slide but leave the tissue section covered by a droplet of the washing buffer.

6. Overlay tissue with the appropriate conjugated antiserum (for example, goat anti-human-IgG and complement; rabbit anti-human-fibrinogen); place in moist chamber and incubate for 30 minutes at 37 C.

7. Remove slides and wash in phosphate buffer for 5 minutes with three changes.

8. Cover-slip slides using glycerine (glycerine 9 parts, phosphate buffer 1 part) as the mounting medium.

Pelvic Organs. Intravascular formalin injection or freezing methods have been used to harden pelvic organs in their natural position.[20] The vascular system of the pelvis can be injected from the internal iliac artery. Corrosion specimens are prepared by the usual techniques.

The urinary bladder can be fixed in the distended position by injecting formalin solution through a catheter. Urine in the bladder must be removed first. The urinary bladder is left intact until fixation is completed. The upper half of the bladder is then removed and the base of the bladder is exposed. This technique is particularly recommended in cases of benign prostatic hyperplasia with urethral obstruction or urinary bladder tumors in the area of the trigone. Some tumors or abscesses are better exposed by frontal sections through the base of the urinary bladder and prostate.

Most pathologists do not routinely dissect the penis and the male urethra. Congenital urethral valves, strictures, and tumors are the main indications for study. The penis, with or without surrounding skin, should be left attached to the urinary bladder. This can be achieved by either sawing out a portion of the pubic bone or by pulling the penis through the pubic arch.

These maneuvers require preparatory dissection of soft tissues and appropriate incision of the skin of the penis. The urethra should be opened lengthwise in the anterior midline. Histologic sections through urethra and corpora cavernosa are usually taken in a frontal plane — that is, perpendicular to the axis of the urethra.

Urethral valves can best be located by injecting radiopaque material into the urinary bladder. The urethra should then be opened along the dorsal midline against the direction of the flow of urine. This will help prevent laceration of the delicate valves.

Fixation of the corpora cavernosa can be achieved by injecting formalin solution or gelatin-formalin through the vena dorsalis penis.

The pregnant uterus can be fixed by first puncturing the uterus through the anterior abdominal wall and replacing the amniotic fluid with formalin solution. After the prefixed uterus has been opened, the fetus is perfused with formalin solution through the umbilical cord. If one intends to preserve uterus and fetus as one specimen, a formalin-gelatin mixture is injected into the cavity of the uterus.

In some institutions the placenta is routinely discarded. The autopsy pathologist should discourage such practices and should refuse to perform autopsies on stillbirths and neonates unless he has the opportunity to study the placenta also. The following procedures for gross examination are suggested.[5]

If the placenta cannot be studied shortly after delivery, it should be stored in a closed container in the refrigerator. The examination begins with the reconstruction, in a tank of saline, of the fetal membranous bag.

This allows one to ascertain the original position of the placenta by demonstrating the site of the uterine cornua and the point of rupture of the membranes. The narrowest width of membranes is measured. If there are no velamentous vessels, the bag is trimmed from the placenta. A sausage-shaped roll of membrane is fixed for histologic study, with the site of the rupture innermost. The cord is then measured and inspected superficially and on gross sections to count the number of vessels. A segment of the umbilical cord is fixed for histologic study. After the cord is cut near its insertion, the placenta is weighed and measured. The placenta should be kept moist. The fetal and maternal surfaces are inspected. The yolk sac is searched for, particularly in twins (see below). If cotyledons are missing, milk injections or other injection procedures help to differentiate true tissue defects from artifacts of handling. The placenta is then cut into thin slices with a long-bladed knife. Blood is wiped off and the cut surfaces are inspected. Grossly abnormal areas are placed in Bouin's solution for histologic study; after a few hours, the tissue is trimmed and refixed. Routinely, one section is taken from the margin of the placenta and one from near the center where chorionic vessels can be included.

Benirschke and Driscoll[5] refer to special techniques. These include rapid frozen sections of the umbilical cord in cases of respiratory distress of the newborn (the findings of perivascular inflammation usually rule against the presence of hyaline membrane disease), preparations for electron and fluorescence microscopy, study of nuclear sex chromatin, tissue culture, and vascular injection and corrosion techniques.

The examination of placentas in multiple pregnancies requires special precautions. A longitudinal strip is cut from the portion of fusion or approximation of the membranous sacs, leaving the placenta intact, and a roll is prepared for histologic study. (One also can prepare "T section"—that is, an area of fused twin placenta with dividing membranes extending above which may show two amnions or two amnions and two chorions. Unfortunately, T sections interfere with subsequent vascular injection.) The dividing membranes are then peeled apart with the aid of forceps. If two chorions are present, separation attempts will disrupt villous placental tissue. The placenta is now weighed and measured.

Vascular injection is necessary to separate the vascular beds of the fused dichorionic placenta. Injections also are used to decide whether vascular communications exist and to determine their nature and number. Because of artifactual villous disruptions, usually only selected areas can be injected, using green saline or other injection media. Shunts seem to be absent in all dichorial twins but will be seen in almost all monochorial twin placentas. The "vascular equator" can be identified after the amniotic membranes have been stripped. At various sites in this area, green saline is injected into arteries near presumed common vascular channels. About 30 to 50 ml of saline usually is necessary at each site to determine whether fluid returns to the same infant or its partner through anastomoses. During the injection, blood must be allowed to escape from where the umbilical cords have been cut near their insertions.

REFERENCES

1. Adlung J, Gürich H-G, Ritter U: Über Veränderungen am Pankreasgangsystem: makroskopische, mikroskopische und klinische Untersuchungen. Med Welt, February 22, 1969, pp 387–391
2. Andrews WHH, Maegraith BG, Wenyon CEM: Studies on the liver circulation. II. The micro-anatomy of the hepatic circulation. Ann Trop Med Parasitol 43:229–237, 1949
3. Bauer FW, Robbins SL: A postmortem study comparing renal angiograms and renal artery casts in 58 patients. Arch Pathol 83:307–314, 1967
4. Benda C: Eine makro- und mikrochemische Reaction der Fettgewebs–Nekrose. Virchows Arch [Pathol Anat] 161:194–198, 1900
5. Benirschke K, Driscoll SG: The Pathology of the Human Placenta. New York, Springer Verlag, Inc., 1967
6. Brites G: A new method of mounting calculi. J Tech Methods 12:29–31, 1929
7. Chomet B, Gach BM: Demonstration of esophageal varices in museum specimens. Am J Clin Pathol 51:793–794, 1969
8. Chomet B, Hart LM, Reindl FJ: Demonstration of esophageal varices by simple technique. Arch Pathol 69:185–187, 1960
9. Coons AH: Fluorescent antibody methods. In General Cytochemical Methods. Edited by JF Danielli. New York, Academic Press, 1958, p 399
10. Dukes C, Bussey HJR: Preparation and mounting of museum specimens of intestinal tumours. J Tech Methods 15:44–48, 1936
11. Dymock IW, Gray B: Staining method for the examination of the small intestinal villous pattern in necropsy material. J Clin Pathol 21:748–749, 1968
12. Elfving G, Teir H, Degert H, Makela V: Mucosal hyperplasia in the gallbladder demonstrated by plastic models. Acta Pathol Microbiol Scand 77:384–388, 1969
13. Gang NF: A rapid method for the isolation of glomeruli from the human kidney. Am J Clin Pathol 53:267–269, 1970
14. Goyal RK, Glancy JJ, Spiro HM: Lower esophageal ring (first of two parts). N Engl J Med 282:1298–1305, 1970
15. Holley KE, Hunt JC, Brown AL Jr, Kincaid OW, Sheps SG: Renal artery stenosis: a clinical-pathologic study in normotensive and hypertensive patients. Am J Med 37:14–22, 1964
16. James TN: Anatomy of the Coronary Arteries. New York, Hoeber Medical Division, Harper & Row, 1961
17. Kelty RH, Baggenstoss AH, Butt HR: The relation of the regenerated liver nodule to the vascular bed in cirrhosis. Gastroenterology 15:285–295, 1950
18. Loehry CA, Creamer B: Post-mortem study of small-intestinal mucosa. Br Med J 1:827–829, 1966
19. Loeschcke H, Otto R: Methoden der morphologischen Untersuchung des Verdauungsapparates, Pankreas. In Handbuch der biologischen Arbeitsmethoden. Vol VIII, part 1 (1). Edited by E Abderhalden. Berlin, Urban & Schwarzenberg, 1924, pp 661–674
20. Loeschcke H, Weinnoldt H: Methoden zur morphologischen Untersuchung des Genitalapparates, Nebennieren. In Handbuch der biologischen Arbeitsmethoden. Vol VIII, part 1 (1). Edited by E Abderhalden. Berlin, Urban & Schwarzenberg, 1924, pp 651–660
21. Luna A, Meister PH, Szanto PB: Esophageal varices in the absence of cirrhosis: incidence and characteristics in congestive heart failure and neoplasm of the liver. Am J Clin Pathol 49:710–717, 1968
22. Mann JD, Wakim KG, Baggenstoss AH: Alterations in the vasculature of the diseased liver. Gastroenterology 25:540–546, 1953
23. Mentzer SH: Methods of preparing gall-bladders and calculi for study and museum display. Int Assoc Med Mus 11:37–40, 1925
24. Michels NA, Siddharth P, Kornblith PL, Parke WW: Routes of collateral circulation of the gastrointestinal tract as ascertained in a dissection of 500 bodies. Int Surg 49:8–28, 1968
25. Mitra SK: Hepatic vascular changes in human and experimental cirrhosis. J Pathol 92:405–414, 1966
26. Mitra SK: The terminal distribution of the hepatic artery with special reference to arterioportal anastomosis. J Anat 100:651–663, 1966
27. Osathanondh V, Potter EL: Development of human kidneys as shown by microdissection. I. Preparation of tissue with reasons for possible misinterpretations of observations. Arch Pathol 76:271–276, 1963
28. Pulvertaft RJV: Museum techniques: a review. J Clin Pathol 3:1–23, 1950

29. Reiner L: Mesenteric vascular occlusion studied by postmortem injection of the mesenteric arterial circulation. *In* Pathologic Annual: 1966. Vol 1. Edited by S Sommers. New York, Appleton-Century-Crofts, Inc., 1966, pp 193–220

30. Reiner L, Rodriguez FL, Platt R, Schlesinger MJ: Injection studies of the mesenteric arterial circulation. I. Technique and observations on collaterals. Surgery *45*:820–833, 1959

31. Robbins SL, Fish SJ: A new angiographic technic providing a simultaneous permanent cast of the coronary arterial lumen. Am J Clin Pathol *42*:156–163, 1964

32. Scheidt RA: A stationary probe-enterotome for routine autopsies. Am J Clin Pathol *36*:139–141, 1961

33. Schmincke A: Methoden zur morphologischen Untersuchung der Milz. *In* Handbuch der biologischen Arbeitsmethoden. Vol VIII, part 1 (1). Edited by E Abderhalden. Berlin, Urban & Schwarzenberg, 1924, pp 599–634

34. Stemmermann GN, Hayashi T: Intestinal metaplasia of the gastric mucosa: a gross and microscopic study of its distribution in various disease states. J Natl Cancer Inst *41*:627–634, 1968

35. Tracy RE, Overll EO: Arterioles of perfusion-fixed hypertensive and aged kidneys. Arch Pathol *82*:526–534, 1966

36. Trueta J, Barclay AE, Daniel PM, Franklin KJ, Prichard MML: Studies of the Renal Circulation. Springfield, Illinois, Charles C Thomas, Publisher, 1947

37. Wakefield EG, Mayo CW, Feldman WH, Welch CS: Permanent fixation of the entire alimentary tubes of mammals: illustration of a practical application. J Tech Methods *18*:66–70, 1938

38. Wilson JB: Vascular patterns in the cirrhotic liver. Edinburgh Med J *58*:537–547, 1951

39. Wilson JP: Post-mortem preservation of the small intestine. J Pathol *92*:229–230, 1966

40. Woolf AL: Techniques of post-mortem angiography of the stomach. Br J Radiol *23*:8–14, 1950.

CHAPTER 6

NERVOUS SYSTEM

By Haruo Okazaki

REMOVAL OF BRAIN

In Adults. *Incision of Scalp.* The head is elevated slightly with a wooden block or a metal headrest attached to the autopsy table. The hair is parted with a comb along the line of the primary incision. The latter is made through an imaginary coronal plane connecting one mastoid with the other over the convexity (Fig. 6-1). If the incision is made too anteriorly, it will be disfiguring. On the other hand, if it is placed too posteriorly, the forward reflection of the scalp will be difficult. Some prefer placing a narrow, pointed knife, with the cutting edge facing upward, underneath the scalp and cutting the scalp from below to avoid cutting the hair. This slow and

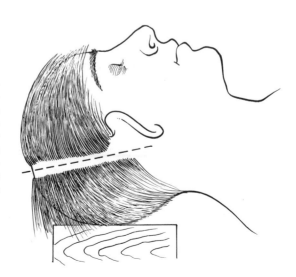

Figure 6-1. Dotted line indicates **coronal plane of primary scalp incision.** It starts on right side over mastoid just behind earlobe and passes over palpable posterolateral ridges of parietal bones to reach opposite mastoid. This line is slightly tilted backward from plane parallel with face.

awkward maneuver is not necessary if the hair first is parted. A sharp scalpel blade can then be used to cut through the whole thickness of the scalp from the outside. It is advisable to start the incision at the right side of the head (the "viewing-side" in most American funeral parlors) just behind the earlobe, as low as possible without extending below the earlobe, and to extend it to the comparable level at the other side. This will make reflection of the scalp considerably easier.

The anterior and posterior halves of the scalp are then reflected forward and backward, respectively, after short undercutting of the scalp with a sharp knife which permits grasping of the edges with the hands. The use of a dry towel draped over the scalp edges facilitates further reflection, usually without the aid of cutting instruments. If the reflection is difficult, a scalpel blade can be used to cut the loose connective tissue that lags behind the reflecting edge as the left hand continues to peel the scalp. The knife edge should be directed toward the skull and not toward the scalp. The anterior flap is reflected to a level 1 or 2 cm above the supraorbital ridge. The posterior flap is reflected down to a level just above the occipital protuberance.

Sawing of Cranium. Opening of the cranium is best performed with an oscillating saw. Some of the commonly used saw cuts are illustrated in Figure 6–2. We routinely use the method illustrated in Figure 6–3, which is designed to minimize slippage of the skull cap during restoration of the head by the embalmer. The temporalis muscle should be cut with a sharp knife and cleared from the intended path of the saw blade. Ideally, sawing should be stopped just short of cutting through the inner table of the cranium, which will easily give way with the use of a chisel and a light blow with a mallet.

Inexperienced prosectors commonly dip the blade deep into the brain substance. Therefore, it is recommended that the extended index finger of the right hand, which holds the neck of the oscillating saw, be used to gauge the distance of the blade penetration. The oscillating blade should be moved from side to side during cutting to avoid deep penetration in a given area. We currently use a model (Lipshaw Co.) which is equipped with a guard (see chapter 7) and can be used by relatively inexperienced personnel without fear of deep penetration.

It is recommended that the frontal point of sawing start approximately two fingerbreadths above the supraorbital ridge. While the lateral aspects of the skull are being cut, turning the head to the opposite side permits the brain to sink away from the cranial vault, thereby diminishing the chance of injury to the brain.

When the dura is left intact, as in the method described above, peeling the skull cap away from the dura is relatively easily accomplished. Ideally, the sawing should be stopped as soon as the blade reaches the inner table of the skull, which will easily give way with light taps on a broad chisel inserted at several points along the line of sawing. A twist of the same chisel placed in the frontal saw line will then permit placement of the fingers inside the skull cap. A blunt hook may be used to pull the skull cap away from

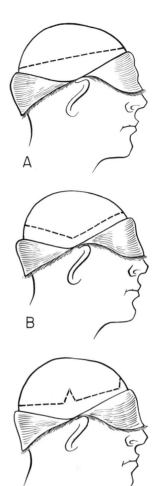

A

B

C

Figure 6–2. Some of the commonly used methods of **skull cap removal.** A, Saucer or circular method. B, Wedge method. C, Triple notch method.

the underlying dura. A hand inserted between the skull and the dura (periosteum) helps the blunt separation of these while the other hand is pulling the skull cap. If this is found to be impossible for some reason, such as firm adherence of the dura to the skull aggravated by inadvertent cutting of the dura by the saw, the dura can be incised along the line of sawing and the anterior attachment of the falx to the skull can be cut between the frontal lobes. The posterior portion of the falx can be cut from inside after the skull cap is fully reflected. The dura is then peeled off the skull cap. The superior sagittal sinus may be opened with a pair of scissors at this time.

Detachment of Brain. The frontal lobes are gently raised and the olfactory bulbs and tract are peeled away from the cribriform plates. The optic nerves are cut as they enter the optic foramina. Under its own weight, the brain is allowed to fall away from the floor of the anterior fossa, but the brain must be supported with the palm of the left hand. The pituitary stalk

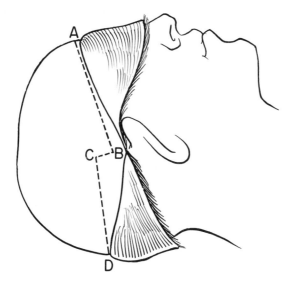

Figure 6–3. Lines of saw cuts for skull cap removal. Frontal point A is approximately two fingerbreadths above supraorbital ridges. Temporal point B is at top of ear in its natural position before scalp reflection. Point C is approximately 2 cm above B. Occipital point D is approximately two fingerbreadths above external occipital protuberance (inion). If A is too low, there is danger of cutting into roof of orbit; if B is too low, saw will enter petrous portion of temporal bone. Either of these will make removal of skull vault difficult. When D is too low, saw line will be below posterior attachment of tentorium.

is cut, followed by the internal carotid arteries as they enter the cranial cavity. Cranial nerves III, IV, V, and VI are severed as close to the base of the skull as possible. Subdural communicating veins are also severed. Next, the attachment of the tentorium along the petrous ridge is cut on either side with curved scissors. At this time, do not allow the brain to drop backward excessively since this will cause stretch tears in the cerebral peduncles.

Continue cutting cranial nerves VII, VIII, IX, X, XI, and XII. One should make it a habit to follow the numerical sequence of these cranial nerves, one by one, to force accurate identification and observation of these structures. The vertebral arteries are severed with scissors as they emerge into the cranial cavity. Then, cut across the cervical part of the spinal cord as caudally as possible but avoiding too oblique a plane of section.

The brain can then be reflected further back, using the right hand to deliver the brain stem and cerebellum from the posterior fossa, without causing excessive stretching pressure at the rostral brain stem level, along with the falx and the dura. Pull the brain away from the base of the skull after cutting the posterior attachment of the tentorium. The latter will remain in its anatomic position until further examination of the removed brain is carried out. Examination of the base of the skull will be described in a subsequent section of this chapter.

In Fetuses and Infants. When the sutures are not closed and the cranial bones are still soft, Beneke's technique is used to open the cranium. The scalp is reflected as in adults. Starting at the lateral edge of the frontal fontanelle, the cranium and dura on both sides are cut with a pair of blunt scissors along the line indicated in Figure 6–4 A. This is necessitated by the fact that, in this age group, it is often difficult to separate the skull from the underlying dura in the manner described for adults. This cut leaves a midline strip approximately 1 cm wide, containing the superior sagittal sinus and the falx, and an intact area in the temporal squama on either side, which serves as a hinge when the bone flap is reflected. The older the infant, the narrower the sagittal strip will be because of advance in ossification toward the midline.

An alternate method of cutting, which follows the cranial suture lines, is illustrated in Figure 6–4 *B* and *B'*. With this method, fracture lines will be created along these bone flaps on their reflection, and an optional cut along the posterior base of the frontal bone on either side will facilitate the procedure. The falx is then sectioned in a manner similar to that described for adults.

Stowens[16] described a modification of Beneke's method of folding out the bone flaps with the dura left intact. This is done by incising the skull lightly along the cranial sutures and at the fontanelles. By reversing the scalpel and passing it under the bones, the bones are separated from the underlying dura. The reflection of the bone flaps is carried out after

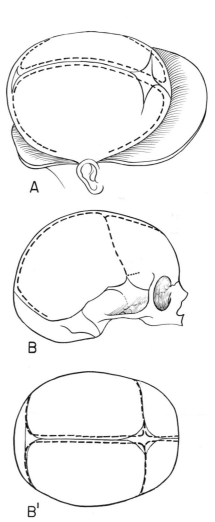

Figure 6–4. Two methods of **opening calvarium in fetus and neonate.** In method shown in B and B', reflection of frontal bone flaps will result in fracture lines along their base. Optional cut may be made into posterior portion of these flaps as indicated by dots in B.

making a small nick at the base in each of the bones. This procedure is similar to the method illustrated in Figure 6–4 *B* and *B '*. The dura is then cut as near to the base of the skull as possible. This method has the advantage of protecting the usually friable surface of the infant brain from damage during its removal.

To minimize damage to the brain, the following procedure may be adopted. The opening of the scalp and calvarium and the sectioning of the falx are accomplished with the body in a sitting position, the head being supported by an assistant. Inspection of the tentorium and vein of Galen is accomplished in this position by gently separating the parieto-occipital lobes. After the tentorium is sectioned, the body is suspended upside down by the assistant, the brain being supported during the movement by the left hand of the prosector. The brain is cut away from the base of the skull in this upside-down position, which minimizes movement of the brain and therefore minimizes damage to the brain substance and its surfaces. Stowens makes use of the bone flaps, replacing them in their normal position on one side and supporting the head with the hand on this side, while the freeing procedure is carried out on the other side. This is repeated on the opposite side. The brain is not touched directly during these procedures and, when all attachments are severed, it is allowed to fall free.

Pros and cons of Beneke's method of leaving the tentorium and removing the cerebral hemispheres from the brain stem and cerebellum were discussed by Towbin.[21] We favor keeping the brain as intact as possible at this stage without omitting inspection of the tentorium and neighboring structures during the removal procedure.

REMOVAL OF SPINAL CORD

In Adults. Removal of the spinal cord, which has been traditionally neglected by general pathologists, can be accomplished very easily within 10 to 15 minutes by the use of an oscillating saw as described below and should be part of every autopsy.

Posterior Approach. Although occasionally favored by some neuropathologists, the posterior approach is used by us only on special occasions such as excision of an occipital encephalocele, in situ exposure of an Arnold-Chiari malformation, or removal of a spinal meningomyelocele (described below).

Anterior Approach. The anterior approach is simple and quick and does not require turning the body over. It also permits removal of the spinal cord and peripheral nerves in continuity when indicated. Adequate examination of the vertebral bodies is an added advantage.

Kernohan's hemivertebral section method,[7] devised as a quick anterior approach with the advantage of providing rigidity to the spinal column, has a serious drawback of not exposing one side of the spinal cord. Consequently, it restricts removal of the spinal cord, roots, and dural covering. A method of complete removal of these structures will be described below.

After evisceration is completed, the first cut is made across the uppermost part of the thoracic region (T1 or T2). The head is dropped back by removing the head support or placing a wooden block behind the back under the midthoracic region, which straightens the spinal column and facilitates the procedure to be described. The next cut is placed on either side of the upper thoracic spine, caudal to the first, for approximately 10 to 15 cm along the line indicated in Figure 6–5. The sawing should be stopped as soon as one feels a "give," so as not to cut into the spinal cord. This plane of section placed over the proximal end of the ribs is lower than that described by McGarry,[10] which is placed at the angle between the vertebral bodies and the ribs. Our method has the advantage of creating a wider opening for the spinal cord and of giving easier access to the spinal ganglia and the peripheral nerves. The freed portion of the thoracic spine readily snaps up toward the prosector at this point (Fig. 6–6), especially when the spine straightening procedure described above is used.

It is not recommended to make a saw cut along one side all the way down to the lumbar area, since one cannot be certain if the line of cut is being placed properly. Cutting both sides of the spine for short distances eliminates this uncertainty. If the upper thoracic spine fails to snap up, due to faulty sectioning, this can be readily remedied at this early stage by placing another cut. Grasping the freed spine with the left hand and pulling toward the prosector makes the caudal extension of the cuts easier.

As one proceeds toward the lumbar area, the angle of the blade should be changed, adjusting to the shape of the vertebrae as illustrated in Figure 6–5. The muscles in this area should be cut away from the spine, down to the level of emerging nerves but without dividing them prior to sawing. It is easy to divide the lumbar spine at the L4-L5 interspace with a slightly curved, short knife. Since removal of the L5 body with the rest of the spine is often difficult because of the angulation of the spine at this level, L5 can be removed separately from the sacral bone with relative ease. In most instances, transecting the cauda equina roots at either L4 or L5 is sufficient.

The task of freeing the rest of the cauda equina from the sacral bone is more time-consuming, largely because of the difficulty in manipulating the saw in this narrow region. It can be achieved by removing a wedge of bone near the midline with an oscillating saw blade and removing the remaining

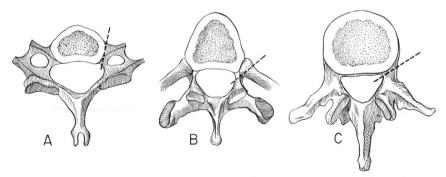

Figure 6–5. Anterior approach to spinal cord. Dotted lines indicate planes of saw cut adjusted to shapes of different levels of vertebral column. **A,** Cervical. **B,** Thoracic. **C,** Lumbar.

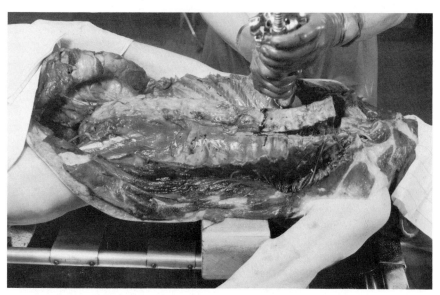

Figure 6–6.   Initial phase of anterior approach to spinal cord. Hyperextension of neck or placement of block behind midthoracic spinal region helps by allowing rostral end of sawed spine to snap up. Without block, special attention has to be paid to follow natural lordotic curvature of midthoracic spine; otherwise, opening will be too narrow to permit extraction of spinal cord at this level.

lateral portion of the sacral bone with a rongeur to avoid damage to the nerve roots in the foramina. Fortunately, this necessity arises infrequently.

Now, the exposed portion of the spinal cord and the cauda equina encased by the dura mater can be lifted off the bed along with as many spinal ganglia as possible. When indicated, the spinal cord can be removed along with all the spinal ganglia and the nerves of the lumbar plexuses and beyond by extending the process of freeing these structures from the bony and soft tissue encasement more peripherally (Fig. 6–7). It often is advisable to tie a string to one of the lumbar roots for future identification.

The remaining cervical spinal cord can be removed by Kernohan's extraction technique,[7] described below, without removing the cervical spine. The cord thus removed usually is without a single cervical spinal root, not to mention the posterior spinal ganglia. Therefore, when examination of these structures is indicated, it is necessary to extend the dissection of the spine upward. The carotid arteries are pushed to the side and the cervical plexuses are exposed in the same manner as used in the lumbar area. The spine is then cut along the plane shown in Figure 6–5 on either side up to the level of the C2-C3 interspace, where it is transected with a scalpel blade (Fig. 6–8 *upper*). Alternately, the cervical spine is simply reflected cephalad and fractured away (Fig. 6–8 *lower*) when there is no necessity of preserving the evidence of antemortem lesions such as fractures or hypertrophic ridges.

A slight lateral tilting of the blade facilitates the removal of the spinal ganglia in this region. An excessive tilting, however, often results in cutting into the spinal cord itself. Another common mistake is to deviate the line of cutting toward the midline cephalad, ending up with a pointed tip. This easily results in damage to the underlying cervical cord. In order to make the insertion of the oscillating saw blade underneath the skin flap easier, we have modified it by cutting off the top portion of the circular blade. It is important to make the primary chest incision shoulder to shoulder and to free the skin flap from the underlying muscles and connective tissue to provide adequate exposure of the neck region.

In order to remove the upper cervical cord and its roots from the bony canal still intact, one has to approach from the cranial cavity to free the dural attachment from the foramen magnum as high as possible. First, one makes a circular cut here. The dura is then peeled off from the bones caudad. Holding the freed dura taut with a hemostat or forceps makes this procedure easier. Usually, no special tools are required other than a pair of long scissors. We have on occasion made use of semicircular chisels as shown in Figure 6–9 *left*. The same instrument can be used from below.

If and when the remaining portion of the spine is to be removed, we use a wire-saw (Fig. 6–9 *right*) passed through the spinal canal or a jigsaw with a long blade to complete the section. While the latter instrument may injure the spinal cord when used prior to its removal, the wire-saw can be used safely with the cervical cord still in place. This will permit removal of the cervical spine in one piece.

If difficulties are encountered in reaching the high cervical level, it is advisable to cut across the cervical spine at a lower level and to extract the spinal cord by Kernohan's method after cutting the dura circumferentially

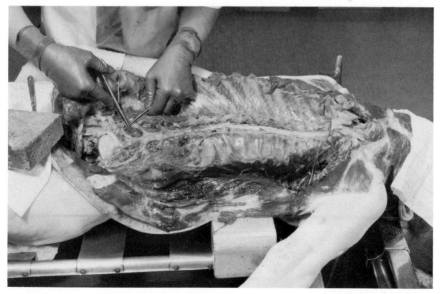

Figure 6–7. Freeing of lumbar roots and lumbar plexus. It is convenient at this time to place a tie around the L5 or L4 root for future identification of spinal cord segments.

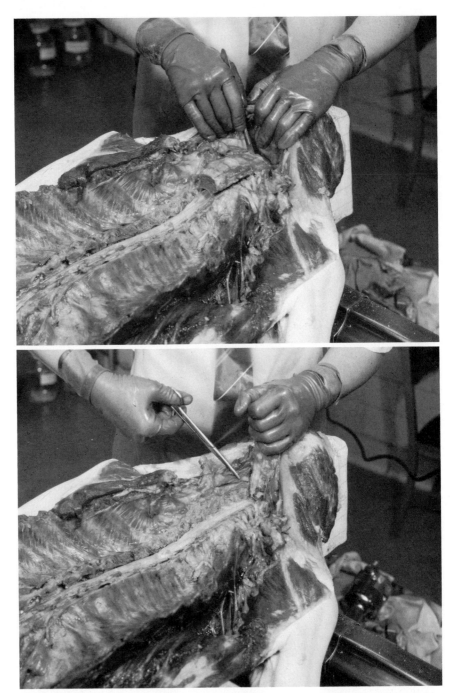

Figure 6-8. Removal of cervical spine. *Upper,* Scalpel blade is used to separate bone block at an intervertebral disk. *Lower,* Bone block to be removed is reflected upward forcefully to break off at high cervical level. This method is faster but not suitable when examination of cervical spine (for fracture, disk protrusion, etc.) is necessary. Notice continuity of cervical roots with spinal cord.

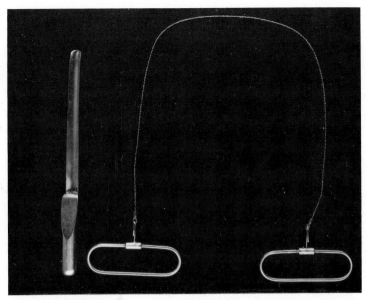

Figure 6–9. *Left,* Lightweight chisel made of stainless steel pipe, 3/4-inch (about 1.9-cm) diameter, for separating dura from upper cervical spine. *Right,* Wire-saw used for removing upper cervical vertebral bodies. Wire is passed through spinal canal to extend saw cuts initiated in lower cervical spine by oscillating saw blade.

at the exposed edge and opening it longitudinally along the midline below this level. The spinal cord and dura are wrapped in a moist towel (Fig. 6–10 *upper*). The right hand grasps the lower portion of the spinal cord and provides a gentle, steady, caudad pull while the fingers of the left hand are placed close to the top of the exposed spinal cord to minimize angulation at this point (Fig. 6–10 *lower*). It is possible to remove most of the spinal roots from the cervical enlargement by this method.

In Infants. *Anterior Approach.* The basic principle is the same as in adults. The incomplete calcification of the spinal column permits the use of a scalpel blade instead of an oscillating saw blade.

Combined Approach. When complete removal of a meningocele, meningomyelocele, or other condition related to a midline fusion defect is desired, it is best to combine the anterior and posterior approaches. After evisceration, the body is turned over and an incision is made around the meningomyelocele or other defects to allow its en bloc removal with the entire spinal column and cord. The latter task can be approached either posteriorly by extending a midline incision over the spinous processes or anteriorly. In either case, the ribs are separated from the spine and the sacral bone is cut away from the rest of the pelvic bones. An appropriate transection is made across the upper thoracic spine and the entire block is freed from soft tissue attachment. For retaining the continuity of the cervical spine, the posterior approach obviously is the method of choice. The method can be used regardless of the position of the midline defect. A similar approach can be used for the removal of an occipital meningocele or en-

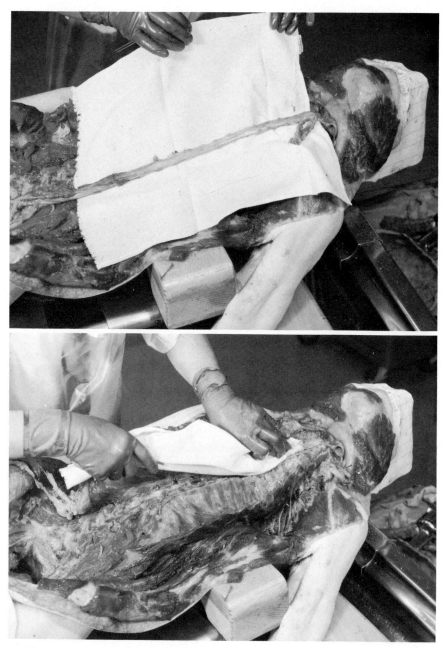

Figure 6–10. Spinal cord extraction. *Upper,* Moist towel is placed underneath freed spinal cord. *Lower,* Towel is wrapped around spinal cord. Left fingers are placed over rostral end of towel to direct force of gentle but steady caudad pull provided by right hand. Placing right thumb at rostral end and pulling spinal cord at this level results in severe squeezing artifact of this segment.

cephalocele. In the case of an Arnold-Chiari malformation, exposing its posterior aspect within the bony cavity is desirable, and this is accomplished by cutting off the posterior portion of the occipital bone combined with laminectomy of the upper cervical spine after the usual opening of the skull.

EXAMINATION AND REMOVAL OF STRUCTURES AT BASE OF SKULL

Venous Sinuses, Ganglia, and Dura. The venous sinuses, including the cavernous sinuses, are opened with curved scissors after removal of the brain. The gasserian ganglia can be removed at this time. The dura at the base of the skull should be thoroughly stripped. This procedure is essential for exposing fracture lines. A heavy use of chisel and hammer should be avoided before the dural stripping so as not to create artifactual fracture lines. When removal of the cavernous sinuses along with their contents in natural relationship is desired, as in a case of aneurysm of the internal carotid artery, a method similar to that described below for the in situ removal of the pituitary gland can be used.

Pituitary Gland. It is advisable to excise all around the margins of the diaphragma sellae before knocking off the posterior clinoid with a small chisel. The tip of the chisel is placed at the crest of the dorsum sellae. The chisel can be directed either posteriorly (downward) over and nearly parallel to the midline anterior fossa or nearly perpendicular to it. The perpendicular placement permits viewing of the pituitary during the procedure but requires a tap over the broad side of the chisel near the tip instead of a tap on the end of it. If the diaphragma is not freed first, the tension on it may result in squeezing of the contents of the pituitary fossa. A pair of forceps is applied to the edge of the diaphragma and the pituitary is dissected out, with a sharp blade, away from the base of the fossa. The pituitary gland may be removed along with its bony encasement — for example, in a case of pituitary adenoma. This can be accomplished by making saw cuts along the lines indicated in Figure 6–11 and lifting the entire block off the base of the skull. With normal pituitary glands, removal from the fossa becomes more difficult after fixation, because of enlargement of the glands and firmer adhesion of the dura to the sellae.

In order to preserve the gland for histologic examination, it is best to cut the pituitary gland after fixation.

Sheehan[12] described a method of removing the hypothalamus and the pituitary gland and its bony encasement in continuity, which may be required in certain special cases. Essentially the method consists of slicing off all the brain tissue except for the hypothalamus and pituitary gland which are left in situ. The block is lifted with the cavernous sinuses and posterior lining of the sella attached. A less drastic compromise method for greater preservation of the cerebral tissue is to remove frontal lobes only along the coronal plane at the level of the lamina terminalis and free the pituitary from the pituitary fossa by sharp dissection and, if necessary, with

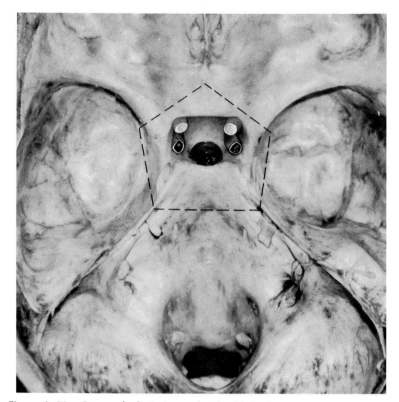

Figure 6–11. Removal of pituitary gland with its bony encasement. Pentagonal block is cut out along lines indicated, with saw blade directed roughly perpendicular to bone surfaces.

use of a small rongeur to chip some of the bones. The remainder of the brain removal technique is the same.

Because of the critical shortage of human growth hormone, it may be advisable to donate those pituitary glands which show no indication of pathologic alterations (see chapter 14). The National Pituitary Agency, Suite 503-7, 210 West Lafayette St., Baltimore, Md. 21201, should be contacted for further detail.

Paranasal Sinuses and Nasopharynx. Various paranasal sinuses can be entered intracranially for inspection or removal of specimens for histologic observation. The ethmoid sinuses can be approached by tearing down the cribriform plate with a chisel and mallet. By continuing the chiseling, the maxillary sinuses can be similarly entered. The frontal sinuses are entered by chiseling away their posterior walls close to the midline. The sphenoidal sinuses can be inspected after the anterior wall and the floor of the pituitary fossa have been chiseled away. If the block of bone containing the pituitary fossa is removed (Fig. 6–11) by using an oscillating saw, the sphenoidal sinuses are exposed even better. The nasopharynx and the throat can be entered by extending this dissection.

For more extensive removal of these structures, Szanto[17] described two methods that can be used for special cases. He also gave an excellent review of other approaches to the nasopharynx from the cranial cavity, the oral cavity, and the neck. Most of these techniques are obsolete, however, because of their disfiguring effects.

Ear. Even when there is no indication for removing the auditory and vestibular apparatus in one piece, it is still a good practice to look into the middle and inner ear, particularly in the presence of an inflammatory process within the cranial cavity. This can be done simply by the use of a large rongeur over the posterolateral portion of the petrous ridge. It often is possible to locate a primary focus of infection within the ear structures. When a total removal of the ear is indicated, our method of removal is identical or very close to that described in the pamphlet from the Temporal Bone Bank.[19] The use of an oscillating saw facilitates the procedure.

The cut is made along the lines indicated in Figure 6–12 *A*. The block of bone thus sectioned is lifted with a bone-holding forceps, and the connective tissue bands anchoring the block are cut with curved scissors. Violent use of chisel and hammer is to be avoided in freeing the temporal bone. Ligation of the internal carotid artery stump or, simpler still, plugging the stump with clay is helpful for the embalmer. Alternately, a bone-plug cutter attached to the vibrating saw (Fig. 6–12 *B*) can be used. The Temporal Bone Bank recommends the use of 20% formalin solution, approximately 400 ml, for fixation in a refrigerator for 1 day and fresh 10% formalin solution daily for 2 days. When placed in a refrigerator, the specimen can be saved indefinitely.

Eye. Removal of the eye can be accomplished intracranially or externally. The external method is carried out by cutting the conjunctival attachment to the bulb with scissors and severing all the attachments to the globe, including the optic nerve, posteriorly. This method, while simple, does not permit exposure of all the orbital content and its removal. Because of the limited amount of tissue removed, however, restoration is effected simply by insertion of a prosthesis (Fig. 6–13).

The intracranial approach is carried out by breaking and lifting the orbital plate by a chisel and hammer or an oscillating saw (Fig. 6–12 *C*). In this way, most of the orbital content can be visualized and removed when necessary. The freeing of the globe from the conjunctival attachment is done similarly with scissors but, in this approach, more care has to be exercised to avoid injury to the eyelid from behind. Some pathologists suggest that in many instances only the posterior half of the eyes need to be examined, but we disagree. There is no advantage in leaving the anterior half of the globe in the process. Since the eyelids are going to be closed by the embalmer, restoring the lost volume of the orbital content is simple, and much is gained by removing the globe in toto. Preliminary injection of 1 or 2 ml of 10% formalin solution into the eyeball through the sclera has been recommended.[18] Mayer[8] injects 10% formalin solution into the globe posterior to the insertion of the rectus muscles.

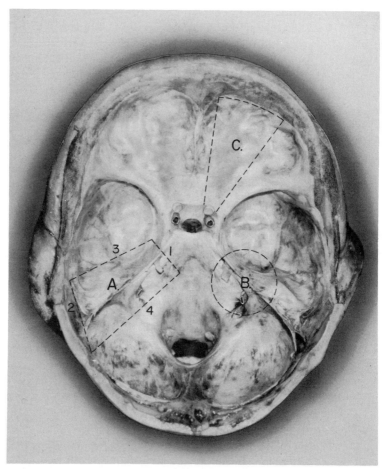

Figure 6–12.   Removal of inner and middle ear and eye. *A,* Line *1* is placed as near apex of petrous bone as possible, roughly at right angle to superior edge of petrous bone. Line *2* is over mastoid region, as close to lateral wall as possible. Line *3* is placed, with blade held vertical to floor of middle fossa, approximately 2.5 cm away from superior ridge of petrous bone. Line *4* is horizontal "undercut," blade being held as near floor of posterior fossa as possible. *B,* Circle indicates block to be removed with bone-plug cutter. *C,* Dotted lines indicate area of bone removal to approach orbital content intracranially.

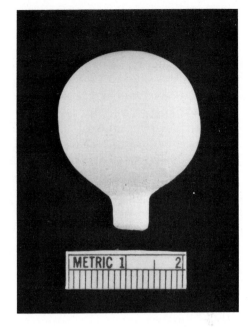

Figure 6–13. Prosthesis for eye, used to replace globe. It is made of "Coecal Buff" dental stone (Coe Laboratories, Inc., Chicago, Ill.) cast in a Silastic mold.

The removed eye is placed in a jar containing an ample amount of 10% formalin solution. There is no need to use cotton or any other material in the jar.

FIXATION

The best routine fixative which allows the widest choice of stains for the nervous tissue is formalin, usually as a 10% solution (see chapter 9).

Immersion Methods. For detailed anatomic studies of the nervous system it is best to fix the specimen, with a minimum of prior handling, in a large amount of freshly prepared 10% formalin solution. We use plastic buckets which hold 8 liters (see Fig. 13-1). (These are readily available at local stores at a considerably lower price than traditional glass or earthenware jars which, in addition, are heavier and more easily breakable.) The most commonly used method of suspension of the brain, to prevent distortion during fixation, is by a thread passed underneath the basilar artery in front of the pons. A minor degree of pulling of the vessel away from the brain substance is inevitable. If this is critical, as in the case of pontine infarcts and other lesions in this region, a thread can be passed under the internal carotid or middle cerebral arteries on both sides, provided, of course, that no pathologic lesions in this region are suspected.

If there is reason to object to these vascular suspension methods, the dorsal dura can be used as an anchoring point. A thread is passed through the short dural flaps on either side of the falx, and the brain is suspended right-side-up. However, minor degrees of pulling of the parasagittal brain tissue with a subsequent deformity (abnormally pointed dorsal midline surface of the brain) may occur by this method. Generally, the vascular suspension methods result in less parenchymatous deformity than the dural method in our experience. Also, accurate weighing of the brain is hindered at the time of autopsy by the latter method. While this method is seldom used by us, the brain may be suspended upside down with a pair of threads tied to the edge of the entire dorsal dural flaps on either side. Whatever the method used, the ends of the thread(s) are tied to the attachments of the bucket handle, care being taken not to allow the specimen to touch the bottom or sides of the bucket. Another safe method makes use of the plastic brain support described below for perfusion (Fig. 6–15). Placing several holes in the dome-shaped receptacle will ensure proper fixation of the contact surface of the brain. In order to avoid tipping over in the fixative, the plastic container may be suspended by four pieces of wire from the top of the bucket. It may also be provided with broad side flaps which are bent down to act as "legs" resting on the bottom of the bucket.

We do not recommend the method described in the AFIP manual,[22] in which a string is tied loosely around the midbrain. In fact, we do not approve of any method based on tying a thread around any portion of the brain substance, such as the stump of the medulla, nor do we find recommendable sectioning the corpus callosum for alleged improved entry of fixative into the ventricle.

Replacement of the formalin solution within the first 24 hours is desirable, particularly when the specimen is very bloody, but is not mandatory in our experience with the large amount of fixative we use. However, when the fixative becomes very bloody, prompt replacement with fresh solution prevents undue discoloration of the specimen.

The time required for complete or satisfactory fixation before dissection is approximately 10 to 14 days by this method. At earlier times there is a greater chance of finding the central portion of the specimen still pinkish in color, while the consistency may be satisfactory.

Perfusion Methods.   One may elect to perfuse the brain with fixative through the arterial stumps prior to further fixation by immersion as described above. This has the advantage of shortening the fixation time required and of ensuring adequate fixation of deeper portions of the brain. When it is necessary to dissect the brain at the time of autopsy, this preliminary perfusion fixation is helpful by increasing the consistency of the specimen for easier dissection and by decreasing the surface wrinkling and tissue warping which are inevitable.

Variable amounts of formalin solution can be injected. The larger the amount (for example, 1,000 ml), the better for quick fixation, but the brain is more likely to show both gross and microscopic artifacts when too much fluid is perfused. Large lakes of accumulated fluid, particularly in the areas weakened by a pathologic process (infarct, hemorrhage, metastasis), as well as asymmetry of the specimen due to uneven perfusion can result. Even without these gross distortions, one may see annoying perivascular zones of tissue rarefaction microscopically due to overperfusion, in addition to unnatural dilation of small blood vessels. Consideration also should be given to the possibility of obscuring or destroying any evidence of vascular occlusion by emboli or thrombosis. The weight changes induced by perfusion fixation are described in the Appendix.

In practice, injection of 150 ml of isotonic saline followed by 150 ml of 10% formalin solution, as suggested by Tedeschi,[18] causes the least problems. This can be accomplished by manual operation of a syringe connected to the tubing system (Fig. 6–14). For easy handling and better preservation of the contour of the specimen, we use a plastic holder and support (Fig. 6–15) during the procedure. Complete or satisfactory fixation for dissection can be obtained in 7 to 10 days. However, earlier dissection may be possible if one can tolerate some degree of incomplete fixation which is manifested mainly by central areas of softness and pink coloration.

For perfusion of a large amount of fixative, an embalmer's pump may be used (Fig. 6–16). For a simple gravity-feed method, one may use an infusion bottle raised 5 or 6 feet above the specimen.

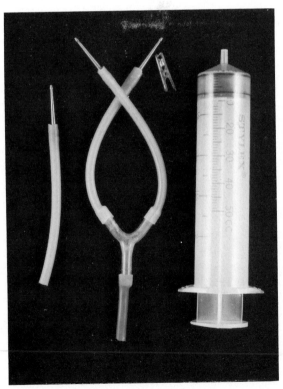

Figure 6–14. Simple manual perfusion fixation kit. The tubes of the double system are crossed over to make insertion into the carotid artery stumps easier. The single tubing is inserted into a vertebral artery, the contralateral artery being clamped. These two systems can be combined by a proximal glass Y-tube connection, but this combination will be more cumbersome to handle.

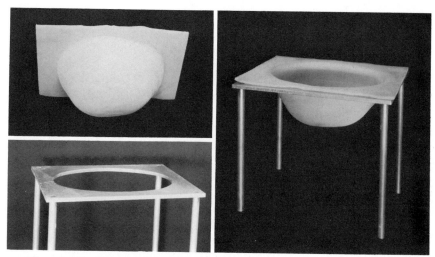

Figure 6–15.   Plastic support for brain (receptacle is 20 by 17 cm oval and 9 cm deep), for transportation and arterial perfusion (*Left Upper*) which in turn rests on metal support (*Left Lower*). *Right,* Complete unit.

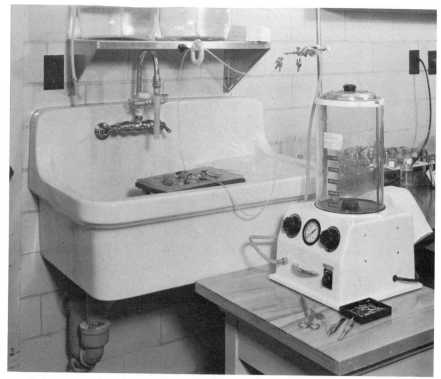

Figure 6–16.   Pressure embalming machine (Turner Co., Cedar Rapids, Ia.) used for perfusion of brain with large (1,000 to 2,000 ml) amount of 10% formalin solution after preliminary flushing with isotonic saline. For this purpose, lowest possible pressure is used. Note use of plastic support shown in Figure 6–15.

DISSECTION OF BRAIN AND SPINAL CORD

It is not necessary to use a very large knife to dissect the brain. We prefer an autopsy knife about 25 cm long and 2 cm wide.

Dissection of Fresh Brains. *In Adults.* While the most exacting examination of brain lesions in terms of anatomic correlation with clinical symptoms can only be achieved when the brain is sectioned after adequate fixation, at times the brain must be dissected in the fresh state, particularly when microbiologic and chemical investigations are of prime importance or when immediate diagnosis is absolutely necessary. (One price of this speed is the certain prospect of distortion of the cut surface during subsequent fixation.) As a compromise, we prefer to limit fresh dissection to three or four coronal cuts through the cerebral hemispheres, leaving more complicated anatomic structures such as the basal ganglia and upper brain stem (thalamus and midbrain) as undisturbed as the circumstances permit. This preliminary dissection usually reveals the presence of large lesions directly or indirectly by distortion of the ventricular system or other anatomic landmarks.

Further judiciously selected sections may be made into the primary slices of the brain tissue to expose the hidden but suspected lesions. The central portion of the cerebral hemispheres is left connected with the brain stem, and this block is suspended by a string as described above. It may be necessary to sever the brain stem and cut into the infratentorial structure; one horizontal cut through these structures usually suffices for preliminary examination. Even with more numerous cuts, one should not be satisfied solely with fresh dissection of the brain since many small lesions are easily missed and subtle lesions such as an early infarct, even though large, can be overlooked. Every brain should be reexamined with new dissection after adequate fixation.

Preliminary perfusion or cooling the brain, preferably in a contoured support as described above, in a refrigerator for about 30 minutes will afford an increased consistency to the brain and make regular dissection easier. The brain suspected of harboring diffuse, roughly symmetric lesions—as in lipidoses, "degenerative diseases," "dysmyelinating" disorders, other inborn or acquired toxic-metabolic diseases, or widespread infectious conditions—may be bisected along the sagittal plane, one half being further sectioned and submitted for chemical or microbiologic investigation while the other is retained for later sectioning and histologic examination. It is important that this latter half is fixed either by suspension or by letting it lie on its midsagittal plane to avoid undesirable distortions.

We find no use for the classical Virchow method of fresh dissection. Any brain subjected to this method would look, after adequate fixation, like a book immersed in water and subsequently dried.

In Fetuses and Infants. Fetal and infantile brains are best kept intact until after proper fixation because of their pronounced softness and ease of bruising unless there is an overriding necessity to secure unfixed specimens for chemical or microbiologic investigations. The method used by us is essentially similar to that described for adult brains. However, use of 10% formalin solution often does not afford a desirable degree of consistency to fetal or infantile brains. We find the use of a 20% formalin solution containing 1% glacial acetic acid quite satisfactory, without the additional measure of hardening such as provided by one or two changes of grades of alcohol as described in the AFIP manual.[22]

DISSECTION OF FIXED BRAIN

After a careful inspection of the external surface of the brain, the arteries at the base of the brain may be exposed through tears made into the arachnoid membrane and followed for a short distance distally to check for evidence of pathologic conditions such as thrombosis, embolism, or aneurysm. This procedure should be omitted when there is a possibility of disturbing pathologic processes which may be present in this region.

After adequate external examination, the first step is to separate the brain stem and the cerebellum from the cerebral hemisphere (Fig. 6–17). It is essential to section through the midbrain along a flat surface perpendicular to the neuroaxis. For this purpose, with the brain placed upside down, the scalpel is held in a pen-holding position with the right hand resting on the ventral aspect of the frontal lobes, to provide the proper angle. The blade is held toward the prosector with its tip in front of the cerebral peduncle a few millimeters above the tip of the mammillary body. After

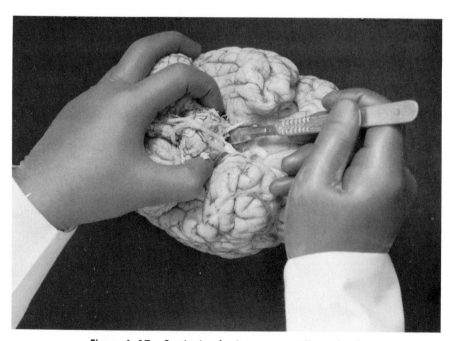

Figure 6–17. Sectioning brain stem at midbrain level.

stubbing into the midbrain, the blade is brought toward the prosector. It is then flipped over and moved forward along the same plane. The frequently used method of placing a knife over the temporal lobe and cutting into the midbrain from the side should be avoided since this will result in a roof-shaped midbrain. This makes the evaluation of midbrain deformity due to supratentorial processes difficult and its complete cross-sectional representation on histologic slides impossible. A gentle pull with the left hand on the brain stem and cerebellum during the procedure helps to complete the sectioning.

Attempts to sever the midbrain too rostrally often result in an uneven cut or in difficulty in cutting cleanly through because the cerebral peduncles widen rapidly in the rostral portion. In order to avoid this, one may place a preliminary section close to the pontoencephalic junction; then, under direct visualization, a parallel slice of the midbrain can be removed more rostrally.

The most commonly used method, and the safest for any contingencies, for dissection of the cerebral hemispheres is a coronal method. We prefer a free cutting method to that which relies on a cutting apparatus. Before making any sections, it is advisable to mark the central sulci by carefully cutting into the leptomeninges bridging over them with the tip of a scalpel blade, without injuring the underlying brain substance. This gives a valuable point of reference on multiple coronal sections. Alternative approaches to sectioning of the cerebral hemispheres are depicted in Figure 6–18.

As an initial step, we prefer placing the brain right-side-up, since this gives more stability to the specimen and therefore consistency to planes of section from case to case (Fig. 6–19). The dissection may be carried out with the frontal lobes either to the left or right of the prosector. Preoccupation with cutting a slice off with a single motion of the knife often results in cutting the specimen with undue pressure directed toward the cutting board, with little slicing motion and, consequently, squashing or tearing of various structures. The vessels are often dragged into the softer brain tissue. Multiple slicing excursions of the knife blade without undue pressure are more important in obtaining a clean cut surface. The preferred thickness of the slice is approximately 1 cm. It also is important to examine each new cut surface before the next slice is made so that any necessary adjustment can be made in the plan of dissection. The slices are displayed on the board, with the right side of the specimen on the right side of the prosector. This corresponds to viewing one's own brain from behind. This is also consistent with the pathologist's approach to the brain in the autopsy room, contrary to the clinician's approach to a living patient which is face to face. There should be no overlapping of the slices displayed, and this requires a relatively large cutting board. Sufficient space for display is mandatory for adequate examination of the brain.

There are several different approaches that can be used in routine dissection of the brain stem and cerebellum (Fig. 6–20).

The brain stem is best sectioned perpendicular to its axis, and consid-

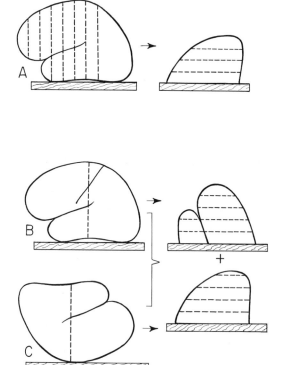

Figure 6–18. Schematic representation of various **coronal dissection methods for cerebral hemispheres.** *A,* Section starts from frontal lobes and is carried through parietal lobe, when remaining posterior portion is laid on board on its coronal cut surface to gain stability. Subsequent cuts are made parallel with the board, either from the dorsal (preferred personally) or ventral aspects (see Fig. 6–19). *B,* Initial cut is made through midpoint in precentral sulcus, and both halves are placed on the coronal surfaces for further dissection. *C,* Initial cut is placed through given structure at base of brain—for example, mammillary bodies. Subsequent procedure is same as in *B.*

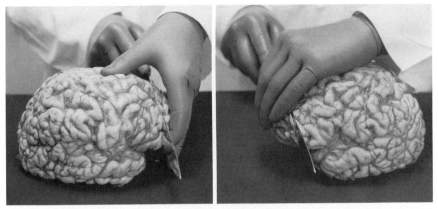

Figure 6-19. Sectioning of cerebral hemispheres. When freehand technique is used, frontal lobes can be directed either to left or right of prosector. In both methods, slice to be cut away should be supported by fingers of left hand to prevent "free-fall" of slice, which often results in uneven cut or inadvertent tear in structure.

eration should be given to the fact that it is slightly curved. Consequently, the plane of section should be adjusted. The cerebellum can be sectioned on horizontal planes or on planes perpendicular to the folial orientation, with the converging point in front of the cerebellum. The latter method gives the best histologic orientation of the cortical structures. A combination of both methods also can be used, as in *B* of Figure 6-20.

Display of the brain stem and cerebellum should be consistent with the principle used for the cerebral hemispheres. There are two options to achieve this end (Fig. 6-22). The choice between the two is largely individual and either method can be suitably used under different circumstances.

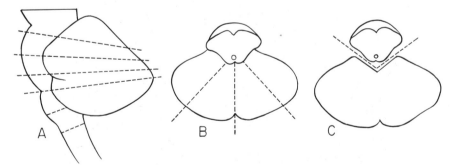

Figure 6-20. Approach to **routine dissection of brain stem and cerebellum.** *A,* Brain stem and cerebellum are dissected together by series of cuts roughly perpendicular to neuroaxis. For consistency, base line is made through pontomedullary junction and posterior ridges of cerebellar hemispheres. For actual cutting, see Figure 6-21 A. *B,* Midline incision is made in vermis, and wedge of tissue is removed from each cerebellar hemisphere. Hemispheres are further sectioned through vertical planes perpendicular to external lines of cerebellar cortex. Brain stem and rest of cerebellum are sectioned as in A. For actual cutting, see Figure 6-21 B. *C,* Cerebellum is separated from brain stem. Latter is sectioned as in A. Cerebellum is sectioned either horizontally or vertically as in *B.* For actual cutting, see Fig. 6-21 C.

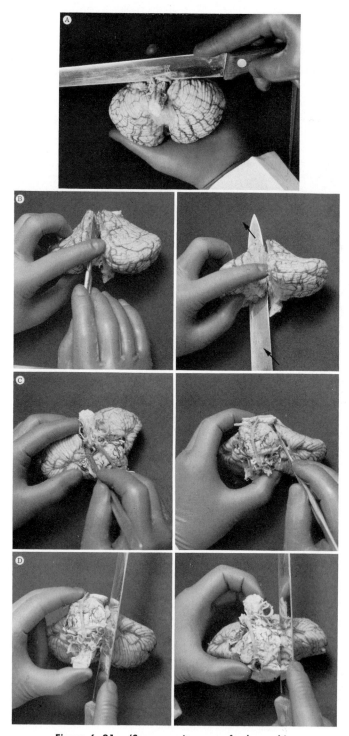

Figure 6–21.   (See opposite page for legend.)

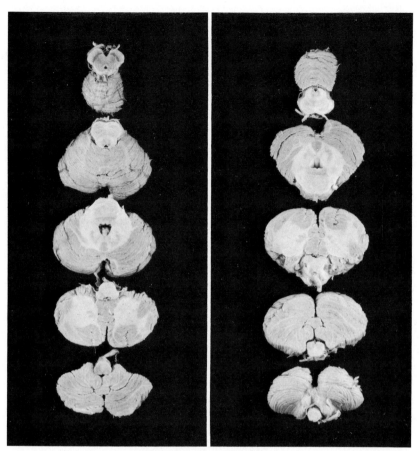

Figure 6–22. Display of brain stem and cerebellum. Slices can be displayed with either their rostral aspect (*Left*) or caudad aspect (*Right*) up. Display should be consistent with that of cerebral hemispheres, and right side of specimens should be on the prosector's right to avoid confusion.

Figure 6–21. Practical hints in dissecting brain stem and cerebellum. *A,* Primary horizontal plane is best made with tissue held in palm of left hand. Subsequent sections are made with tissue flat on board. *B,* Wedge removal method. *Left,* Midline incision is made into vermis with scalpel blade without cutting into floor of fourth ventricle. Then autopsy knife is inserted into fourth ventricle from below with blade tilted approximately 45° laterally; tip of knife should be placed just below inferior colliculi. *Right,* Wedge of tissue is cut out with movement of knife blade upward and outward (*arrows*). *C, Left,* Knife blade inserted from below to sever inferior cerebellar peduncle and lower half of middle cerebellar peduncle. Note pressure of forefinger holding medulla away from blade. *Right,* Then, blade is inserted from above to sever superior cerebellar peduncle and upper half of middle cerebellar peduncle. These two planes of section meet at very broad angle. *D,* Modification of method shown in C. Specimen is held right-side-up (*Left*) or upside-down (*Right*) and brain stem is cut off with single stroke of knife. Note that finger pressure holds medulla away from knife.

DISSECTION OF SPINAL CORD

For routine examination, series of cross sections are preferred. It is advisable to leave the dura intact in most instances to keep the spinal cord strung up. With a sharp scalpel blade, the spinal cord is sectioned approximately at 1.0-cm intervals. Occasionally, longitudinal sections can be made to emphasize the rostral, caudal extent of the lesion, such as in traumatic contusion. However, it often is difficult to get a straight plane of section. In most instances, the cross-sectional extent of the lesion at any given segmental level is more important in understanding the clinical symptoms. A combination of the two methods may be used by taking a cross-sectional slice at the point of maximal damage and slicing the rest longitudinally along the frontal plane.

SELECTION OF TISSUE BLOCKS
FOR HISTOLOGIC EXAMINATION

Brain. When the lesions are obvious, selection of the appropriate blocks for histologic examination is relatively simple. It is imperative to include some recognizable structures from the surrounding, presumably normal, areas. When there are no gross lesions despite the presence of clinical neurologic signs or symptoms, one must be familiar with the topographic distribution of the lesions expected in a given disease or syndrome to be able to select appropriate sections. There is no substitute for thorough familiarity with the clinical history of the patient and some basic knowledge of where the lesions are to be expected.

It is generally agreed that it is difficult to define what constitutes adequate selection of sections in "routine normal cases." There are no universally accepted standards to be followed, but it would be good practice to be consistent topographically for any given section. We have been choosing the areas shown in Figure 6–23 as more or less minimal requirements, and the reasons for such selection are given there. It is best to keep the whole brain until the microscopic examination is completed and the clinicopathologic correlation is made.

In most cases, the size of the sections can be limited to be suitable for the standard 1- by 3-inch glass slides. We have been using several different tissue capsules, as shown in Figure 6–24, for sections to be processed in an automatic processing machine.

One practical recommendation is to leave original brain slices as little "mutilated" as possible. If photographs are taken of cross-sectional surfaces, we prefer to take tissue blocks from the same surface of the adjoining slice since photography may have to be repeated. It also is recommended to partially slice the brain slab thinner up to the area of block removal and to use the knife blade to protect the lower half of the slab while the vertical cut is made into the upper slab. Alternately, if one is adept in cutting, complete thin slices can be made and laid on the cutting board before blocks are

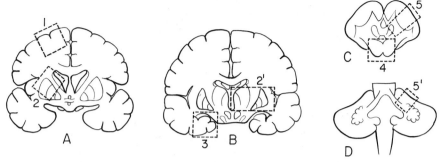

Figure 6–23. Selection of tissue blocks. *A*, 1 = Superior and middle frontal gyri. This is an arterial border ("watershed") zone most likely to harbor small ischemic lesions. This also may reveal atrophic or "senile" changes such as senile plaques or Alzheimer's neurofibrillary tangles. **2** = Basal ganglia. Vascular changes and their effects on parenchyma are likely to be found here, as are other "degenerative changes." ***B*, 2** = Basal ganglia together with thalamus. **3** = Hippocampus and adjacent neocortex. This is often a sensitive indicator of anoxic-ischemic changes. Alzheimer's tangles, senile plaques, and the "aging" changes make their first appearance here. ***C, D*, 4** = Pons. Vascular (particularly small arterial) changes are found more frequently here than in other portions of brain stem. **5, 5'** = Cerebellum. Ischemic and toxic metabolic conditions are often reflected in cerebellar cortex.

removed. It is not a good practice to hold a thick slab and to try to undercut a centrally located block through one of the vertical cuts, since this will invariably result in an uneven "dig" into the remaining tissue.

Peripheral Nerves.   The cervical and lumbar plexuses can be removed totally in continuity with the spinal roots and ganglia as outlined above for removal of the spinal cord, but this is somewhat time-consuming for the average autopsy.

A quicker method is to cut the nerves as they emerge from the intervertebral foramina and to sample selected nerves as the clinical signs dictate. Routinely, lengths of the sciatic and femoral nerves or any other portions of the lumbosacral plexuses proximal to their exits from the pelvic and abdominal cavities can easily be removed without creating new incisions. Similarly, sampling of the brachial plexuses and their distal extensions can be achieved from the supraclavicular axillary regions. Care should be exercised to preserve the brachial arteries for embalming.

In cases in which detailed clinical studies were performed on the peripheral nervous system, an effort should be made to secure the affected nerves at autopsy. This often requires additional sections in the extremities. When incisions are made in the extremities for sampling of muscles, as described in the next section, the nerves innervating them can be removed conveniently. In a diffuse neuropathic condition, one may select the sciatic nerve and its distal ramifications for detailed studies. In this case, the body is turned over and an incision is made in the back of the thigh to free the sciatic nerve which has been previously severed at its pelvic exit. The incision may be extended caudally to allow the removal of the peroneal and tibial nerves in the leg. More conservatively, a 15-cm longitudinal incision in the popliteal region exposes these nerves at their

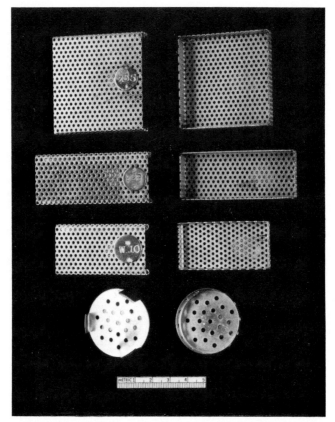

Figure 6–24. Tissue capsules. Various sizes of tissue capsules for use in automatic processing machine. Most sections can be made to fit in round cap, which is commercially available (Technicon Corp.). The lower three capsules are designed for tissues to fit on regular 1- by 3-inch histologic slides. Top one was prepared by our Engineering Department for larger sections.

bifurcation. Care should be exercised not to section the arteries in the vicinity so that embalming will not be interfered with.

One of the more easily accessible peripheral nerves is the sural nerve, which has been extensively studied clinically by means of biopsy. Therefore, its removal at autopsy through a small incision behind the lateral malleolus gives an excellent base for comparison. Details of the removal and fixation technique were described by Dyck and Lofgren.[5] The region close to the stump of the specimen should be avoided for histologic study because of severe crush artifacts frequently seen here. The fixative of choice for routine examination is 10% neutral formalin solution.

A useful adjunct to diagnostic studies of the peripheral nervous system is provided by a fiber-teasing method which has become a standard procedure in many research laboratories. After fixation, a portion of nerve is stained with 1% osmium tetraoxide and macerated in 60% glycerol, and individual fibers are teased out under a dissecting microscope. It is possible by this method to determine whether demyelination is segmental or wallerian in type. More recently, a modification of the teased-fiber technique which permits light and electron microscopic examination of isolated nerve fibers was described by Dyck and Lais.[4] Since prolonged fixation in formalin interferes with osmification, it is advisable to commence the procedure as soon as possible after preliminary fixation or to ship the specimens to a research laboratory equipped to handle them. For best preservation of the material, in these cases, autopsies should be performed no later than 6 hours after death.

Skeletal Muscle. In the absence of specific diseases affecting the neuromuscular system, histologic study of the skeletal muscle is often neglected. It is advisable to store or section at least one or two samples of skeletal muscle in the "routine" autopsy. The iliopsoas muscle is most easily accessible and offers an easy opportunity to see the effects of general systemic disease on the skeletal muscles.

In cases of known or suspected neuromuscular diseases, more extensive sampling is required. Adams et al[1] described sampling and subsequent methods of handling. In cases of primary myopathies, the selection has to be based on clinical findings and the status of the muscles at the time of autopsy. Sections should be taken from muscles that are severely affected, that show early but active involvement, and that are grossly uninvolved. Beckwith[2] presented a list of muscles to be sampled in cases of neurogenic muscle atrophy. Table 6–1 lists muscles which are relatively easily accessible without major procedures and will give a reasonably adequate diagnostic sampling.

The specimen should be cleanly excised or neatly trimmed to about 3.0 by 1.0 by 0.5 cm. Placing the specimens on a piece of cardboard does not completely prevent shrinkage of the tissue during fixation. A corkboard with two narrow strips of cork fastened to it provides ridges to which mul-

TABLE 6–1. SUGGESTED MUSCLES FOR SAMPLING AT AUTOPSY

Muscle	Comment
Extraocular muscles	Obtained through orbital plate intracranially or anteriorly with or without the globe
Tongue	Removed with pharyngeal and laryngeal tissues; small pieces can be removed through mouth
Sternocleidomastoid; diaphragm; pectoralis major	No new incision required; pectoralis major is preferred over deltoid due to possibility of previous intramuscular injections into deltoid
Biceps; triceps	Removed through incision in axillary aspect of upper arm or by subcutaneous extension of primary incision into arm
Forearm muscles	Skin incision for these is generally objected to by morticians, particularly in females; incision in ulnar side of palmar aspect of forearm is least objectionable
Intercostal; psoas major	No new incision required
Quadriceps	Removed through incision in ventral aspect of thigh
Anterior tibialis; gastrocnemius	Removed through incision in lateral aspect of lower leg

tiple muscle samples can be pinned. This eliminates the problem of poor fixation of the underside of the specimens. Pieces of wooden applicator stick may be used to support smaller pieces of muscle, which are tied to it with suture material at both ends. Although objected to by some, 10% neutral formalin solution is a most satisfactory all-purpose fixative, particularly if staining of the nervous tissue in the specimen is considered. Engel[6] recommended that additional pieces be fixed in Bouin's solution for a better result with trichrome stains and that fresh-frozen cryostat sections be made for Gomori's trichrome stain and for hematoxylin and eosin stain after 2 minutes' fixation in 10% formalin solution on a cover slip.

Teasing the removed specimens lengthwise after fixation, rather than cutting with a knife blade, sometimes produces a better longitudinal arrangement of the muscle on histologic slides. As with peripheral nerves, both cross and longitudinal aspects of the muscle should be represented.

SPECIAL TECHNIQUES

Postmortem Angiography.   The importance of adequate examination of the extracranial portions of the cerebral arteries has been recognized in recent years. The simplest method consists of injecting water through the proximal stumps to test patency. Since this test is significant only when there is a complete occlusion and gives no information when the vessels are merely narrowed, its usefulness is limited.

Many postmortem angiographic studies of cerebral arteries have been described.[15] Since we remove the neck vessels in all but a few cases, angiographic studies are not performed routinely. When indications for them do arise, we use a relatively simple technique. After the external carotid arteries are clamped, 5 to 10 ml of warmed barium sulfate-gelatin suspension[11] is injected into the common carotid arteries and roentgenograms are made in the autopsy room. The vertebral arteries can be injected similarly at their origins. A reverse method of injecting from the intracranial stumps of the internal carotid arteries also has been described.[3]

A method using a 40% solution of potassium iodide in Karo corn syrup, injected at approximately systolic pressure, was described.[14] The contrast medium temporarily distends the injected vessels and then dissipates rapidly, thereby not interfering with satisfactory embalming of the face and with proper evaluation of the arteries and brains by the pathologist.

For the opacification of the intracranial cerebral arteries, we prefer to inject them after removal of the brain, in a manner similar to that described by Wollschlaeger et al,[23] so that direct or indirect observation of the lesions can be made first. The medium we routinely use is barium-gelatin suspension, referred to previously, with or without addition of red or blue dye. When a cerebral aneurysm or vascular malformation is suspected but not immediately visualized by external inspection with careful washing out of the blood in the basal subarachnoid space, we prefer to inject the opacifying material before attempting to "dig out" the lesion. Often, successful roentgenographic demonstration (Fig. 6–25) of the lesion eliminates the necessity of excessive "picking" of the brain substance. After roentgenogra-

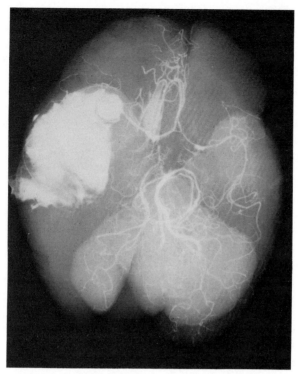

Figure 6–25. Usefulness of **postmortem angiography** is demonstrated by this case in which large temporal lobe hematoma is associated with ruptured saccular aneurysm of right middle cerebral artery at "trifurcation."

phic demonstration of these lesions, the brain is best left intact until adequate fixation is effected. We also have found postmortem angiography to be useful in cases of surgically treated vascular lesions—for example, clipping of an aneurysm—in order to demonstrate patency or obstruction of the vascular system beyond this point.

Venography. Injection of the venous system in situ or after removal of the brain appears to have little diagnostic use although its value in providing background information for neuroradiologists cannot be minimized. Particularly, studies of the deep cerebral venous system have been given increasing attention in recent years in association with the progress of clinical neuroradiology in demonstrating the fine vasculature of this system in life and in arriving at information of great localizing value. It mostly involves injection of radiopaque material into the straight sinus or vein of Galen, preferably before removal of the brain from the cranial cavity, through a burr hole. The external venous system of various cranial sinuses and the superficial cerebral veins can be readily examined directly.

Ventriculography. Outlining the ventricular system of the brain by injection of various materials has been attempted in the past mostly for preparation of anatomic specimens. Since correlation of the autopsy findings with those obtained by pneumoencephalography and ventriculography can be readily accomplished by a standard dissection, we have not found this casting method particularly useful in the practice of diagnostic neuropathology. Those who wish to make casts of the ventriculogram should consult Tompsett and Tedeschi.[20]

Removal of Neck Vessels. For fear of interfering with subsequent embalming, complete removal of the neck vessels is not often performed in the United States in "routine" autopsies or even when there is clinical evidence or demonstrable pathologic lesions of cerebrovascular disease. In our institution, it has been customary to remove the neck organs and arteries after the embalming procedure which is performed in rooms adjoining the autopsy room by private morticians. In some institutions, the common and internal carotid arteries are removed from the neck and a small rubber or plastic catheter is placed in the proximal external carotid artery[15] for subsequent embalming at funeral homes.

After the primary incision, the skin flap is reflected over the face, subcutaneous tissue being severed by blunt dissection with the aid of scissors. Keeping the neck straight or slightly overextended helps the approach to the arteries. The common carotid arteries are followed upward by blunt dissection, with occasional snips of scissors, up to the bifurcation. Then, the external and internal (medially located) arteries are isolated and the dissection is continued along the latter up to as close to the base of the skull as possible. The cavernous and petrous portions of the arteries are freed from the bony enclosure intracranially by chiseling or rongeuring the bone away. The carotid canal may be enlarged and the artery freed from the soft tissue in this region. This can be accomplished by removing a vertical strip of bone mesial to the canal and just above the entrance of the vertebral artery. This is preparatory for the complete removal of the latter. Use of an oscillating saw in part will facilitate the procedure. Then, the neck arteries can be pulled down from below.

Dissection of the vertebral arteries is a little more time-consuming.[13] First, the parts of the occipital and temporal bones above the lateral and posterior parts of the atlas are removed intracranially by chiseling along the line shown in Figure 6–26. We utilize the common bony defect for the intracranial freeing of the carotid and vertebral arteries. The posterior process of the superior articular surface of the atlas which hides the artery is chiseled away. The artery is then dissected free from the dura to the transverse process of the atlas. Second, in the neck (Fig. 6–27), the transverse foramina of the cervical spine up to the C3 level are opened with a chisel directed medially; the transverse processes are broken aside, exposing the vertebral artery. The chisel should now be directed upward and laterally to follow the course of the artery in C2. Because of the fibrous fixation of the artery to the transverse process of the atlas, the process is chiseled off medial to the artery and removed with the latter.

The removed arteries are examined either before or after adequate fixation. A method of perfusion of the neck arteries under constant pressure (120 to 150 mm Hg) was described by McCormick and Stein.[9] It was claimed that this method can preserve the vessels in the shape and degree of distention present in the systolic phase. Longitudinal sections of these vessels reveal the nature and extent of an atheromatous process, but the

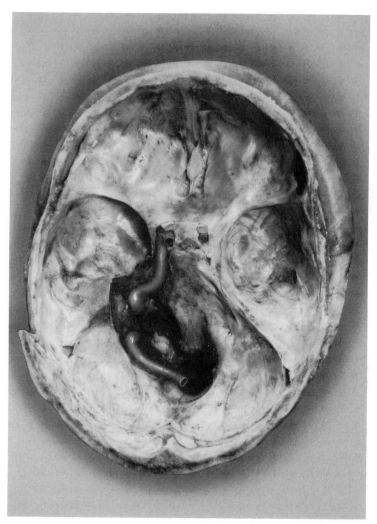

Figure 6–26. Intracranial freeing of internal carotid and vertebral arteries. Portion of basal cranial bones to be removed is shown. Horizontal portion of carotid artery is exposed first down to carotid canal. Latter is exposed along with entrance of vertebral artery.

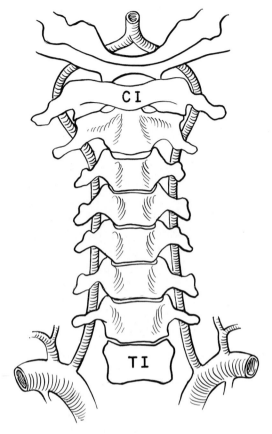

Figure 6–27. Course of vertebral arteries in neck.

degree of narrowing of affected arterial segments cannot be assessed by this method. Also, when the process is extensive, this method of opening will create artifactual fractures on the surface of plaques, and evaluation of the condition of the luminal surface will be difficult. Some of the more fragile atheromatous material will be lost. Of course, when occlusion is complete, this method of opening cannot be continued without destroying the pathologic process. To avoid these difficulties and to demonstrate the degree of luminal narrowing or the presence of thrombotic occlusion, the cross-sectional method is preferred. In general, routine use of the cross-sectional method causes less regret.

REFERENCES

1. Adams RD, Denny-Brown D, Pearson CM: Diseases of Muscle: A Study in Pathology. Second edition. New York, Hoeber Medical Division, Harper & Row, 1962
2. Beckwith JB: Sampling of muscle at autopsy in cases of lower motor neuron disease. Am J Clin Pathol *42*:92–93, 1964
3. Choi SS, Crampton A: Atherosclerosis of arteries of neck: postmortem angiographic and pathologic study. Arch Pathol *72*:379–385, 1961

4. Dyck PJ, Lais AC: Electron microscopy of teased nerve fibers: method permitting examination of repeating structures of same fiber. Brain Res *23*:418–424, 1970

5. Dyck PJ, Lofgren EP: Method of fascicular biopsy of human peripheral nerve for electrophysiologic and histologic study. Mayo Clin Proc *41*:778–784, 1966

6. Engel AG: Personal communication

7. Kernohan JW: Removal of the spinal cord by the anterior route: a new postmortem method. Am J Clin Path *3*:455–458, 1933

8. Mayer LL: Autopsy of the eye. Am J Ophthalmol *53*:681–683, 1962

9. McCormick WF, Stein BM: Technique for study of extracranial arteries. Arch Pathol *74*:52–56, 1962

10. McGarry P: A quick, simple method of removal of the spinal cord. Arch Pathol *83*:333–335, 1967

11. Schlesinger MJ: New radiopaque mass for vascular injection. Lab Invest *6*:1–11, 1957

12. Sheehan HL: Neurohypophysis and hypothalamus. *In* Endocrine Pathology. Edited by JMB Bloodworth Jr. Baltimore, Williams & Wilkins Company, 1968, pp 12–74

13. Solberg LA: A method for postmortem dissection of the vertebral arteries. World Neurol *3*:765–768, 1962

14. Stein BM, McCormick WF, Rodriguez JN, Taveras JM: Radiography of atheromatous disease involving the extracranial arteries as seen at postmortem. Acta Radiol [Diagn] (Stockh) *1*:455–467, 1963

15. Stein BM, Svare GT: A technic of postmortem angiography for evaluating arteriosclerosis of the aortic arch and carotid and vertebral arteries. Radiology *81*:252–256, 1963

16. Stowens D: Pediatric Pathology. Second edition. Baltimore, Williams & Wilkins Company, 1966, pp 12–14

17. Szanto PB: A modified technic for the removal of the nasopharynx and accompanying organs of the throat. Arch Pathol *38*:313–320, 1944

18. Tedeschi CG: Neuropathology: Methods and Diagnosis. Boston, Little, Brown and Company, 1970

19. Temporal Bone Banks Program for Ear Research: Technique for acquiring and preparing the human temporal bone for the study of middle and inner ear pathology. Trans Am Acad Ophthalmol Otolaryngol *70*:871–878, 1966

20. Tompsett DH, Tedeschi CG: Museum preparations of brain and spinal cord. *In* Neuropathology: Methods and Diagnosis. Edited by CG Tedeschi. Boston, Little, Brown and Company, 1970, pp 419–449

21. Towbin A: Neonatal neuropathologic examination. *In* Neuropathology: Methods and Diagnosis. Edited by CG Tedeschi. Boston, Little, Brown and Company, 1970, pp 215–224

22. US Department of Defense. Army Department: Autopsy Manual. Washington DC, US Government Printing Office, 1960

23. Wollschlaeger G, Wollschlaeger PB, Lucas FV, Lopex VF: Experience and result with postmortem cerebral angiography performed as routine procedure of the autopsy. Am J Roentgenol Radium Ther Nucl Med *101*:68–87, 1967

CHAPTER 7

SKELETAL SYSTEM

DISSECTION AND REMOVAL OF BONE SPECIMENS

Routine preparation of gross and microscopic bone specimens can be carried out only on a limited scale. However, portions of rib with costochondral junction, sternum, vertebral body or iliac crest, and sternoclavicular joint should be removed and permanently saved in every autopsy. Specimens suggested for study in cases of metabolic or other systemic bone and joint diseases are indicated below. The site of a circumscribed neoplastic or inflammatory bone lesion can be determined from clinical or roentgenologic examination. Circumscribed osteolytic processes in the ribs or in the calvarium can often be identified by viewing these specimens against a bright light.

Specimens consisting of both bone and soft tissue may be difficult to prepare for satisfactory preservation. The best method is to freeze the fixed specimen and to cut the solidly frozen tissue with a band saw. The sliced specimen is placed in a tank of alcohol. The layer, on the cut surface, of frozen fat and sawdust is removed with a brush or will float off spontaneously. The alcohol treatment will also restore the color in specimens fixed in Kaiserling I solution.[1]

Sawing. At one time, the handsaw, hammer, and chisel were the only tools available and, although considerable skill and effort are needed, they permit preparation of excellent specimens.

Oscillating Saws. We use a Stryker autopsy saw (Stryker Corporation, Kalamazoo, Mich.). The blade of this saw cuts bone by high-speed oscillation. Blades of various shapes with round cutting edges can be attached to the arbor, depending on the size and location of the bone specimens to be removed.

For the anterior removal of the spinal column (see page 162), Stryker's reciprocating saw with a straight blade is preferred. This saw cuts to a depth of 7.6 cm. Blades of special lengths are available.

Another useful electric autopsy saw with various types of extra blades

195

is produced by the Lipshaw Manufacturing Company (Lipshaw electric autopsy saw no. 450; 7446 Central Ave., Detroit, Mich.). This model has an adjustable guide attached to the handpiece, which controls the depth of the saw cut. A heavy-duty motor is separated from the instrument by a cable (the Stryker saw has the motor in the handpiece) and is turned on and off with a foot switch.

Temporal bones are removed with a trephine (Schuknecht temporal trephine, Stryker Corporation). According to the specifications, this trephine cuts about 4.5 cm deep and removes a specimen about 3.7 cm in diameter.

A disadvantage of oscillating saws is the production of bone dust, both in the air and in the structures of the cut surface. Inhalation can be prevented by wearing a mask or by using Stryker's bone-dust collector which can be attached to the autopsy saws. Bone dust on the cut surface can in part be brushed off, but histologic sections must be from deep within the block to avoid the dust particles.

All oscillating saws become hot after prolonged use. Occasional greasing of the moving parts is advisable.

Band Saws. Band saws are required if one wishes to prepare even sections through large bones such as the femur or the spinal column. They also are preferred for cutting small specimens into thin slices for histologic preparations. For years we used a large "Jim Vaughan" band saw (electric meat, fish, and bone cutter, Jim Vaughan Company, 739-740 Franklin Street, Chicago, Ill.), but we have had equally good results with a smaller model (Craftsman; Sears Roebuck and Co.). Dorfman[5] uses a large (254.0 to 355.6 mm) metal-cutting band saw with a speed of about 610 cm/sec and also a smaller variable-speed scroll saw for finer control with more delicate specimens.

Preparation of Histologic Specimens. To achieve optimal fixation with minimal exposure to decalcifying agents, bone specimens for histologic study should not be thicker than 3 mm. However, bone dust from sawing may have been ground into all levels of such a specimen, so that somewhat thicker sections may be required. Thin sections are easier to prepare with a band saw, which also grinds less bone dust into the section than does an oscillating saw. Brushing and flushing of the cut surfaces with saline and submerging the specimen in alcohol help to remove superficial bone dust. Excellent results can also be achieved by freezing the specimens in water and then sawing them in a solid block of ice until pieces of the desired shape and thickness are obtained. The plane of the saw sections will usually be perpendicular to articular, periosteal, or other surfaces.

Sampling Procedures. *Ribs.* These are sawed with a band saw, usually in a horizontal plane. The section should include costal cartilage, costochondral junction, and bony rib.

Sternum. A sagittal midline slice through the manubrium is usually saved. Fragments of bone marrow can be dug out with a sturdy knife. These fragments should contain only cancellous bone so that minimal decalcification time is required.

Vertebrae. We prepare a sagittal saw section through the center of a vertebra after the anterior half of the spinal column has been removed for exposure of the spinal cord. Intervertebral disk tissue should be part of the slice selected for histologic study, particularly in the presence of degenerative diseases, ochronosis, or ankylosing spondylitis. In this latter condition, costovertebral and costotransverse joints should be included.

Iliac Crest. This site is particularly recommended for the study of metabolic bone disease. A slice of iliac crest tissue can easily be removed with an oscillating hand saw. The plane of sawing should be perpendicular to the iliac crest surface.

Calvarium. This is an important bone to study in metabolic bone diseases, neoplastic involvement (myeloma, metastatic carcinoma, and histiocytosis), and certain hemolytic anemias (thalassemia). A strip of calvarium should be removed so that it includes the external and internal tables and the diploë.

Bones of Extremities. Removal of the femur requires a long lateral skin incision. The knee joint is exposed by flexing the knee and cutting the quadriceps tendon, the joint capsule, and the cruciate ligaments. The muscular attachments are dissected from the shaft of the femur, starting at the distal end and continuing toward the hip. The capsule of the hip can be palpated and then incised by flexing and rotating the femur.

If only the femoral head, neck, and trochanter region are needed, essentially the same procedure is used except that the femoral shaft is sawed off about 10 cm below the trochanter major.

The upper femoral shaft and the bone marrow in this region are usually exposed from an anterolateral incision. A 5-cm portion of the anterior half of the femoral shaft is then removed with an electric saw. The continuity of the bone can thus be preserved.

The humerus can be dislocated anteriorly in the humeroscapular joint. In this way the muscle attachments of the proximal humerus can be dissected away from the whole circumference of the bone without additional skin incisions. The upper shaft of the humerus is then exposed and sawed off. For removal of the complete bone, a skin incision down to the elbow is necessary.

The bones of the distal extremities, particularly of the hands and feet, should be exposed from the plantar surfaces.

DISSECTION AND REMOVAL OF JOINTS

The best joint sections are prepared by shelling out the whole joint and sawing across the proximal and distal bones, staying far enough from the joint space so as not to cut into the joint capsule. The whole specimen is then sawed, usually in the frontal plane. Good saw sections should include articular cartilage, synovium, meniscus, capsule, epiphysis, metaphysis, and a small portion of diaphysis of the adjacent long bones.

Complete removal and sectioning of the intact joint might be impractical because of the size of the specimen, prosthetic problems, or legal reasons. In these instances the joint space can be exposed and specimens of articular cartilage with adjacent bone, joint capsule, synovium, and disks or meniscus can be excised for histologic study. The joint space can be palpated, incised, and exposed by bending the joint in the direction opposite to the site of the intended incision.

In the presence of infectious arthritis, both exudate and synovial tissue should be cultured (see page 214).

For the identification of crystals in gout and pseudogout,[11] a small drop of synovial fluid or exudate is placed, with a 1-mm bacteriologic wire loop, on a clean glass slide and is immediately covered. The cover slip is rimmed with clear nail polish to prevent the specimen from drying. The crystals can be analyzed with the polarizing microscope.

Sternoclavicular Joints.   These joints are easily accessible and should be saved routinely. Study of them is recommended in all cases of rheumatoid arthritis and related diseases.[14] The area around the joint is freed from soft tissue. The sternum is split in the midline and halfway across the side where the joint is to be removed. This cross section is made about 1 cm below the level of the joint. The clavicle is sawed apart about 1 cm lateral from the joint space. The specimen is now sawed with a band saw in a horizontal plane to expose the joint spaces and disks.

Acromioclavicular and Humeroscapular Joints.   These can be reached and excised from the conventional skin incisions.

Laryngeal Joints.   These, and particularly the cricoarytenoid joint, are very useful in the study of rheumatoid arthritis and related diseases. Good sections of these small joints can be prepared by sausaging the formalin-fixed larynx into 3- to 5-mm parallel slices. The cricoarytenoid joint is found at or just beneath the level of the vocal cords.

BONE MARROW PREPARATIONS

Sections.   Sections of sternum, vertebrae, and iliac crest usually show abundant red bone marrow. Good fixation is essential—for instance, in Zenker's fixative containing 10% glacial acetic acid.

Excellent bone marrow preparations can be made by injecting, shortly after death, 10 ml of Zenker-formic acid (see page 236) into the sternum. The fixative is injected slowly and the marrow is infiltrated from two puncture sites which should be about 4 cm apart.[10] At the time of the autopsy the marrow is removed and embedded in the usual manner. Obviously, other sites and other fixatives also can be used.

Exposure to decalcifying agents should be kept at a minimum by careful end-point determination (see below) or can even be avoided altogether if marrow can be squeezed out from cancellous bone fragments. Such fragments can be dug out, with a sturdy knife, from the vertebral bodies or sternum. Marrow also can be squeezed from ribs with a pair of pliers.

Smears.   Despite suggestions to the contrary,[8] it is often possible to obtain well-preserved smear preparations of bone marrow as well as of the spleen and lymph nodes. Best results are usually obtained when the post-mortem period is less than 3 hours.[8] However, cellular detail is occasionally retained up to 15 hours after death. We use a stronger solution of Wright's stain (0.6%) than is ordinarily used. Smears are made in the usual way.

PROSTHESES

Skeletal contours and continuity of tubular bones or of the spinal column must be restored at the end of the autopsy. An assortment of wooden prostheses should be available for insertion in place of the removed bone. A simple substitute is a wooden rod with two nails sticking out at both ends. The heads of the nails are first sawed off and then inserted into the wooden rod. The tips of the nails are than driven into the proximal and distal portions of the bone. Complete segments of the spinal column can be replaced by prostheses of this kind. Wooden spokes may serve this purpose. The technique and tools for this procedure have been described in detail by Selin et al.[13] For replacing the hip, angular metal rods are useful. Plaster of Paris provides a good prosthesis for the calvarium. Simple wood dowels or plastic tubing is recommended as replacement for bones and joints of the fingers and toes.

DECALCIFICATION PROCEDURES

Decalcification is required for preparing histologic sections of bone, dentin, cementum, calcified vessels, and calcifications in lesions such as granulomas and tumors. Much of the following is taken from the excellent book on decalcification techniques by Brain.[3]

Acid decalcifying agents are used alone (nitric, hydrochloric, trichloroacetic, formic, phosphoric, picric, sulfurous, or acetic acid) or as mixtures—for example, nitric or hydrochloric acid with alcohol, potassium alum, or sodium chloride solution. The most important complexing agent is ethylenediaminetetraacetate (EDTA); these compounds also work in neutral or alkaline solutions (see below). Commercially available decalcifying fluids include Cal-Ex (Fisher Scientific Company) and Decal (distributed by Scientific Products). These decalcifying fluids act most rapidly. Exact endpoint determination is essential because staining properties will be lost if fluid is not washed out immediately after decalcification is completed.

Decalcification time depends on numerous factors such as the size and texture of the specimen, the type and temperature of the solution, and the use of agitation and electrolysis. A small specimen in an acid bath which is exposed to the heat and agitation of the Autotechnicon will be decalcified in little more than 2 hours[7]; a protective acid-resistant insert must be used. The speed of decalcification can also be increased by electrolysis. The specimen is placed in acid decalcifying fluid with platinum electrodes; the acid serves as the electrolyte. Ultrasound will also increase the speed of decalcification; in this method, 4N formic acid is used as decalcifying fluid.

To achieve histologic slides of the best quality, the decalcification process should not be unnecessarily prolonged. Piercing or bending the specimens usually permits one to judge roughly when decalcification is complete. Another indicator is the decrease or disappearance of CO_2 bubbles from the specimen. There are many qualitative and quantitative chemical (titration) methods for end-point determination of decalcification.[3]

> (*Example of chemical end-point determination.*[9]) Draw approximately 5 ml of decalcifying fluid (from bottom of container) which has been in contact with the tissue for 6 to 12 hours. Add 5 ml each of 5% ammonium hydroxide and 5% ammonium oxalate. Mix and let stand for 15 to 30 minutes. A cloudy or milky solution, caused by precipitation of calcium oxalate, indicates that the specimen is not thoroughly decalcified. The decalcifying solution should be changed and the test repeated at a later time until the precipitate oxalate does not form. This test can be performed as frequently as necessary.

Serial roentgenograms permit the most precise control of the decalcification process. For small specimens, dental films can be used.

Nitric Acid Decalcification.[3]   The decalcifying fluid is a mixture of 63 ml of concentrated nitric acid (sp. g., 1.42; 70% w/w) and 937 ml of water. For very fatty bone specimens, the water can be replaced by 95% alcohol.

1. Minimize the thickness of the specimen and, whenever possible, keep it less than 3 mm.

2. Into a 250-ml flask with a wide neck, insert a piece of lint so that it covers the bottom of the flask.

3. Place the specimen on top of the lint. Add 200 ml of the decalcifying fluid (1 part of bone to 50 to 100 parts of acid is the suggested ratio). Seal the flask with tinfoil or plug it with cotton wool. The temperature of the solution should be maintained between 18 and 22 C.

4. Do not change the fluid. Gently agitate it by hand for a few seconds, two or three times a day.

5. Follow the progress of demineralization by using a chemical method or roentgenography.

6. On completion of decalcification, pour off the decalcifying fluid. Carefully place the specimen in a processing basket. Transfer the identification tag and insert a cork into the open end of the basket.

7. Wash the acid from the tissues by floating the basket in a beaker containing 500 ml of water. Change the water at least four times at 1-hour intervals or until the washing fluid is about pH 7.0. Alternatively, place the basket in a pipet washer and wash in water continuously for 2 to 4 hours depending on the thickness of the specimen.

Ethylenediaminetetraacetate Decalcification.[3]   To make the decalcifying solution, add 100 gm of ethylenediaminetetraacetate disodium salt (EDTA, Versene, Sequestrene) to approximately 600 ml of water and then add 280 ml of 1N sodium hydroxide solution so that, when all of the solid has dissolved, the resulting solution is at pH 7.4 Dilute to 1 liter.

1. Minimize the thickness of the specimen and, whenever possible, keep it less than 3 mm.

2. Into a 250-ml flask with a wide neck, insert a piece of lint so that it covers the bottom of the flask.

3. Place the specimen on top of the lint. Add 200 ml of the decalcifying fluid. Seal the flask with tinfoil or plug it with cotton wool. Decalcification may be carried out at a temperature between 5 and 60 C.

4. Do not change the fluid. Gently agitate it by hand for a few seconds, several times each day.

5. Follow the progress of demineralization with roentgenograms.

6. On the completion of decalcification, pour off the decalcifying fluid and carefully place the specimen in a processing basket. Transfer the identification tag and insert a cork into the open end of the basket.

7. Wash the tissue by immersing the basket in a beaker containing 500 ml of water. Change the water three or four times at intervals of 1 hour. Alternatively, place the basket in a pipet washer and wash continuously for 2 to 4 hours depending on the thickness of the specimen.

Decalcification by Formic Acid-Ion Exchange Resin.[9] The formic acid solution is 10.0 ml of 90% formic acid plus 90.0 ml of distilled water. To each 100 ml of this solution add 10.0 gm of a strong cationic exchange resin such as Ionac C-242 or Dowex 50-X8.* Place the specimen into this decalcifying fluid. The ion exchange resins have no deleterious effects after the decalcification is completed. It is preferable to change solutions daily. If speed is essential the solution can be warmed but to not more than 40 C. Wash the specimen thoroughly after decalcification.

PREPARATION OF UNDECALCIFIED SECTIONS

The preparation of undecalcified bone sections has been improved greatly in recent years, mainly prompted by the use of tetracycline as a bone-labeling agent. With experience, beautiful sections of cortical and cancellous bone can be prepared with this technique. Bean and Banks[2] described an elegant method which requires, for fixed specimens, only about 1 week. The dehydrated specimens are embedded in Paraplast, a purified paraffin plastic embedding medium (Aloe Scientific Company). Sections are cut with a Jung model "K" motorized sliding microtome. A Jung no. 3 or no. 4 knife is used.

MACERATION OF BONE

Maceration of bone yields instructive specimens which are esthetically satisfying and of unlimited durability.

---

* Ionac is available from A. H. Thomas Company, P.O. Box 779, Philadelphia, Pa. Dowex is available from any distributor of J. T. Baker Chemical Company products or from Lapine Scientific Company, 6001 S. Knox Avenue, Chicago, Ill.

The specimens shown in Figures 7–1, 7–2, 7–3, and 7–4 were prepared by the antiformin maceration technique.[4]

Method of Antiformin Maceration. 1. Clean attached soft tissues mechanically from bone (avoid knife marks).

2. Immerse specimen in a glass jar with 3% anti-formin solution.* Place the jar in an incubator (embedding oven) at 70 to 80 C for 3 to 4 hours. The time of incubation may be less with small or more with large specimens.

3. Decant antiformin and flush specimen with hot water. The remaining fragments of soft tissue are removed by blowing compressed air through the specimen and by scratching them from the surface of the bone with a knife. Occasionally, the specimen has to be incubated again in 1 or 2% antiformin. Check the progress every 30 minutes. Repeat step 3.

4. Bleach bone with 3% hydrogen peroxide solution in an incubator at 70 to 80 C. Bleaching time is 12 to 24 hours. Flush in hot water.

5. Place specimen on cotton and dry at room temperature.

6. Place specimen in ether for about a week. This is to remove fat which has remained in the bone. The duration of ether treatment depends on the amount of fat in the tissue. Subsequently, the specimen is air dried.

---

* (1) Antiformin stock solution: sodium hypochlorite, 10% solution, 1,400 ml; distilled water, 1,400 ml; potassium hydroxide, 45% (w/w), 4,200 ml. For maceration of bones, 1, 2, and 3% dilutions of this stock solution are prepared. (2) Antiformin stock solution after Edwards and Edwards:[6] sodium hydroxide, 15%, 1 part; chlorinated soda, 1 part (150 gm of sodium carbonate, 100 gm of calcium hypochlorite, and 1,000 ml of distilled water). For maceration of fresh bones, 10% dilutions of this stock solution are prepared.

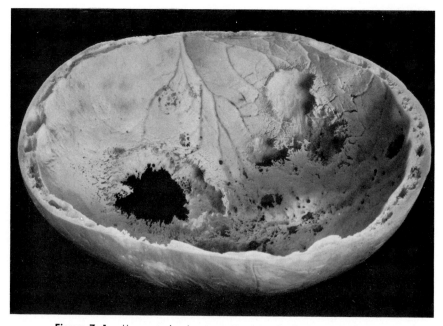

Figure 7–1. Macerated calvarium. (Courtesy Prof. Dr. E. Uehlinger.)

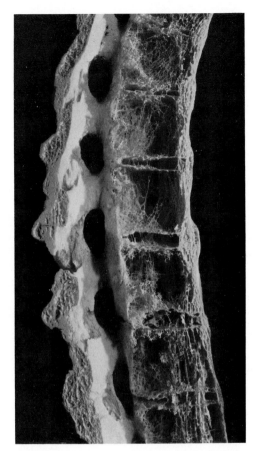

Figure 7-2. Macerated spine, sagittal section. (Courtesy Prof. Dr. E. Uehlinger.)

Specimens can also be degreased with carbon tetrachloride or tetrachlorethylene. These are excellent fat solvents. Beware of the vapors; they are very toxic.

Other Methods. Maceration also can be achieved by prolonged putrefaction, by treatment with 0.25N NaOH at 90 C, or by autoclaving with 1N NaOH.[12] Repeated checking and mechanical removal of soft tissues are essential in all methods.

A slow but safe method is to boil the specimen until only the bone is left. This method is particularly recommended if one is dealing with a very valuable specimen.

Enzymatic maceration[6] is carried out with 0.1% papain in isotonic saline. The specimen is incubated for 24 hours at 37 C, washed, and bleached in hydrogen peroxide.

For Study of Exhumed Bones. Boiling is the method of choice. Maceration may permit otherwise unobtainable diagnoses, not only in medicolegal autopsies on bodies that had been buried for months and years but also for historic and prehistoric material. For instance, Ullrich von Hutten (a knight, revolutionary, and poet, 1488 to 1523) was thought to have suf-

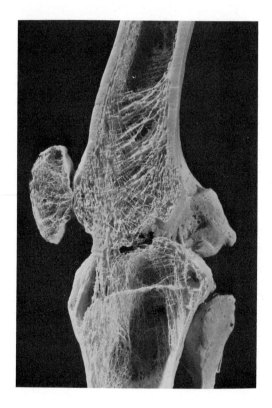

Figure 7–3. Macerated knee joint, sagittal section. (Courtesy Prof. Dr. E. Uehlinger.)

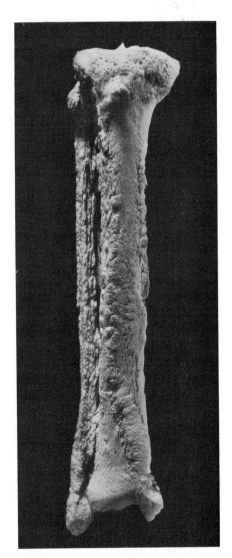

Figure 7–4. Macerated tibia and fibula. (Courtesy Prof. Dr. E. Uehlinger.)

fered from syphilis of the skeletal system. Uehlinger[15] macerated the disinterred bones and concluded that the unfortunate rebel had polyostotic sclerosing osteomyelitis, not syphilis.

REFERENCES

1. Baker SL: A freezing method for preparing museum specimens composed of bone and soft tissue. J Tech Methods 20:42–47, 1940
2. Bean DA, Banks HA: A rapid technic for the preparation of large microscopic sections of decalcified and undecalcified bone. Am J Clin Pathol 48:277–280, 1967
3. Brain EB: The Preparation of Decalcified Sections. Springfield, Illinois, Charles C Thomas, Publisher, 1966
4. Bürgi J: Personal communication
5. Dorfman H: Pathology of Arthritis and Rheumatic Diseases. Syllabus of Short Course, International Academy of Pathology, San Francisco, California, 1969
6. Edwards JJ, Edwards MJ: Medical Museum Technology. London, Oxford University Press, 1959
7. Glenn GC, Davis CJ Jr: Decalcification of bone in 2 hours with the Autotechnicon. Am J Clin Pathol 48:363–364, 1967
8. Jeanneret H: La moelle osseuse en clinique et à la salle d'autopsie: Etude comparative. Schweiz Med Wochenschr 70:351–357, 1940
9. Luna LG: Hints on Histologic Technic. Short course, International Academy of Pathology, St. Louis, Missouri, 1970
10. Oettgen HF: Zur methodischen Verbesserung der morphologischen Knochenmarksuntersuchung an der Leiche. Zentralbl Allg Pathol 94:232–236, 1955
11. Phelbs P, Steele AD, McCarty DJ Jr: Compensated polarized light microscopy: identification of crystals in synovial fluids from gout and pseudogout. JAMA 203:508–512, 1968
12. Pulvertaft RJV: Museum techniques: a review. J Clin Pathol 3:1–23, 1950
13. Selin G, Schlyen S, Jaffe HL: Vertebral column: methods for removal, reconstruction, and gross sectioning. Arch Pathol 55:245–252, 1953
14. Sokoloff L, Gleason IO: The sternoclavicular articulation in rheumatic diseases. Am J Clin Pathol 24:406–414, 1954
15. Uehlinger E: Personal communication

CHAPTER 8

SPECIAL METHODS

With C. Terrence Dolan, Arnold L. Brown, Jr.,
and Jack L. Titus

AUTOPSY MICROBIOLOGY

By C. Terrence Dolan

   Obtaining Specimens.   The accuracy of any microbiologic study depends on starting with a proper specimen. For example, one might receive a lymph node specimen which the histologic report describes as containing caseating granuloma but which grossly is only adipose tissue; a microbiologic study of such a specimen probably would be fruitless. It is the responsibility of the pathologist to send a specimen which is representative of the lesion and which, if possible, is taken aseptically. When the presence of infection is strongly suspected, the entire specimen might be sent to the microbiology laboratory where a proper sample for microbiologic study can be removed aseptically, and then the remainder can be returned to the autopsy pathologist for histologic sections.
   It is generally thought that cultures of embalmed tissue are useless. Weed and Baggenstoss[60] carried out a microbiologic study of such tissue and were able to isolate several pathogens. Clearly, embalming bodies prior to autopsy studies will decrease the probability of but not entirely prevent isolating microorganisms.
   If the lesion is large, several specimens should be taken from various areas because the organisms may not be evenly distributed throughout the lesion.[59] Specimens should be taken from the walls of abscesses as well as from the necrotic debris in the center of the lesion. Tuberculoma-like lesions should be sampled from the center of the caseation as well as from the granulomatous wall. If "sulfur granules" are found in pus, they should be carefully washed in sterile beef heart infusion broth to remove any as-

207

sociated organisms. One portion of the granule is crushed on a slide for Gram and acid-fast stains and the other portion is cultured.

Direct smears should be made, especially of specimens which have been inadvertently contaminated at the autopsy table. These are stained with Gram's, Grocott's modification of Gomori's methenamine-silver, and Kinyoun's acid-fast stains. This combination will stain the organisms most commonly seen in postmortem studies. They also are of special importance in interpreting the culture results of contaminated specimens as they will indicate the predominant organism.

The specimen should be cultured as soon as possible after it is taken. If this is not feasible, storage under refrigeration will maintain the viability of almost all of the aerobic organisms and many of the anaerobic organisms for at least a few days. Certain strains of fastidious fungi and anaerobic bacteria do not tolerate storage well.

General Technique of Processing Tissues for Culture. Techniques for removing specimens aseptically from specific sites will be discussed later; the general techniques of processing tissue will be discussed here.

A portion of tissue, representing at least 6 cm^3 with a serosal or capsular surface intact, should be submitted for microbiologic study. Routinely, we do not recommend that a tissue specimen be taken aseptically in the autopsy room unless it is smaller than 6 cm^3, because the chance of contamination is much greater there than in the microbiology laboratory. After it is removed, the specimen is placed in a sealed plastic container (Fig. 8–1) and sent immediately to the laboratory or stored in a refrigerator at 4 to 6 C. On arrival of the specimen in the laboratory, the capsular or serosal surface is thoroughly seared with an ordinary soldering iron. A 20-cm-long scissors and forceps, sterilized in an electric hot cup containing boiling water, are used to handle the tissue. On a rare occasion, a spore-forming organism has survived in the boiling water, but this has never amounted to more than one to three colonies on a culture plate. Presterilized instruments also can be used, but the sterilization in boiling water is less expensive and more convenient, especially if an instrument is inadvertently contaminated.

A 1-cm cube of tissue is cut aseptically from the center of the submitted specimen. If indicated, three imprint smears are taken of the cut surface left by the removed specimen. Also, a block of tissue can be removed for formalin fixation and histologic sectioning. The cube of tissue is minced with the scissors in a sterile mortar. A small amount of sterile 60-mesh Alundum (aluminum oxide) is added to the mortar to aid in pulverizing the tissue with the pestle. Sterile beef heart infusion broth is added to make a 10 to 20% suspension. This suspension then is placed in a sterile dropper bottle from which all media and animal inoculations are performed. Instead of a pestle and mortar a small conical grinder can be used for small bits of tissue.

When a specimen is known to be contaminated and is too small for searing, we place it in the boiling water bath for 2 to 3 seconds to kill as many of the surface contaminating organisms as possible. However, care

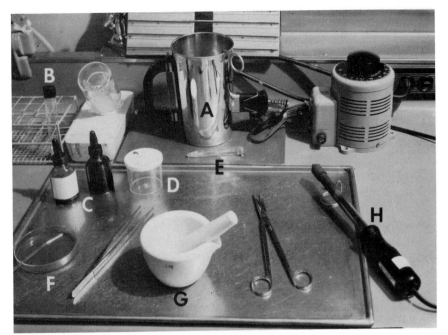

Figure 8-1. General equipment for processing autopsy tissues for culture. A = electric hot cup; B = Alundum; C = dropper bottles for specimen suspension and heart infusion broth; D = specimen container; E = conical grinder; F = glass hockey-stick on blood agar plate; G = pestle and mortar; H = soldering iron.

must be taken to avoid cooking the tissue through, as this will destroy the significant organisms.

Special Techniques for Processing Tissues and Body Fluids for Culture. *Lungs, Liver, Spleen, and Kidney.* Specimens from these tissues are best sent in 6-cm³ cubes with a pleural or capsular surface intact, so that it can be adequately seared and a portion removed aseptically. On occasion, not suspecting an infection, the pathologist may cut into an abscess while sectioning tissues. When this occurs, two approaches can be used. In the first, from one half of the abscess three smears are made, for Gram's, Kinyoun's acid-fast, and Grocott's modification of Gomori's methenamine-silver stains. From the other half, pus is taken, for culture, with a sterile curette; this should include central necrotic material as well as some of the wall of the cavity. The culture should be labeled to indicate that it has been contaminated. The laboratory will then make streak plates and, by correlation of the smear and culture results, a reliable decision can usually be made as to the etiologic agent or agents.

The second technique would be used if the abscess is large enough and there is a capsular or serosal surface intact opposite to the cut surface. In this approach, the capsular or serosal surface is seared and a portion of the abscess wall and necrotic center is removed aseptically. Care must be taken to avoid including material from the contaminated cut surface.

Pleural, Pericardial, and Peritoneal Fluids. If an effusion is suspected, it is best to remove the fluid through the body wall rather than attempting to take a sample aseptically after the cavity is opened. A sterile 20-ml syringe with a 15- or 18-gauge needle is used, and precautions are taken to prepare the skin by adequate cleansing with soap and water and then iodine and alcohol. If the specimen is removed after the body is opened, it is important that it be cultured immediately, that streaking of agar plates be used, and that three direct smears are made for the usual stains.

Pericardial fluid can be aspirated through the chest wall or after the thorax is opened. If the latter approach is used, the pericardial surface is seared before the needle is inserted.

Loculated fluids are best aspirated before the body is opened, but frequently they are difficult to locate until the chest or abdominal cavity is exposed. However, aspiration may be performed through the exterior body wall even after the cavity has been opened. If aspiration is performed within the open body cavity, it is best to sear the surface of the loculated fluid wall before obtaining the fluid.

All fluids are concentrated by centrifuging for 15 minutes at 2,000 rpm, and cultures and smears are made from the sediment. Filtering through a Millipore filter (0.45-μ grid) can be used, but the fluid may contain appreciable sediment making it difficult, if not impossible, to filter.

Lymph Nodes. Short of using total aseptic autopsy technique, there is no satisfactory method of removing lymph nodes aseptically for culture. Fortunately, in the majority of instances, lymph nodes are usually cultured for fungi and acid-fast bacteria, which allows the use of antibiotics and NaOH treatment to inhibit contaminating bacteria. In a few instances, when the lymph nodes are large enough, we have put them into boiling water for 2 to 3 seconds to decontaminate the exterior surface, at least partially, but care must be taken to avoid heating the specimen through and killing the infecting organisms.

Intestine. The best approach is to tie off 20-cm segments of bowel and send these immediately to the laboratory. There, the serosal surface is seared and the bowel is opened aseptically. A portion of the bowel wall is removed and pulverized into a suspension for culture. A sample of the lumen contents is also taken for culture and smears. If ulcers are present in the mucosa, a portion of one should be taken for culture and four smears should be made. The smears are stained with Gram's, Kinyoun's acid-fast, Grocott's modification of Gomori's methenamine-silver, and Bodian's stains. The last stain is particularly useful for demonstrating the trophozoite of amoeba. The silver stain demonstrates fungi and also will stain the cysts of amoeba.

Urinary Bladder and Urine. Removal of urine for culture is best accomplished by aspirating the bladder contents in situ with an 18-gauge spinal needle after the anterior superior surface of the bladder is seared. A bladder tissue specimen can be removed aseptically by searing the surface of the bladder and cutting out the appropriate specimen with sterile instruments.

Blood. One of the most common methods used in aspirating blood for culture at autopsy is to insert an 18-gauge needle attached to a 20-ml syringe into the right atrium. The epicardial surface of the atrium is exposed by reflecting the pericardium and is sterilized by searing. If a clot is encountered, blood may be aspirated from the ascending aorta, left atrium, or either ventricle using a similar technique. Also, the iliac veins or vena cava can be aspirated if an adequate specimen is not obtained from the heart.

A recent report[50] has indicated that the most "practical and efficacious" method of obtaining cultures is intracardiac aspiration through the closed chest. In this technique, the third costal space adjacent to and to the left of the sternum is seared after the skin is reflected. An 18-gauge spinal needle with a 20-ml syringe attached is inserted into the heart. Ten milliliters of blood is aspirated; if difficulty is encountered, the needle is withdrawn partially and reinserted. Manipulation of the bowel should be avoided prior to obtaining the blood cultures as this will increase the number of false-positive blood cultures.

Heart Valves, Pericardium, and Myocardium. 1. Heart valves. Every practicing pathologist has had the experience of opening a heart and finding an unsuspected endocarditis. Aseptic removal of vegetations or valve tissue in this situation is virtually impossible because the methods used in opening the heart will undoubtedly contaminate the valves. However, a specimen still should be taken and labeled as being contaminated. In addition, three smears should be made from the valve vegetation and sent to the laboratory with the tissue specimen. The specimen should be processed and the plates streaked as soon as possible to minimize the opportunity of the contaminating organisms to overgrow the infecting organisms. Correlation of the culture results with the smears and with fixed sections stained with Kinyoun's acid-fast, Gram's, and Grocott's modification of Gomori's methenamine-silver stains will usually allow the identification of the infecting organism.

In the case of a known endocarditis, the following technique can be used. The major vessels are clamped to prevent contamination of the interior of the heart, and the heart is removed. In this technique it is necessary to have two prosectors for aseptic removal of valve tissue. Each valve is opened separately. To examine the mitral valve, the heart is placed on its anterior surface. An approximately 3- by 10-cm rectangular area is seared just to the left of ventricular and atrial septums and extending over the posterior surface of the left atrium and ventricle. A sterile scalpel then is used to incise the atrium and ventricle in the center of the seared area of epicardium. One prosector holds the heart on each side parallel with the incision and bends the heart, so as to open the incision and expose the left atrial and ventricular cavities. Clamps can be used to facilitate this exposure. As is frequently the case in endocarditis, the myocardium may be hypertrophied, so that the rectangular seared area and cut should be as long as possible to facilitate adequate exposure of the valve. The valve is carefully examined with sterile forceps, scissors, or scalpel, and representative tissue samples are removed and sent for cultures (Fig. 8–2).

The aortic, pulmonary, and tricuspid valves are examined in a similar

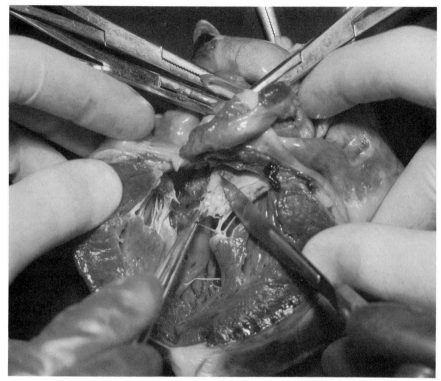

Figure 8–2. Aseptic exposure of mitral valve for obtaining valve tissue for culture. Alternatively, clamps attached to walls of incision can be used by assistant to facilitate exposure.

fashion; however, in the case of the aortic and pulmonary valves the searing is extended onto the aorta and pulmonary vessels well above the valves to allow adequate exposure. The tricuspid valve is opened posteriorly, similar to the mitral valve, but the searing and incision are to the right of the atrial and ventricular septums.

2. Pericardium. After the chest is opened and the sternum and anterior half of the ribs are removed, the pericardial sac can be inspected to determine if there is any evidence of infection. If removal of pericardial fluid is desired, it can be aspirated aseptically as described above. Removal of pericardial tissue is best accomplished after searing well beyond the confines of the specimen to be obtained. The tissue then can be removed aseptically with sterile forceps and scissors.

3. Myocardium. Myocardial tissue can be removed before or after the valves are examined, as long as care is taken to avoid contamination of the endocardial surface adjacent to where the myocardial tissue is to be removed. A 1-cm³ portion is obtained by first searing the epicardial surface and then cutting out the block of tissue with a sterile scalpel and forceps. Decontamination of the endocardium by searing has been rarely successful, so we prefer to avoid contamination. In the event the myocardium

is contaminated, it is possible to sear the epicardial surface and cut out a portion of myocardium which does not include the endocardium. This is best accomplished with a small sterile forceps and scissors. An alternative approach would be to submerge a large portion of myocardium in boiling water for 2 to 3 seconds before removing the tissue and then streaking the tissue suspension on plates for culture. Frequently, cultures of myocardium are for viruses, so the antibiotics used in the tissue culture medium may inhibit the contaminating organisms.

Cerebrospinal Fluid and Brain Tissue. In cases of meningitis of undetermined etiology, it is important to remember that removal of the calvarium with an electric saw is hazardous, particularly if the case proves to be tuberculous meningitis. In this instance, a hand saw is recommended.

1. Cerebrospinal fluid. The most reliable method of removing uncontaminated cerebrospinal fluid is by a spinal or cisternal tap as performed antemortem. Care must be taken to prepare the skin by adequate cleansing with soap and water and then with tincture of iodine and alcohol; the alcohol must be allowed to evaporate. Aseptic removal of cerebrospinal fluid may not be possible after the calvarium is removed because contamination readily occurs when the calvarium is sawed. However, with a sterile syringe or dropper it may be possible to aspirate uncontaminated cerebrospinal fluid from the subarachnoidal space. This is done by carefully reflecting the dura to expose the untouched superior surface of the parietal and occipital lobes. Even if contamination occurs, fluid should be obtained and labeled as contaminated. Also, direct smears of the fluid should be included with the specimen to facilitate interpretation of the cultures.

2. Brain tissue. Aseptic removal of brain tissue for culture is difficult not only from a technical point of view but also because it is desirable to fix the brain by perfusion. To obtain tissue for culture without significantly impairing the perfusion of the brain, we recommend that a 1-cm cube of brain be removed from one cerebral hemisphere or from the area appearing abnormal. During removal of the calvarium, care must be taken to avoid contaminating that portion of the brain to be cultured. If the dura is left covering this area, it is carefully reflected before the specimen is taken because it usually becomes contaminated on its external surface during the removal of the calvarium. If the brain surface is contaminated, searing the surface before the specimen is taken is sometimes successful. It is difficult to sterilize the surface with searing because the contaminating bacteria may be implanted deep in the sulci.

If a brain abscess is suspected, it may be advisable to remove a tissue specimen from deep in the brain, even though this will interfere with perfusion fixation. In this instance, the tissue is removed with sterile forceps and scissors aseptically after the brain surface is seared. Pus from the cavity, collected with a sterile dropper, and three direct smears should be included for study. Another method, which is less satisfactory, is to aspirate the abscess with a 20-ml sterile syringe fitted with a 15- to 18-gauge spinal needle. Several aspirations should be attempted if the first does not yield enough material for culture and smears.

In cases of meningitis, the inferior surface of the base of the brain will frequently yield suppurative fluid which can be aspirated with a sterile dropper after the brain is reflected posteriorly.

3. Spinal cord tissue. Aseptic removal of spinal tissue for culture is not an easy procedure. With a Vim-Silverman biopsy needle, a sterile specimen of the cord can be obtained by inserting the needle through the spinal column posteriorly in the thoracic region. The skin must be properly prepared. An alternative is to take at least a 5-cm portion of cord, submersing it in boiling water for 2 to 3 seconds to decrease the contamination. Fortunately, in the majority of cases, brain specimens will be adequate for diagnosis of infections of the nervous system without study of the spinal cord. If spinal tissue is cultured, it usually is studied for viruses, so the antibiotics present in tissue culture medium may be adequate to suppress the growth of contaminating bacteria and yeasts.

Bones. 1. Petrous bone and middle ear. If an infection of the middle ear is extensive, aspiration can be accomplished by a sterile 20-ml syringe with a 15- to 18-gauge needle attached. The dura overlying the middle ear should be seared before the needle is inserted. If the bone is too firm for insertion of this needle, a bone-marrow aspirating needle can be used. After the bone in the middle ear is sawed and removed, it is virtually impossible to obtain an uncontaminated specimen, but one could then resort to the method used in studying a contaminated specimen—that is, making three direct smears for special stains and sending the specimen labeled as contaminated.

2. Other bones. In a case of osteomyelitis with a draining sinus tract a specimen is removed by first cleansing the external orifice thoroughly with alcohol. After the alcohol has evaporated, a sterile curet is inserted into the tract and vigorous curettage is performed to remove material from the lining of the tract. The use of swabs for removal of a specimen is not recommended because in many cases the swab will not contain the infecting organism.

In closed osteomyelitis, the lesion usually has been located by x-ray, so that a specimen can be obtained with a Vim-Silverman needle. If a saw cut has been made through the lesion, it is virtually impossible to obtain an uncontaminated specimen, but again the three direct smears will be useful in interpreting the culture results.

3. Joints. The skin is prepared by cleansing with soap and water and then with iodine and alcohol. Joint fluid is aspirated by inserting a 15- to 18-gauge sterile needle attached to a 10-ml syringe into the synovial cavity. If no fluid is aspirated, a few milliliters of nutrient broth can be injected and aspirated as synovial washings.

Selection of Type of Cultures To Be Requested. The cultures are selected on the basis of the clinical history of the patient and the gross and microscopic features of the lesions. Table 8–1 shows the appropriate media used for culturing various pathogens; the media are available commercially from BioQuest (Cockeysville, Md.) or Difco Laboratories (Detroit, Mich.). Specimens which are granulomatous and uncontaminated are studied for fungi by making heavy inoculation on brain heart infusion-blood agar

TABLE 8–1. MEDIA FOR CULTURING VARIOUS PATHOGENS

Media	Bacteria Aerobes	Bacteria Anaerobes	Brucella	Nocardia	Actinomyces	Mycobacteria	Fungi
Trypticase soy-blood agar	X						
Phenylethyl alcohol-blood agar	X						
Eosin-methylene blue agar	X						
Thioglycollate broth with serum or ascitic fluid		X					
Thioglycollate broth with trypticase soy and trypticase broth added					X		
Middlebrook 7H10						X	
Lowenstein-Jensen						X	
Beef heart infusion-blood agar in 10% CO_2			X				
Brain heart infusion-blood agar				X			X
Brain heart infusion agar; anaerobic with 10% CO_2					X		

plates with the use of a hockey stick-shaped glass rod (Fig. 8–1) and incubating at 25 to 30 C. Mycobacteria are cultured by inoculation of Middlebrook 7H10 and Löwenstein-Jensen media slanted in tubes and incubation at 35 C in 10% CO_2. The nonfermenting gram-negative bacilli (such as *Pseudomonas pseudomallei*) which may produce granulomatous lesions can be isolated on ordinary trypticase soy-blood agar.

Acute suppurative lesions are generally bacterial in origin. The usual laboratory media such as trypticase soy-blood agar, blood phenylethyl alcohol, and eosin-methylene blue agar at 35 C are recommended. For anaerobic bacteria, thioglycollate broth with serum or ascitic fluid added is the most practical medium, but not all anaerobes will grow in this medium. Reference should be made to a standard text on anaerobic bacteriology for more detailed information.[51]

Suppurative fibrosing lesions are characteristically produced by *Actinomyces israeli* and *Nocardia asteroides*. The former is primarily an anaerobe and is best isolated on brain heart infusion agar incubated anaerobically in 10% CO_2 at 35 C. The latter can be isolated aerobically on trypticase soy-blood agar at 35 C, but it does grow well on brain heart infusion-blood agar. Media containing antibiotics usually are not suitable for isolating either of these organisms. Many fungi are inhibited by certain antibiotics; however, penicillin and streptomycin, each at 20 μg/ml, do not have an inhibitory effect. Recent data suggest[11] that chloramphenicol (16 μg/ml) and gentamicin (5 μg/ml) may be suitable for the isolation of strains of most fungi and *Nocardia asteroides*.

With contaminated specimens or those containing bacteria other than mycobacteria, heavy inoculation should be avoided; streaking of the agar plates is recommended for these specimens.

Animal inoculation is rarely used; however, one can inoculate guinea pigs for the isolation of *Mycobacterium tuberculosis* and mice for the isolation of fungi when specimens are heavily contaminated.

One useful basic text containing the recommended procedures for cultivation of bacteria and the most likely bacterial pathogens to be recovered from specific specimens is Bailey and Scott's monograph.[3] Beneke's *Medical Mycology: Laboratory Manual*[7] is a practical source for the techniques used in isolating fungi and also contains an excellent bibliography. Herrmann[22] has described a practical approach to laboratory viral diagnosis compatible with medical practice.

ELECTRON MICROSCOPY OF AUTOPSY TISSUES

By Arnold L. Brown, Jr.

Effect of Postmortem Changes. One of the basic requirements for the preparation of tissue for electron microscopy is that the specimens be obtained and fixed either during life or within minutes after death. This condition is based on the fact that early autolytic changes, invisible under the light microscope, seriously distort cellular organelles at the levels of resolution obtained by the electron microscope.

Mitochondria are particularly susceptible to postmortem changes. Within minutes they swell, often with rupture of their external membranes and the appearance of vesicles. The endoplasmic reticulum dilates, although ribosomes generally remain attached. Lysosomes disintegrate at varying rates but usually are indistinct shortly after death. Peripheral clumping of chromatin occurs rapidly in nuclei, and nucleoli become blurred within minutes after death.

Other structures retain their characteristic fine structural details long after death. Collagen and smooth as well as striated muscle are the best examples of this. The typical periodicity of collagen can be seen in specimens taken 18 hours after death, and the structure of myofibrils, including myofilaments, is apparent after at least 6 hours of postmortem autolysis. Amyloid also is resistant to postmortem change.

In general, the shorter the time that has elapsed between death and start of fixation, the better preserved will be the fine-structure detail. However, considerable valuable information can be obtained even after several hours of autolytic activity.

Not only is it possible to prepare tissue for study of fine structure at the time of autopsy but also significant information can be gained from formalin-fixed tissues after more than 2 years. Ribosomes, intracellular fibrils, desmosomes, microvilli and the brush border of the outer cell membrane, and centrioles are quite stable.[24]

Fixation. The most commonly used fixative for tissues to be prepared for electron microscopy is glutaraldehyde. A 4% solution in 0.05 M caco-dylate buffer[41] is usually used. As with most of the aldehyde fixatives, pen-etration is rapid. However, tissue blocks should be small, generally about 1 mm³. This is necessary for the slowly penetrating osmium tetraoxide that is used later.

Fortunately, formaldehyde is also an excellent fixative.[2,39] The stan-dard 10% solution of formalin "neutralized" to approximately pH 6.4 is ordinarily used. For later electron microscopic study of routine formalin-fixed autopsy tissue, small blocks of the tissue are thoroughly washed in cacodylate buffer (to 100 ml of distilled water add 1.1 gm of cacodylic acid and 6.16 gm of sucrose, adjust pH to 7.2 with 20% sodium hydroxide) and then put in 1% osmic acid for 1 hour. Various osmic acid solutions are described by Pease.[39] Dehydration can be done in the standard way[39] or by a rapid method developed by Bencosme and Tsutsumi.[5] Any of the usual embedding media can be used although epoxy resin is the most popular.[28]

Thin sections are best double-stained with uranyl acetate and lead ci-trate.

Applications. Perhaps the most useful application of the electron microscope to postmortem tissue is in the classification of sarcomas. Often these tumors are so undifferentiated that precise identification is impos-sible with the light microscope. However, the persistence of the myofila-ments of smooth muscle and the characteristic myofibrillar structure of striated muscle make the distinction between a leiomyosarcoma and rhab-domyosarcoma relatively easy.

As additional studies of the fine structural changes responsible for human disease are reported, the electron microscope will become increas-ingly necessary for meaningful postmortem examinations.

CHROMOSOME STUDY OF AUTOPSY TISSUES

With Jack L. Titus

Indications. Malformations in fetuses and infants represent the most frequent indications for chromosomal analysis. Some of the congenital con-ditions are hereditary. In the absence of a clinical chromosomal analysis, postmortem chromosome studies may provide crucial information for genetic counseling;[54] occasionally, analysis of tissue fibroblasts may yield in-formation in addition to that obtained from culture of blood lymphocytes. Among the chromosomal abnormalities most often found in pediatric au-topsies are those characterized by autosomal trisomic states—Down's syn-drome (trisomy G), Patau's syndrome (trisomy D), and Edwards' syndrome (trisomy E). Aneuploidy of sex chromosomes, as in Turner's syndrome and Klinefelter's syndrome, is found more frequently in adult autopsies. Rarely, structural abnormalities of autosomes are encountered (*cri-du-chat* syndrome, Bloom's syndrome).

Postmortem chromosomal analysis in acquired conditions is primarily a research procedure with the possible exception of cases in which the diagnosis of chronic granulocytic leukemia requires confirmation by demonstrating the Ph_1 chromosome (Philadelphia chromosome).

Tissues Used for Postmortem Chromosome Analysis. Peripheral blood lymphoctyes[61] and thymus cells[4] have been cultured. Tissues successfully used for postmortem culture and chromosome analysis include brain, bone marrow, spleen, small intestine, fibrous tissues, and gonads.[18]

Effect of Postmortem Interval. When blood is withdrawn aseptically within 12 hours after death (more than 24 hours in some cases), about two thirds of the cases may be expected to yield material which can be used for chromosome analysis.[32,53] Fibroblast cultures may grow after similar or even longer postmortem intervals.

Technique of Chromosome Analysis From Postmortem Fibroblast Cultures. The following method[53] has been used in our department for several years and has been successful in most instances.

The skin of the anterior thigh is sterilized with any suitable disinfectant, and a small portion of fascia lata and adjacent muscle is removed in a sterile fashion. This tissue is washed two or three times in balanced salt solution containing antibiotics to remove blood and loose tissue debris and then is cut into small fragments (approximately 1-mm cubes). The fragments are distributed over the bottom of two or three tissue culture flasks which then are put in the 37 C incubator for 10 to 20 minutes. During this period the tissue dries enough to adhere to the surface of the flask but without loss of viability of many cells. The culture medium is then gently added to the flask.

This explant method is simpler and faster than traditional methods utilizing trypsin or other enzymes to dissociate cells and make a cell suspension.

In an interval ranging from 3 days to 2 weeks, cells that resemble fibroblasts may be observed growing out from some of the explants. In a variable period after this, commonly 1 to 2 weeks, sufficient numbers of dividing cells will be present to allow chromosome preparations to be made. Frequently, there will not be enough dividing cells from the original explants; in this case, the cells present may be passed by conventional tissue culture techniques of trypsinization and subculture until reasonably large numbers of dividing cells are present.

At the time of passage of the cells, some are transferred to tubes containing cover slips so that a monolayer of cells may grow on the cover slip. The cover slips are then removed and the cells are stained with the Feulgen technique or cresyl violet for later examination for the presence or absence of the sex chromatin (Barr body) in the nucleus.

Chromosome preparations are made from cultures in which there are many mitoses. If the cells have been recently passed, 24 hours after passage usually is a good time. Colchicine or demecolcine (Colcemid) is added to the culture medium in a concentration of about 1.0 μg/ml. Two to 4 hours after this, the cells are washed three times with balanced salt solution and trypsinized so that a cell suspension is created. Then the cells are treated with a hypotonic solution to swell them. Fixative is added next.

The usual fixative is a 3:1 mixture of methyl alcohol and glacial acetic acid; this must be freshly prepared. Fixation is a critical step, and it is best to use two or three changes of fixative.

Slides are prepared by dropping one to three drops of the fixative suspension of cells on wet, chilled slides and promptly igniting the fixative, after which the remaining moisture is shaken off so that the slide dries rapidly. The slides may be stained by any method. Giemsa stain is satisfactory and yields a permanent preparation after cover slips are applied.

Examination is carried out by oil immersion microscopy. Metaphases in which the chromosomes are well spread and sharp are studied. The chromosomes in at least 30 cells are counted, and more than one slide should be used to make the counts. If different counts are obtained on the 30 cells, it may be necessary to count many more to ascertain the modal number, or numbers, if mosaicism is present. Representative metaphases are photographed and from these photographs, karyotypes are prepared (Fig. 8–3).

AUTOPSY CHEMISTRY

Effect of Postmortem Changes. After death, the nature and concentration of many chemical substances in the body may change rapidly because

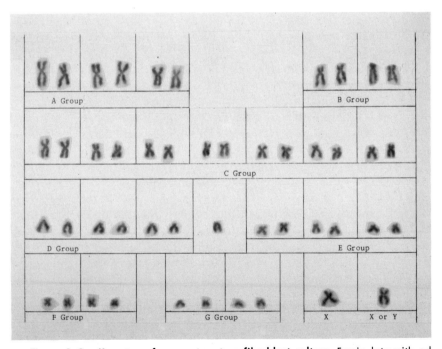

Figure 8–3. Karyotype from postmortem fibroblast culture. Fascia lata with adjacent muscle had been removed for tissue culture $18\frac{1}{2}$ hours after death. This karyotype is from the second passage of the fibroblast culture. It shows trisomy D (Patau's syndrome) in a female; there is an extra D chromosome. The chromosomal diagnosis is 47,XX,D+.

of the unpredictable interplay of such processes as dehydration, diffusion, hemolysis, enzymatic activity, and putrefaction. The length of the post-mortem interval is an important factor influencing these processes.

Chemical and physical changes in the blood occur rapidly after death and may vary from site to site because of close association with autolyzing tissues. Movements of blood after death[14] are also likely to increase the interchange of chemical substances between blood and surrounding tissues. Blood oxygen saturation decreases rapidly after death, usually reaching 10 to 20% after 3 to 4 hours. The oxygen capacity and carbon dioxide content also decrease. The pH decreases to about 6.4 within the first few hours after death and may continue to decrease until protein breakdown produces ammonia (after about 24 hours).[15] There is no relationship to the cause of death.[12] Blood viscosity and hematocrit value begin to increase some time after death, while the osmotic resistance of erythrocytes decreases rapidly.[47] Chemical postmortem changes in various body fluids and tissues are listed in Table 8–2. This table shows that cerebrospinal fluid, vitreous humor, and urine often permit more reliable conclusions as to the antemortem concentrations of chemical substances[38] than does blood. Effusions and exudates in body cavities or stool may be expected to remain unaltered for a longer time after death.

Sampling Techniques. Blood should be withdrawn and serum prepared as early as possible after death (see also page 34). Serum for neutralization tests should be kept sterile and in Dry Ice without preservative; for other immunologic and chemical tests, 0.3% cresol may be added as a preservative and the serum should be kept in a refrigerator.[57] Sampling procedures for cerebrospinal fluid, vitreous humor, and urine are described in chapter 2.

Postmortem Values. *Protein.* The serum protein levels seem to change little after death.[45] In infants a desiccation factor of about 10% has been suggested.[6] Immunoelectrophoresis, paper electrophoresis, and agar precipitation yielded unaltered values in 82% of sera which were removed within the first 10 hours after death. Hemolysis led to an extra gradient in the α_2-β position.[31] Low, normal, or high antemortem immunoglobulin (IgG, IgA, IgM) values also tend to be low, normal, or high for at least 20 hours after death.[8] Paraproteins can be identified after death.[30] The isolation after death of an abnormal amino acid has led to the diagnosis of maple syrup urine disease in a case of sudden death in infancy.[19]

Hormones and Enzymes. Only few systematic studies are available. In cases of choriocarcinoma or related tumors, we have repeatedly determined chorionic gonadotropin in blood and urine and the results corresponded well with the antemortem values. The postmortem detection of insulin in tissue received wide publicity in connection with a famous murder case[52]—extracts of tissue from the injection sites in the buttocks of the victim were shown to cause hypoglycemic shock in mice. Hormones can be isolated both from blood and from endocrine organs. Of special significance for the autopsy pathologist may be the determination of hormone levels in endocrine tumors, such as 5-hydroxyindoles in carcinoid tumors. Such tissues must be kept in the deep freeze until analysis.

TABLE 8–2. POSTMORTEM CHANGES AS COMPARED WITH ANTEMORTEM VALUES*

Substance	Specimen	Change	Reference
Amino acids	Spinal fluid	Increase	48
Ammonium	Serum	None or increase	48
Bilirubin	Serum	None	36
	Urine	None	36
	Vitreous humor	Always <0.1 mg/100 ml	10
Calcium	Serum	Fairly stable	48
	Spinal fluid	Fairly stable	37
	Urine	Fairly stable	
	Vitreous humor	Irregular	10
Carbon dioxide	Blood	Decrease	34
	Spinal fluid	Decrease	34
Chloride	Serum	Decrease	33
	Vitreous humor	None	10
Cholesterol esters	Serum	Decrease	36
Cholesterol, total	Serum	None	36
Cortisol	Blood	None	16
Creatine	Serum	Increase	48
	Spinal fluid	Increase	34
Creatinine	Serum	None	34,48
	Spinal fluid	None or increase	34,48
Enzymes	Serum	Increase first, then decrease	15
	Tissues	Irregular	15
Fatty acids	Subcutaneous tissue	Minimal increase	48
Glucose	Serum, R. ventr. & inf. v. cava	Increase	23,55
	Serum, L. ventr. & peripheral blood	Decrease	15
	Spinal fluid	Decrease	56
	Vitreous humor	Erratic decrease	10
Glycogen	Liver	Decrease	13
	Muscle	Decrease	13
Hypoxanthine	Spinal fluid	Increase	48
Inositol	Spinal fluid	Increase	48
Ketones	Blood	None	21
Lactic acid	Serum	Increase	48
	Spinal fluid	Increase	48
Lipids (see also phosphatides)	Serum	Increase	13
	Tissues	Decrease	26
Magnesium	Serum	None for 24 hr	33
	Skeletal muscle	None	9
Nitrogen, nonprotein	Serum	None or increase	48
	Spinal fluid	None or increase	48
Phosphatides	Serum	None or increase	48
	Tissues	Decrease	26
Phosphorus	Serum	Increase	15,48
Potassium	Serum	Increase	25
	Spinal fluid	Increase	37
	Vitreous humor	Increase	10,25
Proteins	Serum	None for 10 hr	31
Sodium	Serum	Often none but unreliable; may decrease	48
	Spinal fluid	Often none but unreliable	48
	Vitreous humor	None	10
Triglycerides	Tissues	Decrease	26
Urea	Serum	Increase	48
	Spinal fluid	Increase	48
	Vitreous humor	None	10
Uric acid	Serum	Minimal increase	48
	Spinal fluid	Minimal increase	48
Urobilin	Urine	None	36
Urobilinogen	Urine	Decrease	36
Xanthine	Spinal fluid	Increase	48

* Only changes in the first 24 to 48 hours after death are considered.

Tissue breakdown after death releases enzymes into the blood, and their concentrations increase until proteolysis outstrips their production. The subsequent decrease in enzyme activity depends on the speed with which the protein is broken down. Transaminases, lactic dehydrogenase, phosphatases, and amylase accumulate in the serum during the first 2 to 3 days after death.[13,15] After death, the increase in concentration of substrates and coenzymes, such as adenosine monophosphate, and the decrease of adenosine triphosphate indicate that postmortem glycogenolysis and increased cell permeability are important factors which affect the concentration of numerous blood enzymes.[29]

In the liver, glucose-6-phosphatase, nonspecific phosphatase, and phosphoglucose isomerase decrease after death at more or less characteristic rates.[15] In skeletal muscle, great variations are found in the postmortem concentrations of aldolase, glutamic-oxaloacetic transaminase, glutamic-pyruvic transaminase, and phosphoglucose isomerase.[15]

Blood Coagulation Factors. After death, blood coagulation factors change quickly and often unpredictably. Postmortem blood may coagulate intravascularly and in vitro up to several hours after death. Subsequently, the intravascular clots dissolve spontaneously. This may be due to the release of plasminogen activator from the vascular endothelium.[58] The process is probably associated with the desquamation of large clumps of endothelial cells, which I have found in human cadaver blood. In many instances, sudden death, shock, and collapse are followed, after death, by high fibrinolytic activity. The titer of fibrinogen split products in postmortem serum varies over a wide range. We have been unable to relate these titers to the cause of death, the underlying disease, or the postmortem interval. The clinical diagnosis of intravascular coagulation and fibrinolysis syndrome cannot be confirmed simply because high titers of fibrinogen split products are present in the postmortem serum. Thrombin-clottable fibrinogen may be completely lost as early as 5 hours after death.[27,46] Factors II, V, VII, and X show considerable and unpredictable variations when measured between 5 and 41 hours after death.[27] There also are considerable differences in the concentrations of coagulation factors in blood from the right atrium and from the left atrium.

Postmortem Chemical Diagnosis. *Diabetes Mellitus, Hyperglycemia, and Hypoglycemia.* In general, after death blood glucose decreases due to glycolysis, except in hepatic veins, the inferior vena cava, and the right heart chambers where it may be increased due to hepatic glycogenolysis.[23,55]

Examination of cerebrospinal fluid is best for the postmortem diagnosis of diabetes mellitus.[35,56] Hyperglycemia may be diagnosed if the glucose concentration in cerebrospinal fluid and in blood from the left heart chambers is more than 200 mg/100 ml.[20] For the diagnosis of diabetes mellitus, one has to rule out asphyxia, pancreatitis, and glucose administration shortly before death.[34] Blood ketone levels seem to be independent of the length of the postmortem interval, age, or cause of death and can be used for the diagnosis of diabetic ketosis. If the ketones are expressed as acetone, the control values vary between 0.5 and 3.4 mg/100 ml.[21] Diabetic acidosis is characterized by the presence of acetone in the spinal fluid and by a decrease in spinal fluid carbon dioxide. Protein, sugar, and acetone may be present in the urine.

Hypoglycemia cannot be confirmed at autopsy unless the blood is examined within 2 hours after death. Glucose in the vitreous humor may decrease rapidly after death and seems to be of little use for the post-mortem diagnosis of hypoglycemia.[10]

The differential diagnosis of fatal diabetes and hypoglycemia should be based on the determination of both cerebrospinal fluid glucose and lactic acid values.[56] This method takes into account the breakdown after death of glucose to lactic acid. Characteristic cerebrospinal fluid levels are shown in Table 8–3.

Uremia. Creatinine determination in blood from a left heart chamber or in cerebrospinal fluid is the most reliable postmortem renal function test. The cerebrospinal creatinine values increase somewhat after death and reach a maximum after about 10 hours. Cerebrospinal urea values of more than 200 mg/100 ml associated with creatinine values of more than 4 mg/100 ml, in the presence of corresponding urinary findings (casts, protein), indicate fatal uremia.[34]

Jensen[24a] concluded that postmortem concentrations of creatinine exceeding 8.4 mg/100 ml in the serum and 4.5 mg/100 ml in the spinal fluid, of urea exceeding 388 mg/100 ml in the serum and 329 mg/100 ml in the spinal fluid, and of inorganic sulfate exceeding 27 mg/100 ml in the serum and 14 mg/100 ml in the spinal fluid constitute strong evidence of renal insufficiency.

Postmortem Liver Function Tests. Serum bilirubin and urinary urobilin are the most useful substances for evaluation of hepatic function;[36] their postmortem concentrations appear to be quite stable. Alkaline phosphatase and other enzymes are of little value when determined after death. Serum cephalin flocculation increases and cholesterol esters decrease.[36]

TABLE 8–3. COMBINED GLUCOSE AND LACTIC ACID VALUES IN CEREBROSPINAL FLUID FOR POSTMORTEM DIAGNOSIS OF FATAL DIABETES MELLITUS OR HYPOGLYCEMIA*

Glucose plus lactic acid (mg/100 ml)	Diagnosis
<56	Hypoglycemia
<76 and *presence* of certain conditions†	Hypoglycemia
<177	Rules out decompensated fatal diabetes mellitus
177–304	Not diagnostic
305–362 and *absence* of certain conditions†	Decompensated fatal diabetes mellitus or idiopathic lactic acid acidosis
>362	Decompensated fatal diabetes mellitus

* Data from Traub F: Methode zur Erkennung von tödlichen Zuckerstoffwechselstörungen an der Leiche (Diabetes mellitus und Hypoglykämie). Zentralbl Allg Pathol *112*:390–399, 1969.

† Malignant tumors, respiratory insufficiency, inflammatory processes with toxic circulatory failure, renal uremia, pernicious anemia, hemorrhage, pulmonary emboli, or inflammatory cerebrospinal diseases.

AUTOPSY ROENTGENOLOGY

Roentgenology provides the most important supplement of modern autopsy technology. Its potential role in training, diagnosis, and research was outlined half a century ago.[40] The recent establishment in our department of a Radiologic Pathologic Anatomy Research Facility has permitted us to use roentgenologic techniques extensively for these purposes.

Many applications of postmortem roentgenograms are described in chapters 2 through 7. In medicolegal cases, roentgenograms are used primarily for identification purposes and for the search for bullets and other foreign bodies which might be impossible to find by any other method.[44] The diagnosis of gas embolism,[42] pneumothorax, pneumomediastinum, and pneumoperitoneum (Fig. 8–4) may be greatly facilitated by postmortem roentgenography, without which these conditions may be totally missed. Lesions of bones and joints are particularly difficult to evaluate at autopsy without the help of roentgenograms. Vascular anomalies or occlusions may necessitate postmortem angiography. The uses of tech-

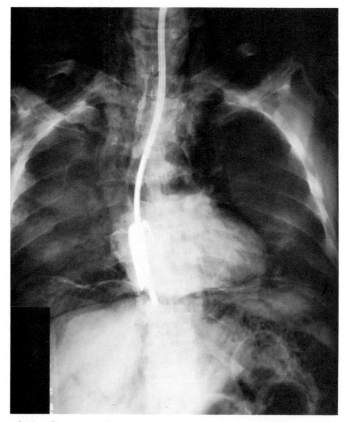

Figure 8–4. Pneumoperitoneum in postmortem roentgenogram, showing large amounts of gas in abdomen (particularly under right diaphragm), gas in portal veins, Miller-Abbott tube in esophagus, and air in mediastinum.

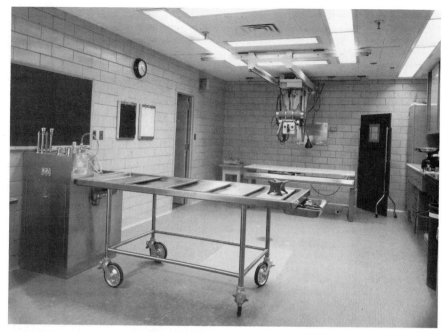

Figure 8–5. Autopsy room modified for roentgenologic examination. In the background is a Machlett Super Dynamax Tube and a Picker x-ray table. In adjacent room to the left, a 300-ma Keleket x-ray machine with a 125-kv generator is installed. In the foreground is a mobile autopsy table (Brason) with separate service island.

niques such as coronary, pulmonary, mesenteric, and cerebral angiography are presented in chapters 3 through 6.

In cases in which no autopsy permission has been granted, postmortem roentgenograms may help to clarify the cause of death. In a series of 34 cases, the postmortem roentgenograms showed a progression of a pulmonary disease process in 12 cases when compared with the last available antemortem film. [43]

We use a modified and shielded autopsy room, as shown in part in Figure 8–5. A Machlett Super Dynamax Tube (1-mm and 2-mm focal spots) has been installed. We are using a Picker x-ray table. A 300-ma Keleket machine (125-kv generator) is in an adjacent room. Films are processed in a small darkroom with a Kodak RP X-OMAT processor, which permits one to monitor injection procedures by reviewing films while the injection is still under way.

We are using this facility for chest roentgenography prior to most autopsies, for roentgenographic surveys in medicolegal cases, and for a number of special studies, mostly associated with vascular injection. These studies are carried out either on isolated organs or in situ. In the latter case, the autopsy is done on the x-ray table or on the mobile autopsy table.

The modifications of an autopsy room with shielding and new installations may be forbiddingly expensive. However, less elaborate setups also

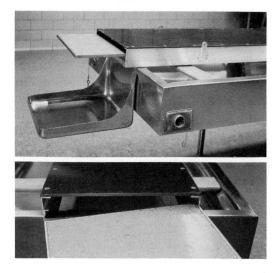

Figure 8–6. Autopsy rack for postmortem roentgenography with transportable x-ray machines. This rack measures 198 by 40 cm and consists of an aluminum frame with channels (*Lower*) which permit the x-ray cassette to slide to the desired position. The cassette is inserted at the end of the rack and can be moved by hand from below. The rack is covered with x-ray Bakelite, 0.64 cm thick. The Bakelite seams are watertight so that autopsies can be carried out on this rack and cleaning is necessary only from the outside.

are available. For years we worked with an old transportable Keleket machine and had satisfactory results. The most cumbersome part of this method is bringing the cassette into proper position. We therefore designed a special rack which was sturdy enough to carry bodies and to do autopsies on. It consists of an aluminum frame with channels at the inside, for sliding cassettes back and forth, and a top layer of x-ray Bakelite (Fig. 8–6).

A special problem is the preparation of postmortem roentgenograms with the body in the erect position. X-ray tables have been designed for this purpose.[1] If one wishes to simulate inspiratory thoracic roentgenograms, a needle with a stylet should be inserted into the trachea before the body is hoisted into the erect position. This can be done with a special autopsy table or with the help of an orthopedic traction apparatus with straps around the occiput, chin, and axillae. After the body has been suspended the stylet is removed. The weight of the abdominal organs will suck air through the needle and cause diaphragmatic excursion.[17]

If only roentgenograms of specimens are desired, low-cost cabinet-type installations are available.* Built-in shielding decreases external radiation to safe levels.

Special methods and indications for postmortem roentgenography have been presented in chapter 2 in regard to medicolegal autopsies and in chapters 3 through 7 in regard to the preparation of organs and organ systems for study and display. The atlas by Schoenmackers and Vieten[49] can be recommended as a guide for the preparation of technically outstanding postmortem angiograms.

---

* Faxitron 805–55, Field Emission Corporation, Melrose Ave. at Linke St., McMinnville, Ore.

REFERENCES

1. Allred WL, Garland LH: A simple and efficient table for postmortem chest roentgenography. Am J Roentgenol Radium Ther Nucl Med *33*:839–841, 1935
2. Ashworth CT, Stembridge VA: Utility of formalin-fixed surgical and autopsy specimens for electron microscopy. Am J Clin Pathol *42*:466–480, 1964
3. Bailey WR, Scott EG: Diagnostic Microbiology: A Textbook for the Isolation and Identification of Pathogenic Microorganisms. Third edition. St. Louis, C. V. Mosby Company, 1970
4. Bain AD, Gauld IK: The use of thymus and spleen in the demonstration of chromosomes postmortem in foetuses and infants. Br J Exp Pathol *45*:530–532, 1964
5. Bencosme SA, Tsutsumi V: A fast method for processing biologic material for electron microscopy. Lab Invest *23*:447–450, 1970
6. Benditt EP: Discussion. In Sudden Death in Infants. (Publication No. 1412.) Edited by RJ Wedgwood, EP Benditt. Bethesda, Maryland, US Department of Health, Education, and Welfare, 1966, p 85
7. Beneke ES: Medical Mycology: Laboratory Manual. Second edition. Minneapolis, Burgess Publishing Company, 1966
8. Brazinsky JH, Kellenberger RE: Comparison of immunoglobulin analyses of antemortem and postmortem sera. Am J Clin Pathol *54*:622–624, 1970
9. Chemical pathology: Postmortem may reveal magnesium deficiency. Lab Med *1*:39–40, 1970
10. Coe JI: Postmortem chemistries on human vitreous humor. Am J Clin Pathol *51*:741–749, 1969
11. Dolan CT: Optimal combination and concentration of antibiotics in media for isolation of pathogenic fungi and *Nocardia asteroides*. Appl Microbiol *21*:195–197, 1971
12. Dotzauer G, Naeve W: Die aktuelle Wasserstoffionenkonzentration im Leichenblut. Zentralbl Allg Pathol *93*:360–370, 1955
13. Evans WED: The Chemistry of Death. Springfield, Illinois, Charles C Thomas, Publisher, 1963
14. Fallani M: Contributo allo studio della circolazione ematica post-mortale. [Contribution to the study of the post-mortal blood circulation.] Minerva Medicoleg *81*:108–115, 1961
15. Fatteh A: Estimation of time of death by chemical changes. Med Leg Bull *163*:1–6, 1966
16. Finlayson NB: Blood cortisol in infants and adults: a postmortem study. J Pediatr *67*:248–252, 1965
17. Greening RR, Pendergrass EP: Postmortem roentgenography with particular emphasis upon the lung. Radiology *62*:720–724, 1954
18. Gustavson KH, Hagberg B, Finley SC, Finley WM: An apparently identical extra autosome in two severely retarded sisters with multiple malformations. Cytogenetics *1*:32–41, 1962
19. Hallock J, Morrow G III, Karp LA, Barness LA: Postmortem diagnosis of metabolic disorders: the finding of maple syrup urine disease in a case of sudden and unexpected death in infancy. Am J Dis Child *118*:649–651, 1969
20. Hamilton-Paterson JL, Johnson EWM: Post-mortem glycolysis. J Pathol Bact *50*:473–482, 1940
21. Hansson L, Laiho K, Uotila U: Ketonkörper im postmortalen Blut. Deutsch Z Ges Gerichtl Med *58*:184–189, 1966
22. Herrmann EC Jr: Experience in providing a viral diagnostic laboratory compatible with medical practice. Mayo Clin Proc *42*:112–123, 1967
23. Hill EV: Significance of dextrose and nondextrose reducing substances in postmortem blood. Arch Pathol *32*:452–473, 1941
24. Hübner G, Paulussen F: Die Feinstruktur des Gewebes nach protrahierter Formalinfixierung. Virchows Arch [Zellpathol] *1*:107–119, 1968
24a. Jensen OM: Diagnosis of uraemia post mortem: necrochemical studies. Dan Med Bull *16* Suppl 8:1–93, 1969
25. Lie JT: Changes of potassium concentration in the vitreous humor after death. Am J Med Sci *254*:136–143, 1967
26. Lindlar F: Postmortale Lipidveränderungen und Todeszeitbestimmung. Beitr Gerichtl Med *26*:71–73, 1970
27. Ludwig J, Duckert F: Unpublished data
28. Luft JH: Improvements in epoxy resin embedding methods. J Biophys Biochem Cytol *9*:409–414, 1961

29. Mallach HJ, Laudahn G: Vergleichende Untersuchungen mit enzymatischen Methoden an Vital- und Leichenblut im Hinblick auf die Todeszeit. Klin Wochenschr 42:693–699, 1964

30. Martinez-Tello F, Braun D: Über Anwendungsmöglichkeiten der postmortalen Serum-analyse in der Obduktionsdiagnostik besonders bei Paraproteinosen. Virchows Arch [Pathol Anat] 339:349–357, 1965

31. Martinez-Tello F, Braun D, Sawade H, Haferkamp O: Untersuchungen zum Verhalten der Eiweisskörper aus Leichenseren in der Norm und bei Fällen mit akuter Entzündung mit Nekrose. Virchows Arch [Pathol Anat] 339:337–348, 1965

32. Mold JW: Chromosomes after death (letter to the editor). Lancet 2:107, 1966

33. Moritz AR: Scientific evidence in establishing the time of death. Ann West Med Surg 6:302–304, 1952

34. Naumann HN: Studies on postmortem chemistry. Am J Clin Pathol 20:314–324, 1950

35. Naumann HN: Postmortem blood sugar (letter to the editor). JAMA 157:780, 1955

36. Naumann HN: Postmortem liver function tests. Am J Clin Pathol 26:495–505, 1956

37. Naumann HN: Cerebrospinal fluid electrolytes after death. Proc Soc Exp Biol Med 98:16–18, 1958

38. Naumann HN: Body chemistry after death (letter to the editor). JAMA 171:2278, 1959

39. Pease DC: Histological Techniques for Electron Microscopy. Second edition. New York, Academic Press, 1964

40. Robertson HE: Teamwork between the roentgenologist and the pathologist. J Radiol 3:308–310, 1922

41. Sabatini DD, Bensch K, Barrnett RJ: Cytochemistry and electron microscopy: the preservation of cellular ultrastructure and enzymatic activity by aldehyde fixation. J Cell Biol 17:19–58, 1963

42. Saliba NA, Maya G: Air embolism during pneumoperitoneum refill. Am Rev Resp Dis 92:810–812, 1965

43. Saliba NA, Maya G, Leguizamon C, Pal E, Goldin AG: Postmortem chest radiography. Am Rev Resp Dis 99:903–908, 1969

44. Sanes S, Eschner EG: Roentgen-ray examination in medicolegal autopsies. New York J Med 55:628–633, 1955

45. Schlang HA, Davis DR: Paper electrophoretic studies of postmortem serum proteins. Am J Med Sci 236:472–474, 1958

46. Schleyer F: Quantitative Untersuchungen über den Fibrinogenschwund im Leichenblut. Arch Exp Pathol Pharmacol 211:292–302, 1950

47. Schleyer F: Postmortale Blutviscosität, Blutzellvolumen, osmotische Erythrocytenresistenz und Blutkörperchensenkung in Beziehung zu Leichenalter und Todesursache. Virchows Arch [Pathol Anat] 331:276–286, 1958

48. Schleyer FL: Postmortale klinisch-chemische Diagnostik und Todeszeitbestimmung mit chemischen und physikalischen Methoden. Stuttgart, Georg Thieme Verlag, 1958

49. Schoenmackers J, Vieten H: Atlas postmortaler Angiogramme. Fortschr Geb Roentgenstr 69:1–203, 1954

50. Silver H, Sonnenwirth AC: A practical and efficacious method for obtaining significant postmortem blood cultures. Am J Clin Pathol 52:433–437, 1969

51. Smith LDS, Holdeman LV: The Pathogenic Anaerobic Bacteria. Springfield, Illinois, Charles C Thomas, Publisher, 1968

52. Thorwald J: The Century of the Detective. (English translation by Richard and Clara Winston.) New York, Harcourt, Brace & World, Inc., 1965, pp 403–413

53. Titus JL, Larson SL: Unpublished data

54. Titus JL, Pierre RV: Chromosomal analysis in clinical medicine. Med Clin North Am 54:1009–1027, 1970

55. Tonge JI, Wannan JS: The post-mortem blood sugar. Med J Aust 1:439–447, 1949

56. Traub F: Methode zur Erkennung von tödlichen Zuckerstoffwechselstörungen an der Leiche (Diabetes mellitus und Hypoglykämie). Zentralbl Allg Pathol 112:390–399, 1969

57. US Department of Defense. Army Department: Autopsy Manual, Washington DC, US Government Printing Office, 1960

58. Warren BA: Fibrinolytic activity of vascular endothelium. Br Med Bull 20:213–216, 1964

59. Weed LA: Technics for the isolation of fungi from tissues obtained at operation and necropsy. Am J Clin Pathol 29:496–502, 1958

60. Weed LA, Baggenstoss AH: The isolation of pathogens from tissues of embalmed human bodies. Am J Clin Pathol 21:1114–1120, 1951

61. Weinberg SB, Purdy BA: Postmortem leucocyte culture studies in sudden infant death. Nature (Lond) 226:1264–1265, 1970

CHAPTER 9

AUTOPSY LABORATORY PROCEDURES

STAINING REACTIONS AND AUTORADIOGRAPHY OF AUTOPSY TISSUES

Staining of Gross Tissues. Hematoxylin is used as a differential tissue stain — for example, to outline malignant lesions or to identify changes in the intestinal mucosa. The technique is described in chapter 5.

Eosin also is used as a differential tissue stain. The technique is described in chapter 5.

Fat and Lipoid Stains. Fat stains are used either as differential tissue stains — for example, to outline malignant lesions infiltrating fat tissue — or to identify fat and lipoids in organs or pathologic lesions.

When differential fat staining is desired, the freshly trimmed, fresh or formalin-fixed specimen is immersed in a saturated solution of Sudan III or Scharlach R in 70% alcohol.[11] The fat will stain bright red. Nonfatty structures are decolorized by placing the specimen in 95% alcohol. After the differentiation is complete, the tissue is washed and mounted in formalin solution.

Another method is described in chapter 5.

A method of staining for fat and lipoid in organs or pathologic lesions is described in chapter 3. Scott[18] used Scharlach R in 70% alcohol for gross demonstration of lipoid changes in the adrenal cortex.

Staining of Myelinated and Nonmyelinated Fibers of Brain. With the method of Edwards and Edwards[4] or of Tompsett,[21] satisfactory specimens can be prepared if the procedures are strictly adhered to. Specimens prepared by these methods are primarily recommended for the anatomic museum and will not be described here.

229

Stain for Iron (Hemosiderin). The reaction of Fe^{+++} with ferrocyanide has been used as a differential tissue stain in the brain. However, this method is best known and most widely used for the demonstration of tissue iron in hemosiderosis and hemochromatosis. Slices of liver, pancreas, heart, or lung are treated as described in chapter 5. Positive stains are blue. The intensity of the stain roughly parallels the iron content.

Amyloid Stains.[16] 1. Iodine stain. Immerse the specimen in a solution made up of 1 gm of iodine, 2 gm of potassium iodide, 1 ml of sulfuric acid, and 100 ml of water. Amyloid will turn blue. The specimen is then washed in tap water and mounted in liquid paraffin. This technique is said to prevent fading of the stained amyloid; without sulfuric acid, amyloid will turn brown.

Edwards and Edwards[4] suggested that the specimen should not be washed but should be put in 70% alcohol until the differentiation is complete. The specimen is then removed from the jar and the alcohol is allowed to evaporate. Subsequently, the tissue, which should be almost dry, is placed in liquid paraffin until it is completely soaked, which may take 8 weeks or more. Edwards and Edwards also mount the specimen in liquid paraffin. According to Boyd,[1] liquid petrolatum is the best preservative for iodine-stained amyloid-containing tissues.

2. Congo Red stain.[16] The specimen is fixed in Kaiserling I solution (see later in this chapter) and subsequently immersed for 1 hour in 1% Congo Red. It then is transferred to a saturated solution of lithium carbonate for 2 minutes and differentiated in 80% alcohol. Normal arteries and veins tend to retain their color. The specimen is mounted in Kaiserling III solution (glycerine 300 ml, sodium acetate 100 gm, 0.5% formalin solution to a final volume of 1,000 ml; adjust to pH 8; if necessary, filter to clear the solution). In this instance, sodium bisulfite should not be added prior to sealing the jar.

Calcium Stains.[11] 1. Silver nitrate method. Wash the formalin-fixed specimen under running tap water for 24 hours and then in several changes of distilled water for 24 hours. In a darkroom, immerse the specimen in a 1% solution of silver nitrate in distilled water and stain for 6 to 15 hours. Rinse it in distilled water and then place it in 5% sodium bisulfite solution for 24 hours. The specimen can now be exposed to light, washed, and mounted in 50% alcohol or Kaiserling solution.

2. Alizarin method. Immerse the specimen for 12 hours in a 1:10,000 solution of Alizarin Red S with just enough potassium hydroxide to render the solution basic. For differentiation, transfer the specimen to a solution of equal parts of alcohol and glycerine and expose the jar to sunlight. Alizarin dyes stain calcium pink. After several days, mount the specimen in Kaiserling solution which is made alkaline by adding a small amount (1:1,000) of potassium hydroxide.

Effects of Postmortem Interval on Histochemical Reactions. The effects of postmortem changes have not been systematically evaluated in all organs.

In the heart,[2] glycogen and phosphorylase disappear rapidly, so that no valid results can be obtained. Isocitric dehydrogenase, reduced triphosphopyridine nucleotide diaphorase, β-hydroxybutyrate dehydrogenase, and cytochrome oxidase also disappear relatively rapidly or show marked variability after death. Histochemical studies in normal hearts and in hypertrophic hearts, idiopathic cardiomyopathy, myocardial ischemia, and other myocardial lesions revealed no selective or specific histochemical alterations. However, qualitative gross staining reactions of the diminished endogenous substrates and dehydrogenase activity, as are used for detection of myocardial infarcts of longer than 6 to 8 hours' duration (see chapter 3), seem to be fairly reliable within the usual postmortem intervals.

In the heart and liver of dogs, glycogen disappears rapidly after death.[9] After incubation at 37 C, succinic dehydrogenase activity and DNA content in heart, liver, and kidney are decreased. This is not the case after incubation at 4 C. Alkaline phosphatase does not decrease after death, particularly when incubated at 4 C.[9]

In the rabbit cerebellum, alkaline phosphatase, acid phosphatase, lactic dehydrogenase, glutamic dehydrogenase, hexokinase, and malic dehydrogenase were found to be stable after postmortem intervals of 2 to 6 hours. Phosphofructokinase proved to be unstable.[19]

For any histochemical study on postmortem material, pilot experiments have to be carried out to determine the effect of postmortem changes. The comparison of histochemical reactions in freeze-dried tissues with those in water homogenates at various postmortem intervals is one way in which such pilot studies can be performed.[19]

Autoradiography. Postmortem material can be used for the identification and localization of radioactive material. Postmortem changes have little effect on the quality of the autoradiograms. The demonstration of thorium dioxide contrast medium (Thorotrast) (Fig. 9–1) is probably the

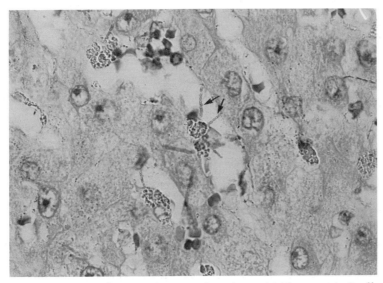

Figure 9–1. Autoradiogram of autopsy liver tissue with Thorotrast in Kupffer cells. Tracks arising from the α-emitting Thorotrast are clearly visible (*arrows*). This autoradiogram was prepared 6 years after the death of the patient. (Hematoxylin and eosin; ×700.)

main application of this method, but autopsy autoradiography may also be employed as a collateral of clinical research. For detection of diagnostic and therapeutic radioisotopes, scanning techniques are usually used (see chapter 10).

The preparation of good autoradiograms requires some experience. Several techniques are available, and the reader is referred to the appropriate textbooks. The following method is given as an example which can be varied in many ways. The slide shown in Figure 9–1 was prepared by the technique described here.

The tissue is fixed in buffered 10% formalin solution and embedded in paraffin. Sections are cut at a thickness of 2 to 5 μ. Autoradiograms are prepared by dipping the slides in nuclear track emulsion (Kodak, Type NTB2). This procedure is carried out in the darkroom. The autoradiograms are stored at 4 C for a period which depends on the expected radioactivity of the specimen. It may be necessary to try various times in order to achieve optimal exposure. In the case of Thorotrast storage in the liver, illustrated in Figure 9–1, the slides were stored for 2 months before being developed. We develop with Kodak D-19 at 24 C for 2 minutes. The slides are then fixed, washed, and stained with hematoxylin and eosin.

FIXATION AND COLOR
PRESERVATION OF TISSUES

Some fixatives are superior for the demonstration of certain histologic details; others are specifically required (or specifically contraindicated) for certain special stains. Special indications are listed with the various fixative recipes. For routine purposes, excellent fixation can be achieved with almost all of the mixtures listed below so that the choice will depend on availability, costs, and technical help.

The smaller the specimen, the sooner will the fixation be completed. The acceptable thickness of tissues is listed with the various fixation mixtures. Larger specimens may remain completely unfixed in the center. The use of small volumes of fixation fluid for large specimens is the most frequent cause of poor tissue preservation. The minimal acceptable volume of fixation fluid is about 15 to 20 times the volume of the specimen.

No matter what type of fixative is used, the tissues should not touch each other or be pressed against the bottom or walls of the jar. Suspension of larger specimens or use of a cushion of cotton for smaller specimens will permit optimal exposure.

If the fixative becomes stained, cloudy, or diluted by blood or other tissue fluids, it must be replaced.

Heating will accelerate the fixation process but, at the same time, will enhance autolytic changes in the unfixed portion of the tissue. Boiling will result in rapid fixation and has been used to prepare rapid-fixed frozen sections. We prefer to use unfixed tissue for frozen sections. Since boiling in saline avoids the chemical effects of fixatives, this method has been used to carry out comparative studies of chemical fixation fluids.

Fixation Mixtures. Many fixatives have been modified by various authors and institutions. However, it seems that the improvements, if any, are minor compared with the results which will be achieved if size and exposure of the specimen and volume and freshness of the fixation fluid are appropriately controlled. Most of the following recipes and specifications are from the textbook by Thompson.[20]

Alcohol. 1. Indications. Preservation of urates, glycogen, sulfhydryl groups of protein, and water-soluble pigments; enzyme studies. If alcohol is used to preserve water-soluble substances, no aqueous staining procedures can be used.

2. Composition. Absolute ethyl alcohol.

3. Procedure. Fix slices, not thicker than 5 to 6 mm, in 20 volumes of absolute alcohol. The fixation time will be about 4 hours. Transfer to 70% ethyl alcohol for another 72 hours. For enzyme studies, 70% alcohol should not be used but instead use two additional treatments (12 hours each) with absolute ethyl alcohol.

4. Storage. Fixed tissue should be stored in 70% alcohol.

Bouin's Fixative. 1. Indications. May serve as a general-purpose fixative but proper use is time-consuming. Excellent for subsequent trichrome staining. Glycogen is retained. Erythrocytes are lysed. Excellent for histologic demonstration of pulmonary edema fluid.

2. Composition. Stock solution:

Saturated aqueous picric acid	750 ml
Formaldehyde solution (36 to 40%)	250 ml.

Preparation of aqueous picric acid for stock solution:

Picric acid (trinitrophenol, USP)	20 gm
Distilled water	1,000 ml.

Heat until picric acid dissolves. Cool and decant supernate. Prepare fixative, just before use, by mixing:

Stock solution	95 ml
Glacial (99.7%) acetic acid	5 ml.

3. Procedure. Fix slices not thicker than 3 to 5 mm. If the tissue is very soft, thin slices can be cut from larger pieces after about 2 hours of fixation. The fixation must be completed in 12 to 24 hours. Transfer to 50% ethyl alcohol for another 6 to 24 hours. The alcohol should be changed when it becomes yellow.

4. Storage. Fixed tissue should be stored in 70% alcohol.

Carnoy's Fixative. 1. Indications. Preservation of nuclei and other structures rich in nucleic acids, protein sulfhydryl groups, and glycogen.

2. Composition.

Absolute ethyl alcohol	640 ml
Chloroform	120 ml
Glacial (99.7%) acetic acid	40 ml.

Prepare fixative just before use.

3. Procedure. Slices up to 1.5 cm in thickness can be fixed. The fixation time will vary between 2 and 20 hours. Transfer into absolute ethyl alcohol.

4. Storage. Fixed tissue should be stored in cedar oil (reagent grade or USP) or lightweight liquid petrolatum.

Formalin Solutions. Formalin is a 36 to 40% solution of gaseous form-aldehyde (HCHO) in water. One usually uses a 10% solution, which is a 4% solution of gaseous formaldehyde in water. The term "formalin" is also frequently used for the 10% solution. Thus, "formalin" and "10% formalin" have become synonymous. The 36 to 40% solution of gaseous formaldehyde in water, or formalin, is then referred to as "concentrated formalin." In some places the 4% solution of gaseous form-aldehyde in water is occasionally, but wrongly, called "4% formalin."

In this book the term "formalin" or "concentrated formalin" means a 36 to 40% solution of gaseous formaldehyde in water. The usual 10% formalin solution is referred to as "10% formalin solution" or "formalin solution." When tissues are referred to as "formalin-fixed" it also means that a 10% formalin solution had been used.

1. Indications. Ten percent formalin solution is the most widely used fixative, recommendable for most purposes, cheap, and requiring little attention. Formalin-calcium solution is used for the preservation of phospholipids, and formalin-ammonium bromide solution is recommended for fixation of central nervous system tissue when impregnation with gold and silver is intended.

2. Composition. Unbuffered formalin (10% solution):

Formalin	100 ml
Tap water	900 ml.

Formalin-saline:

Formalin	100 ml
Sodium chloride	8.5 gm
Tap water	900 ml.

Buffered neutral formalin solution is preferred in many instances because the formation of acid hematin becomes negligible.

Buffered neutral formalin solution:

A crude method is to add an excess of calcium and magnesium carbonate to unbuffered 10% formalin solution.

Formalin solution buffered at pH 6.8 to 7.0:

Dibasic anhydrous sodium phosphate (Na_2HPO_4)	6.5 gm
Monobasic acid potassium phosphate (KH_2PO_4)	4 gm
Formalin	100 ml
Distilled water	900 ml.

Formalin-alcohol:

Formalin	100 ml
Ethyl alcohol, 95%	900 ml
Calcium acetate	0.5 gm
	(added if neutral-ization is required)

Formalin-calcium (Baker):

Formalin	10 ml
Calcium chloride, anhydrous $(CaCl_2)$	1 gm
Distilled water to make	100 ml
Piece of chalk, 3 to 5 cm long.	

Dissolve the calcium chloride in part of the water. Add the formalin and then make to volume with water. Add the chalk to the mixture to maintain the pH, which should be approximately 4.7 to 4.9.

Formalin-formic acid:

Formalin	100 ml
4N formic acid	900 ml.

Formalin-acetic acid-alcohol:

Formalin	100 ml
Glacial (99.7%) acetic acid	50 ml
Ethyl alcohol, absolute	850 ml.

3. Procedure. Fix slices not thicker than 6 mm in 20 volumes of formalin solution. The fixation time will be about 6 to 18 hours. However, the tissues may remain in formalin solution for unlimited periods. Change the formalin solution until the fixative remains clear.

4. Storage. Fixed tissue should be stored in formalin solution.

Glutaraldehyde. 1. Indications. This fixative has been known for some time as suitable for electron microscopy and certain histochemical methods. Recently, phosphate-buffered glutaraldehyde has been advocated as an all-purpose fixative.[3] Glutaraldehyde produces less irritating fumes than formalin, is well suited for perfusion of large specimens, and yields excellent cytologic details. Connective tissue stains are well differentiated. The dye uptake is increased in glutaraldehyde-fixed sections. Sectioning artifacts are less frequent. This fixative is more expensive than formalin.

2. Composition. The final preparation represents a 4% glutaraldehyde solution:

Purified glutaraldehyde, 25%	100 ml
Sorenson's phosphate buffer, 0.1M, pH 7.4	525 ml.

3. Procedure. Fix slices not thicker than 4 mm in 20 volumes of 4% glutaraldehyde solution. The fixation time at room temperature will be 6 to 24 hours. Cold fixation with glutaraldehyde for histochemical enzyme location yields complete fixation after 6 hours but in only the outer 1 mm of tissue.

4. Storage. Use 4% glutaraldehyde solution.

Helly's Fixative. 1. Indications. This is an excellent fixative for bone marrow and organs containing much blood. It is superior to Zenker's fixative in terms of penetration.

2. Composition.

Potassium dichromate ($K_2Cr_2O_7$)	2.5 gm
Mercuric chloride ($HgCl_2$)	5.0 gm
Sodium sulfate, anhydrous (Na_2SO_4)	1.0 gm
Distilled water	100 ml
Formalin	5 to 6 ml.

3. Procedure. Fix slices not thicker than 6 mm in 20 volumes of fixative. The fixation time will be about 12 to 24 hours. Tissues must then be washed for 14 to 16 hours. Transfer to 80% alcohol. Residues of mercuric chloride must be removed from the sections with 0.5% aqueous iodine (5 minutes) followed by 5% aqueous sodium thiosulfate (5 minutes).

4. Storage. Use 70% ethyl alcohol for short-term storage. For long-term preservation, dehydration and storage in thin cedar oil or paraffin embedding has been suggested.

Regaud's Fixative. 1. Indications. For the demonstration of rickettsiae.

2. Composition.

Potassium dichromate ($K_2Cr_2O_7$),	
3% aqueous solution	80 ml
Formalin	20 ml.

3. Procedure. Fix slices not thicker than 4 mm in 20 volumes of fixative. The fixation time will be about 24 to 48 hours. Wash in running water for 24 hours. Transfer to 70% ethyl alcohol.

4. Storage. Store in 70% ethyl alcohol.

Trichloroacetic Acid. 1. Indications. Preservation of sulfhydryl groups and amino groups of protein.

2. Composition.

Trichloroacetic acid (USP crystals)	50 gm
Ethyl alcohol, 95%	750 ml
Distilled water	200 ml.

3. Procedure. Fix slices not thicker than 3 to 5 mm in 20 volumes of fixative. The fixation time will be 16 to 18 hours. Transfer to 95% ethyl alcohol.

4. Storage. Use 70% ethyl alcohol.

Zenker's Fixative. 1. Indications. Similar to Helly's fixative. Recommended for staining of cytoplasmic inclusions and for use with the Feulgen stain.

2. Composition. Stock solution:

Mercuric chloride ($HgCl_2$)	50 gm
Potassium dichromate ($K_2Cr_2O_7$)	25 gm
Sodium sulfate, anhydrous (Na_2SO_4)	10 gm
Distilled water	1,000 ml.

Just before use, the stock solution is mixed with either acetic acid or formic acid:

Stock solution	95 ml
Glacial (99.7%) acetic acid	5 ml

or

Stock solution	95 ml
Formic acid (88%, analytical grade)	5 ml.

3. Procedure. Fix slices not thicker than 6 mm in 20 volumes of fixative. The fixation time will be about 24 hours. Thick specimens should be postfixed for 2 hours in a 2.5% aqueous solution of potassium dichromate. Tissues must then be washed for 14 to 16 hours. Transfer to 80% alcohol. Residues of mercuric chloride must be removed from the sections with 0.5% aqueous iodine (5 minutes) followed by 5% aqueous sodium thiosulfate (5 minutes).

4. Storage. Use 70% ethyl alcohol for short-term storage. For long-term preservation, dehydration and storage in thin cedar oil or paraffin embedding has been suggested.

Fixation by Microwave Heating. This technique is still experimental. Preliminary studies with 1-cm cubes of tissue showed uniform fixation in 90 seconds with minimal shrinkage. An unexplained finding, and a disadvantage of microwave fixation, was the disappearance of erythrocytes and, to a lesser degree, collagen fibers.[13]

Color-Preserving Fixation Mixtures. Most fixatives and fixation mixtures turn the natural color of organs into a uniform gray. In the past, color-preserving fixatives were preferred by many workers. A review of the contemporary literature reveals that there were only a few original color-preserving fluids but that large numbers of modifications were developed and advertised. Modern color photography of fresh specimens and the decline of the pathologic museum have to some extent terminated the search for the ideal color-preserving mixture. None of the color-preserving or restoring mixtures creates truly natural colors. The same holds true for carbon monoxide rejuvenation. Nevertheless, some of the classic recipes and their modifications are presented here.

Jores' Solution. 1. Composition.

Sodium chloride (NaCl)	10 gm
Magnesium sulfate ($MgSO_4$)	20 gm
Sodium sulfate (Na_2SO_4)	20 gm
Formalin solution (2 to 4%)	1,100 ml.

2. Procedure. Fix specimens for 1 to 2 days or longer. Rinse in 95% ethyl alcohol. Leave in 95% ethyl alcohol for 24 hours or until red color has returned.

3. Mounting. Jores mounted specimens in a solution of equal parts of glycerine and water. Two other mounting fluids can be used:

Potassium acetate	100 gm
Glycerine	400 ml
Formalin	20 ml
Water with thymol added	2,000 ml
or	
Potassium acetate	500 gm
Sodium chloride	9.5 gm
Carbolic acid crystals	12.5 gm
Glycerine	1,000 ml
Water	5,000 ml.

Modified Jores' Solution (After Klotz and Maclachlan[10]). 1. Composition.

Chloral hydrate	125 gm
Carlsbad salt	125 gm
Formalin	125 ml
Tap water	4,000 ml.

The composition of Carlsbad salt is:

Sodium sulfate (Na_2SO_4)	22 gm
Sodium bicarbonate ($NaHCO_3$)	20 gm
Sodium chloride (NaCl)	18 gm
Potassium nitrate (KNO_3)	38 gm
Potassium sulfate (K_2SO_4)	2 gm.

2. Procedure. Fix the specimen for 10 days. Wash thoroughly in cold running water for 6 to 10 hours.

3. Mounting.

Cane sugar	3,500 gm
Potassium acetate	160 gm
Chloral hydrate	80 gm
Water with thymol added	8,000 ml.

Kaiserling's Solutions. 1. Composition. The following solutions are among Kaiserling's own final modifications,[8] published 28 years after his original description in 1896.

Kaiserling I:

Potassium acetate	85 gm
Potassium nitrate (KNO_3)	45 gm
Formalin solution (3 to 4%)	4,800 ml.

Kaiserling II:

Ethyl alcohol, 80 to 90% (others[7] prefer 95%).

2. Procedure. Fix specimen for 1 to 5 days in Kaiserling I. Fixation time will vary with the thickness of the organ. Excessive perfusion with Kaiserling I solution will cause loss of natural color because too much blood is rinsed out. Transfer to Kaiserling II for a few hours. Acid hematin will turn into alkaline hematin which approximates the color of hemoglobin.

3. Mounting. Use Kaiserling III solution:

Potassium acetate	200 gm
Glycerine	300 ml
Tap water	900 ml.

Modified Kaiserling's Solutions (After Lundquist[12]). This method was developed in this department to avoid the use of alcohol which tends to add to the stiffening and contraction of the specimens.

1. Composition. Kaiserling I:

Potassium acetate	85 gm
Potassium nitrate (KNO_3)	45 gm
Chloral hydrate	80 gm
Formalin	444 ml
Tap water	4,000 ml.

2. Procedure. Suspend the specimen in 10 to 12 times its volume of fluid. Just after the fixation is completed (avoid overfixation), wash thoroughly in running water and retrim so that all cut surfaces are resurfaced. Transfer to mounting solution for 12 hours. Change solution for permanent mounting.

3. Mounting. Kaiserling III:

Potassium acetate	10 gm
Chloral hydrate	5 gm
Glycerine	10 ml
Tap water	90 ml.

Modified Kaiserling's Solutions (After Wentworth[23]). This method also avoids the use of alcohol but introduces sodium bisulfite ($NaHSO_3$) which is added to the mounting solution.

1. Composition. Kaiserling I:

Sodium acetate	30 gm
Potassium nitrate	15 gm
Formalin	100 ml
Tap water	1,000 ml.

2. Procedure. Suspend the specimen in 10 to 12 times its volume of fluid until thoroughly fixed. Immerse for a few days in Kaiserling III. Retrim so that all cut surfaces are resurfaced.

3. Mounting. Kaiserling III:

Sodium acetate	100 gm
Glycerine	200 ml
Tap water	1,000 ml.

The solution is first heated to boiling to drive out dissolved oxygen and then cooled to not higher than 30 C. Immediately before the lid of the museum jar is sealed, 1 to 2 gm of sodium bisulfite is added to each liter of Kaiserling III mounting solution.

Method of Meiller.[14] 1. Procedure. Fix specimen in 10% formalin solution until fixation is just completed. Avoid overfixation. Wash in running water for 3 to 6 hours. Immerse in 2% ammonium hydroxide for 5 to 10 minutes. Wash in running water for 1 hour.

2. Mounting. Mount in saturated solution of antimony trioxide (Sb_2O_3): Mix about 5 gm of antimony trioxide in 1 liter of water. Filter this solution and to 1 liter of the filtrate add 100 gm of potassium acetate, 100 gm of chloral hydrate, and 50 ml of glycerine. The filtrate is stirred until the chemicals are dissolved.

Method of Wright and Bali (After Faulkner et al[5]). 1. Composition.

Tap water	1,000 ml
Sodium chloride (NaCl)	9 gm
Disodium arsenate ($Na_2HAsO_4 \cdot 7H_2O$)	50 gm
Sodium tetraborate (Borax)	50 gm
Prague powder*	20 gm
Formalin	10 ml
Sodium erythorbate (isoascorbate)	20 gm.

The amount of Prague powder used seems to vary widely from author to author.

2. Procedure. Formalin-fixed (but not overfixed) specimens can be saved in the mounting fluid for years. The color of the specimens will then begin to fade. Addition of sodium erythorbate will restore the colors. There should be no air in the containers. The specimens should not be allowed to dry. The authors placed Ionol (Shell Oil Products) on top of the mounting solution to prevent growth of molds.

Rejuvenation of Old Formalin-Fixed Specimens. **Rejuvenation Fluid.**
1. Composition. The rejuvenation solution is:

Sodium chloride (NaCl)	100 gm
Sodium sulfate (Na_2SO_4)	5 gm
Glycerine	50 ml
Tap water	1,000 ml.

2. Procedure. Sodium chloride and sodium sulfate are dissolved in the water and the solution is filtered. Then the glycerine is added. Just before the jar containing the specimen and this solution is resealed, a few drops of alcoholic camphor are added. There will be a temporary cloudiness of the solution.

Carbon Monoxide Rejuvenation.[17] This method is dangerous because of the risk of carbon monoxide intoxication for those who work with the gassing apparatus. The organ is placed in a jar with isotonic buffered 10% formalin solution or Kaiserling I solution, and gas containing carbon monoxide (illuminating gas) is intermittently bubbled through the solution until the specimen turns red. The gas is continuously collected from the surface of the solution through an inverted funnel and burned. After a few days, the cherry red organ is washed in running water and mounted promptly in:

Cane sugar	40 gm

---

* Griffith Laboratories, Inc., Chicago, Ill.

| Chloral hydrate | 2 gm |
| Distilled water | 100 ml. |

Color Preservation of Special Organs and Lesions. *Chloroma (After Edwards and Edwards[4]).* 1. Procedure. The specimen should be fixed without previous washing and then placed for 24 hours in methyl alcohol. Transfer for the following 24 hours to the following solution:

Sodium bisulfite (NaHSO$_3$)	0.5 gm
Sodium hydroxide (NaOH)	1 gm
Tap water	100 ml.

The container with this fluid should be filled to the brim, and the lid should be sealed with petroleum jelly.

2. Mounting.

Sodium bisulfite (NaHSO$_3$)	0.1 gm
Glycerine	30 ml
Sodium acetate	10 gm
Formalin	0.5 ml
Tap water	70 ml.

Melanoma and Melanotic Tissues. 1. Procedure. Thin slices (about 6 mm) of fixed tissue are kept in methyl alcohol for 12 hours. Transfer into acetone for another 12 to 18 hours and then into xylol for about 2 hours. Remove when shrinkage begins and put into mounting fluid.

2. Mounting. Mount in liquid paraffin.

Specimens With Gouty Changes. 1. Procedure. Fix specimen preferably in an anhydrous fixative such as alcohol. Although urate crystals are freely soluble in water, crystalline deposits are usually identifiable in the center of the specimens even after aqueous formalin fixation. The crystals often also resist the dehydration and staining procedure.[6] For the preservation of the gross specimen, the preparation is dehydrated over 2 weeks in several changes of absolute ethyl alcohol. Transfer into mounting fluid.

2. Mounting. Mount in plastic jar with undiluted glycerine. Seal without leaving air under the lid.

Gallbladders.[15] If the gallbladder can be obtained within a few hours after death the oxidative greenish discoloration will not yet have occurred and can be prevented by the following procedure.

1. Procedure. Place specimen in 3% solution of sodium sulfite* for 20 minutes. Rinse for a few minutes in running water. Place in 10% formalin solution for 12 to 24 hours. Wash thoroughly and mount.

2. Mounting.

Potassium acetate	10 gm
Chloral hydrate	5 gm
Glycerine	10 ml
Tap water	90 ml.

Instead of the sodium sulfite-formalin mixture, a saturated solution of calcium chloride can be used. The specimens should be soaked in this solution for 24 to 48 hours.[16]

---

* If the greenish color of biliverdin has already formed, a 5% sodium sulfite solution is used, to which 1% formalin is added. The specimen is left in this solution for 12 hours. The subsequent steps remain the same.

SHIPPING OF AUTOPSY MATERIAL

Containers. Human tissues or body fluids can be mailed if two containers or bags are used, one within the other.[5] Absorbent material (see below) is placed between the two containers. Paper, plastic, glass, or metal jars and plastic bags are used. Various types of containers and plastic bags are described in chapter 13. Ordinarily, waxed paper or plastic jars are most convenient for shipping autopsy tissues. However, for toxicologic examinations, the inner container should be of glass, particularly when the tissues or body fluids are to be analyzed for volatile substances. Plastics may be permeable to gases, and corrosion of metal containers may interfere with toxicologic studies. Stoppers, corks, and lids should be taped in place.

For use as an absorbent, cotton can be soaked with 10% formalin solution and wrapped around the tissues. Towels and gauze cause marks on tissue surfaces and should not be used for wrapping or covering of tissues. Fixatives should not be used if the material is sent for toxicologic or microbiologic examination. Enough cotton or paper should be placed between the inner container (or plastic bag) and the outer container to take up all liquid in case of breakage or leakage. The absorbent material is also useful for cushioning the inner container.

Shipping of frozen material is recommended for submission for toxicologic and biochemical examinations. Ordinary ice is sufficient if the specimen is transported by a messenger who will replenish the ice if necessary. Dry Ice will be effective for about 24 hours. For longer periods, refilling is required, or the specimen has to be sent in Dry Ice with ether or acetone in a Thermos bottle as described on page 242. The Dry Ice is put around and on top of the specimen and on the inside of the absorbent material. The mailing container should be insulated.

As mailing containers, durable shipping cartons, wooden boxes, or metal containers are used. For frozen material the mailing container should be insulated. Shipping cartons are sealed with strips of gummed paper.

Inside the mailing container, a tag or letter should be placed giving (1) name and address of the submitter, (2) name and address of receiver of the shipment, (3) name, clinic number, and autopsy number and year of the patient from whom the material came, and (4) type of examination requested, together with all pertinent data. If a separate letter has been sent, a copy should always be put into the mailing container. This may help to avoid much confusion and delay. It is a continuing problem for many institutions to receive tissues without any further information, and a frustrating search follows for a misfiled or lost letter to match the shipment.

Letters and addresses in the shipping container should be protected from leaking fluids, for instance by sealing them into plastic.

Mailing containers should be marked on the outside with appropriate warnings such as "Glass, Handle With Care" and "Perishable Material." Additional labels are recommended for medicolegal or microbiologic material (see following page).

Shipping and Labeling of Medicolegal Material. Medicolegal material is sent by messenger, registered mail, railway express, or air express. Care must be taken that the chain of custody remains uninterrupted (see chapter 2). Medicolegal material will often be passed through local police authorities to the state bureau of criminal identification or investigation laboratory. The address for shipments to the laboratories of the FBI is:

Director, Federal Bureau of Investigation
US Department of Justice
Washington, DC 20012
Attention: FBI Laboratory

Specimen labels should contain (1) name and address of the submitter, (2) name and address of receiver of the shipment, (3) description of the container and of the source and nature of its contents, (4) a tag describing the shipment as "Evidence," and (5) if applicable, a request for specific examination.

Containers with medicolegal material should be sealed prior to shipping so that the contents cannot be tampered with. We are using sealing wax imprinted with the thumb of the submitter.

The mailing container should show (1) the name and address of the submitter, (2) the name and address of the receiver, and (3) warning tags such as "Glass, Handle With Care," "Perishable Material," or "Fragile, Rush, Specimen for Toxicologic Study."

Special Shipping Procedures. *Blood and Tissues for Carbon Monoxide Determination.*[22] For blood, 10 ml is placed over 10 mg of lithium oxalate in a screw-cap test tube. The blood is covered with mineral oil, and the cap or stopper is sealed with hot paraffin or plastic tape. Tissues can be packed in rubber containers as described below. They are shipped in Dry Ice in an insulated mailing container.

Brain and Spinal Cord Tissue for Lactic Acid Determination.[22] Lactic acid determination is indicated in cases of suspected hypoxia. A 10-gm sample of brain or spinal cord is removed with minimal handling. Contact with water must be avoided. The tissue is placed into a rubber container (dental rubber dam or a condom can be used) from which all air is expressed. Two knots are tied in the open end of the rubber container. Chips of Dry Ice are placed into a Thermos bottle, and ether or acetone is poured over them. The rubber container with the tissue is dropped into this freezing mixture. The stopper on the Thermos bottle must be perforated to permit gas to escape.

Another method requires only table salt and water. A disassembled Thermos bottle and a salt solution (100 gm of table salt in 300 ml of tap water) are placed in the deep freeze or freezing compartment of the refrigerator overnight. The Thermos bottle is then filled about halfway with chipped ice. The salt solution is poured over the chipped ice, leaving about 2.5 cm of space under the stopper. The Thermos bottle is now stoppered, the cap is screwed on, and the assembled bottle is stored in the deep freeze until needed. For shipment, the tissue is placed in the rubber container as described above and dropped into the ice-salt solution in the Thermos bottle. The Thermos bottle is then sealed and shipped.

Tissues and Body Fluids for Microbiologic Study (by C. T. Dolan). Not all organisms will survive shipping, but the method described here seems to be a reasonable compromise for isolating the majority of human pathogenic bacteria, viruses, and fungi.

Specimen size is of practical importance when shipment through the mail is planned. Several 1-cm^3 portions of tissue should be obtained aseptically and placed in a standard sterile screw-cap test tube. Body fluids obtained aseptically can also be placed in such containers. If the specimen was not taken aseptically, a 6-cm^3 specimen must be obtained with a serosal or capsular surface intact so that proper decontamination can be performed as described in chapter 8. The larger the specimen, the more difficult it is to obtain proper shipping containers, but too small a specimen will not allow proper decontamination by searing.

Postal regulations require that the lid of the container with the specimen be sealed with wax or an appropriate impermeable tape to prevent leakage. This primary container must be placed in a soldered metal mailing container with a screw cap. This second container must be placed into a third one, preferably an insulated container, together with an ice can (a screw-cap can filled with water and frozen). In general, freezing the specimen is not indicated as this may destroy certain viruses and fungi or may render histologic examination difficult. The ice can will provide adequate cooling for 2 to 3 days or more if the container is properly insulated. Appropriate packing material should be used in each container to absorb liquid and provide cushioning for shipment.

The outer shipping container should be labeled "Rush, Perishable, Specimens for Bacteriologic Examination," and the package should be sent air express. The person sending the specimen should call the reference laboratory to inform them when the material is being shipped so that expeditious handling is guaranteed. Any pertinent information concerning the specimen should be included as well as sent separately in a letter.

REFERENCES

1. Boyd W: The preservation of amyloid specimens. Int Assoc Med Mus Bull *8*:77–78, 1922
2. Braunstein H: Effect of postmortem interval on histochemical reactions of the myocardium. Am J Clin Pathol *49*:224–231, 1968
3. Chambers RW, Bowling MC, Grimley PM: Glutaraldehyde fixation in routine histopathology. Arch Pathol *85*:18–30, 1968
4. Edwards JJ, Edwards MJ: Medical Museum Technology. London, Oxford University Press, 1959
5. Faulkner WR, King JW, Damm HC: Handbook of Clinical Laboratory Data. Second edition, Cleveland, Ohio, The Chemical Rubber Co., 1968
6. Gardner DL: Pathology of the Connective Tissue Diseases. Baltimore, Williams & Wilkins Company, 1965
7. Judah EL: Personal modifications in the technique of the Kaiserling methods for colour preservation. Int Assoc Med Mus Bull *8*:62–64, 1922
8. Kaiserling C: Die Herstellung anatomischer Sammlungspräparate. *In* Handbuch der Biologischen Arbeitsmethoden. Vol VIII, part 1 (1). Edited by E Abderhalden. Berlin, Urban & Schwarzenberg, 1924, pp 675–696
9. Kent SP: Effect of postmortem autolysis on certain histochemical reactions. Arch Pathol *64*:17–22, 1957

10. Klotz O, Maclachlan WWG: A modified Jores' method for the preservation of colors in gross specimens. Int Assoc Med Mus Bull 5:59–60, 1915

11. Kramer FM: Macroscopic staining of anatomic and pathologic specimens. J Tech Methods *19*:72–78, 1939

12. Lundquist R: A proposed modification of the Kaiserling method for preserving gross specimens. Int Assoc Med Mus Bull *11*:16–18, 1925

13. Mayers CP: Histological fixation by microwave heating. J Clin Pathol *23*: 273–275, 1970

14. Meiller FH: A method for preserving gross specimens in color. J Tech Methods *18*:57–58, 1938

15. Mentzer SH: Methods of preparing gall-bladders and calculi for study and museum display. Int Assoc Med Mus Bull *11*:37–40, 1925

16. Pulvertaft RJV: Museum techniques: a review. J Clin Pathol *3*:1–23, 1950

17. Robertson HE, Lundquist R: Experiences with the carbon monoxide method of preparing museum specimens. J Tech Methods *13*:33–35, 1934

18. Scott WJM: Gross demonstration of adrenal lipoid changes. Int Assoc Med Mus Bull *10*:27, 1924

19. Smith DE, Robins E, Eydt KM, Daesch GE: The validation of the quantitative histochemical method for use on postmortem material. I. The effect of time and temperature. Lab Invest *6*:447–457, 1957

20. Thompson SW: Selected Histochemical and Histopathological Methods. Springfield, Illinois, Charles C Thomas, Publisher, 1966

21. Tompsett DH: Anatomical Techniques. Edinburgh, E. & S. Livingstone, Ltd., 1956

22. US Department of Defense. Navy Department: Manual of Aviation Pathology. US Naval Aviation Medical Center, Pensacola, Florida, 1962

23. Wentworth JE: Hydrosulphite method of preserving museum specimens. J Tech Methods *19*:79–82, 1939

CHAPTER 10

AUTOPSY OF BODIES CONTAINING RADIOACTIVE ISOTOPES

With Alan L. Orvis

All essential aspects of autopsies on radioactive bodies are summarized in the National Bureau of Standards Handbook No. 65[5] and in Report No. 37 of the National Council on Radiation Protection and Measurements.[2] Much of the following is taken from these informative booklets. The reader also is referred to *Radioactive Isotopes and the Mortician*[3] for a review of the basic principles of radioactive decay and of protection from radiation.

Tables 10–1, 10–2, 10–3, and 10–4 show typical radioactivity contents and exposure that might be expected from bodies containing ^{198}Au, ^{90}Y, ^{192}Ir, ^{131}I, or ^{32}P.

GENERAL SAFETY PRECAUTIONS

Bodies containing tracer quantities of radioisotopes administered for diagnostic purposes generally present no hazard. However, the radiation safety officer (institutions licensed to dispense therapeutic quantities of radioactive pharmaceuticals are required to designate a qualified individual as "radiation safety officer") should be summoned in all cases in which therapeutic doses of radioactive isotopes were given during the 2 weeks prior to death. This is the duty of the house officer who is charged with transferring the body to the morgue. However, the pathologist should make sure that this has been done. Radioactive bodies should be labeled with a magenta and yellow tag or radioactivity form which indicates the type and quantity of radioisotope, time of last administration, and expected

245

TABLE 10–1. PROBABLE RADIOACTIVITY CONTENT OF BODY AT VARIOUS TIMES AFTER VARIOUS DOSES*†

Dose of isotope (mCi)	Days elapsed since treatment							
	1	2	3	4	6	8	10	15
198Au remaining in injected cavity								
150	115	90	69	52	32	20	12	*3*
125	96	75	58	44	27	16	10	*3*
100	77	60	46	35	21	13	8	*2*
75	58	45	35	26	16	10	6	*2*
50	38	30	23	18	11	7	*4*	*1*
40	31	24	18	14	9	5	*3*	*1*
30	23	18	14	10	6	*4*	*2*	*1*
131I remaining in thyroid gland								
60	18	16	14	12	10	8	6	*4*
50	15	13	12	11	9	7	5	*3*
40	12	10	9	8	7	5	*4*	*2*
30	9	8	7	6	5	*4*	*3*	*2*
20	6	5	5	*4*	*4*	*3*	*2*	*1*
10	*3*	*3*	*2*	*2*	*2*	*1*	*1*	*1*
131I remaining in functioning metastases‡								
100	20	18	16	14	12	9	7	*4*
75	15	13	12	11	9	7	5	*3*
50	10	9	8	7	6	5	*4*	*2*
35	7	6	5	5	*4*	*3*	*2*	*1*
20	*4*	*4*	*3*	*3*	*2*	*2*	*1*	*1*

* From US Department of Defense. Army Department: Autopsy Manual. US Government Printing Office, Washington DC, 1960. By permission.

† For values in *italics*, no precautions are necessary except use of surgical rubber gloves. For values *not* in italics, consultation with radiologic safety officer is indicated.

‡ These are maximal values; usual levels are smaller.

TABLE 10–2. RADIATION DOSE TO HANDS IN PERITONEAL CAVITY*

Isotope	Dose (rads/mCi/hr)		
	No gloves	Single surgical gloves	Double autopsy gloves
198Au	0.7	0.4	0.1
32P or 90Y†	0.8	0.5	0.3

* Reprinted from National Bureau of Standards Handbook 65, Safe Handling of Bodies Containing Radioactive Isotopes, July, 1958.

† These values would also be good for any other beta-ray emitter whose radiation energies were 1.5 Mev or greater. For beta radiation of less energy, doses will be markedly less, especially when gloves are used.

TABLE 10–3.   APPROXIMATE TIME FOR HANDS IN PERITONEAL CAVITY
TO RECEIVE 1.5 RADS*

Total activity on surface (mCi)	Time (min)			
	^{198}Au		^{32}P or ^{90}Y	
	Single surgical gloves	Double autopsy gloves	Single surgical gloves	Double autopsy gloves
10	21	64	17	32
20	11	32	8	17
30	7	21	6	11
40	5	16	4	8
50	4	13	3	6
60	4	11	3	5
70	3	9	2	5
80	3	8	2	4
90	2	7	2	4
100	2	6	2	3

* Reprinted from National Bureau of Standards Handbook 65, Safe Handling of Bodies Containing Radioactive Isotopes, July, 1958.

radiation exposure level at the day of the autopsy, embalming procedure, or cremation. Tags or forms must be signed by the radiation safety officer. This should be part of the procedure guide in all hospitals so that any physician who might be called to pronounce a patient dead is aware of this requirement.

Bodies with an isotope content of more than 30 mCi should not be released to the autopsy pathologist or funeral director without special advice of the radiation safety officer, regardless of whether or not autopsy, embalming, or cremation is intended. If an autopsy is required, the radiation safety officer should be consulted in all cases in which the body contains more than 5 mCi of any radioactive isotope.

The autopsy pathologist should wear a rubber apron beneath his operating gown so that the cotton may absorb spilled body fluid. High

TABLE 10–4.   RADIATION EXPOSURE RATES AND EXPOSURES
EXPERIENCED BY EMBALMERS DURING PREPARATION
OF CADAVERS*

Radioisotope in cadaver	Exposure rate (mR/hr per mRe or mCi)		Exposure (mR per mRe or mCi)	
	Average	Maximum	Average	Maximum
^{192}Ir†	1.2	3.2	1.7	7.1
^{198}Au	0.36	0.92	0.48	2.1
^{131}I	0.40	1.0	0.54	2.3

* From Laughlin JS, Vacirca SJ, Duplissey JF: Exposure of embalmers and physicians by radioactive cadavers. Health Phys 15:451–455, 1968. By permission of the Health Physics Society.

† Radon-222 produces the same exposures as ^{192}Ir on this basis.

rubber boots and rubber gloves will prevent contamination of legs, hands, and forearms. The face should be protected by a mask and goggles.

The floor of the autopsy room should be covered by some material to facilitate decontamination. Other exposed objects in the autopsy room might also be covered in this way.

AUTOPSY TECHNIQUE

The radiation safety officer will generally monitor radiation exposure levels during the autopsy. Tissue with intense radiation should be handled only with instruments such as long forceps and long-bladed knives. When removing radioactive body fluids, trocars should not be held by hand during the draining procedure. If the exposure rates are high, pathologists should alternate in doing the autopsy. Wounds sustained during the autopsy and possibly contaminated with radioactive material should be washed thoroughly. The radiation safety officer should be notified.

SPECIAL PROCEDURES

^{198}Au, ^{90}Y, and ^{32}P usually are administered into fluid-filled body cavities. ^{32}P has a considerably longer half-life than ^{198}Au and ^{90}Y, but usually much less of this isotope is given.

The fluids should be removed by a trocar or suction apparatus without coming in contact with the hands of the pathologist. The open cavity is dried with sponges which subsequently are disposed of with special precautions (see below). The radiation dose to the hands in the peritoneal cavity is outlined in Tables 10–2 and 10–3. Hands should never be bare in these situations. Double autopsy gloves are the safest but difficult to work with, particularly in cases in which extensive adhesions and tumor infiltrates make precise dissection necessary. The best alternative is for two or more experienced pathologists to work in the body cavity alternately, for 10 minutes each, using double surgical gloves. Obviously, the same precaution must be taken for the dissection of the organs exposed to the isotopes. Constant monitoring and the use of long-handled instruments are advised. Storage of organs or tissues for several days in the refrigerator or fixative will considerably decrease the emission rate.

^{131}I is given orally or intravenously and will be present throughout the body, although in uneven distribution. If the death occurred immediately after administration of ^{131}I, step-by-step monitoring is advised. Blood and urine will be radioactive and must be drained into appropriate containers. If the death occurred later than 1 day after administration of ^{131}I, areas of high activity can be identified, shielded, and handled with long instruments. Dissection of tissues with high radioactivity should be deferred to allow for radioactive decay while the tissues are stored in thick-walled jars or crocks.

Local application of radioactive material, by interstitial injection of radioactive colloids or implantation of wires or other radioactive material, poses few problems at autopsy. If the radioactive area cannot be avoided it should be removed with a large block of tissue as early as possible in the course of the autopsy. Or the rest of the autopsy should be done first, avoiding the radioactive area, and only at the end of the autopsy should a sample of this area be taken. Monitoring will be necessary after incision of the radioactive area. The radioactive tissues must be stored or handled with gloves and forceps according to the level of radiation.

Occasionally, radionuclides with a relatively long half-life are used, such as metallic ^{192}Ir "seeds" (half-life, 74 days). These are used as permanent implants, similar to ^{222}Rn (half-life, 3.86 days). The exposure rate varies according to the decay scheme of the nuclide. Therefore, a fixed amount of radioactivity as officially recommended does not seem to be an ideal basis for radiation safety precautions, and it has been recommended that safety procedures be based on the exposure dose rate.[1] The radiation safety officer should supervise the pathologist and embalmer when the exposure dose rate on the surface of a body exceeds 30 mR/hr (approximately 1 mR/hr at 1 m). Exposure dose rates are shown in Figures 10–1 and 10–2.

STORAGE OF RADIOACTIVE TISSUES AND BODY FLUIDS

Radioactive tissues and body fluids must be stored in a safe area in appropriately labeled containers with radioactivity warning tags showing

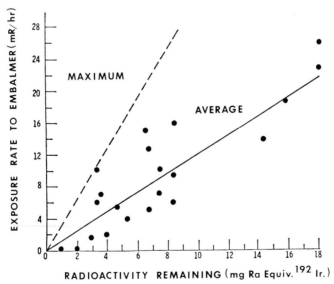

Figure 10–1. Exposure rates to embalmers during handling of radioactive cadavers (^{192}Ir). (From Laughlin JS, Vacirca SJ, Duplissey JF: Exposure of embalmers and physicians by radioactive cadavers. Health Phys 15:451–455, 1968. By permission of the Health Physics Society.)

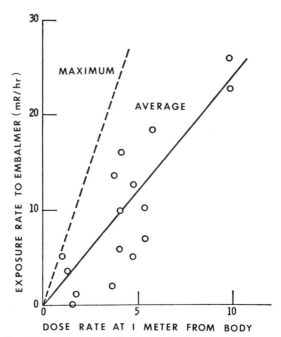

Figure 10–2. Exposure to embalmers and physicians handling radioactive ca-davers. (From Laughlin JS, Vacirca SJ, Duplissey JF: Exposure of embalmers and physicians by radioactive cadavers. Health Phys 15:451–455, 1968. By permission of the Health Physics Society.)

the date, name and clinic and autopsy numbers of the patient, the type of isotope, the radiation levels at a specified date, and the calculated date at which handling of the specimen will be safe.

If sufficient time is available, radioactive tissues should be stored until, as a consequence of radioactive decay, they can be handled without precautions. Suggested time intervals are 3 weeks for ^{198}Au or ^{90}Y, 2 months for ^{131}I, and 4 months for ^{32}P. Precautions must be taken until the radioactivity is 20 mR or less in close proximity to the specimen.

DECONTAMINATION OF CLOTHING, INSTRUMENTS, AND WASTE

Radioactive clothing, instruments, and waste are decontaminated according to the guidelines laid down in the National Bureau of Standards Handbook No. 48.[4] If the radioactivity is low, instruments can be sufficiently decontaminated by repeated soaking in detergents and rinsing in tap water. Gloves are washed before they are removed from the hands. Clothing is best soaked in detergent and stored until the radioactivity level is low enough for safe handling.

Disposable waste is stored in marked containers as described above, according to the directions of the radiation safety officer.

EMBALMING AND CREMATION OF BODIES CONTAINING RADIOACTIVE ISOTOPES

The same precautions followed by morgue personnel must be followed by the funeral director who embalms the body. If the embalming is to be done prior to the autopsy, the referring physician is responsible for warning the funeral director verbally and by an accompanying radioactivity form about possible radiation hazards. The form must be signed by the radiation safety officer who is also charged with instructing the funeral director in how to handle the body safely. If the embalming is to be done after completion of the autopsy, the pathologist must arrange for the radiation safety officer to advise the funeral director. Radioactivity of more than 30 mCi makes embalming in the hospital autopsy room advisable. The procedure should be supervised by the radiation safety officer.

The crematorium personnel must be informed and advised by the house officer or autopsy pathologist who transfers the body and by the radiation safety officer who signs the radioactivity form. Cremation of bodies containing radioactive isotopes is considered acceptable according to present standards if the crematorium does not handle more than 200 mCi of ^{131}I per year and more than 2,000 mCi of ^{198}Au, ^{90}Y, or ^{32}P per year. The crematorium is required to keep appropriate records. Possible exceptions may be ^{192}Ir and ^{182}Ta when they are used for permanent implants. These implants should be removed, prior to cremation, under the supervision of the radiation safety officer.

REFERENCES

1. Laughlin JS, Vacirca SJ, Duplissey JF: Exposure of embalmers and physicians by radioactive cadavers. Health Phys 15:451–455, 1968
2. National Council on Radiation Protection and Measurements: Precautions in the Management of Patients Who Have Received Therapeutic Amounts of Radionuclides. (Report No. 37.) Washington DC, US Government Printing Office, 1970
3. Orvis AL, Van Herik M: Radioactive isotopes and the mortician. Mortuary Management 1957, pp 26–28; 1958, pp 28–30
4. US Department of Commerce, National Bureau of Standards: Control and Removal of Radioactive Contamination in Laboratories. (Handbook 48.) Washington DC, US Government Printing Office, 1951
5. US Department of Commerce, National Bureau of Standards: Safe Handling of Bodies Containing Radioactive Isotopes. (Handbook 65.) Washington DC, US Government Printing Office, 1958

CHAPTER 11

MUSEUM TECHNIQUES

The museum was the pride of the great institutes of pathology of the past. Teaching and research were based on the museum, and these activities, not service, were the foremost purposes of the pathologist. It is therefore not surprising that quite a number of journals and books were dedicated to museum technology, and their study is recommended to those interested in this field.

At present the pathologic museum has declined. The cost of space, maintenance, and administration of the pathologic museum seems to outweigh the disadvantages of replacing museum specimens by color photographs—that is, to represent three dimensions by two. Color photographs are inexpensive, easy to file, and easy to reproduce. Color preservation is not a problem. But even when color photography is used as the only method for teaching and permanent documentation, specimens should be prepared and displayed for photography as if intended for the show case of the pathologic museum. This will greatly enhance the quality of the photographs.

In this chapter only a few basic methods are discussed, and the reader is referred to the review by Pulvertaft[13] and to the excellent and comprehensive books on museum techniques by Tompsett[19] and Edwards and Edwards.[2]

PREPARATION OF SPECIMENS

Preparation of organs and lesions for display has been presented in chapters 3 through 7. The most frequent approach is perfusion fixation, aided in a number of instances by gross staining (chapter 9), use of color-preserving fluids (chapter 9), injection and corrosion techniques, clearing techniques, infiltration of organs, or mummification. Organ models are of great didactic and esthetic value primarily for the teaching of normal anatomy.

253

MOUNTING OF SPECIMENS

Containers. In the past, only thick-walled glass jars were used, and these still can be recommended. Most museum glass jars are quite sturdy. They are inert to fixatives. Cleared specimens which are preserved in benzyl benzoate and oil of wintergreen must be kept in glass jars because plastics will be dissolved.

There are some disadvantages to the use of glass jars. They are heavy, their optical properties often leave something to be desired, and they break easily. In a museum of 2,500 specimens, the average breakage among glass-mounted specimens was 5 per week.[13] The variety of shapes and sizes of glass jars required by an active pathologic museum may be quite costly, and some types may be unavailable altogether. In the latter case, one has to switch to homemade jars constructed of flat glass plates held together by channel and angle irons,[14] or one has to use plastics.

Plastic jars have been used for more than 40 years,[7] and the advent of crystal-clear acrylic resins has made plastics the material of choice. Excellent optical properties, low weight, minimal breakability, toughness, and chemical stability to most mounting fluids are the outstanding characteristics of this material. There are a few disadvantages. Plastics are easily scratched and may have to be repolished on occasion. Benzyl benzoate and oil of wintergreen cannot be used as mounting fluids, and alcohol should be replaced by formalin or glycerine mixtures.[19]

Plastic jars can be prepared in many shapes and sizes. Large sheets of varying thickness (1 mm to 50.8 mm) of plexiglass (Perspex) are available. This polymethyl methacrylate is easy to cut, machine, and glue. Several excellent descriptions of the preparation of bent type and block type plastic jars and the mounting of various types of specimens are available.[2,13,19]

Plastic bags are light, tough, inexpensive, and easy to prepare. Their pliability permits palpation of the specimen. The preservation fluid can be replaced repeatedly if cloudiness develops. Plastic bags are now widely used for teaching, board examinations, and permanent storage. Plastic bag materials and sealing procedures are described in chapter 13.

In the past, we have mounted wet specimens in a partial vacuum without fluid.[9] The preparations were light to handle and easy to seal. However, the dry preservation always caused shrinkage and fading of colors. The method is obsolete.

Mounting Media. Ethyl alcohol and methyl alcohol have been widely used but these craze the surface of plastic containers. If this type of jar is used, a recommended mounting fluid consists of pure glycerine-distilled water-formalin (40%), 25:70:5 (v/v/v). Color-preserving fixatives and mounting fluids are described in chapter 9. We fill our plastic museum jars with Prague solution:

Prague powder*   128 gm
Erythorbic acid (isoascorbic

---

* See page 239.

acid; *L*-ascorbic acid)	25 gm
Distilled water	10,000 ml
Formalin, 40%	1,000 ml
Solution A	4,000 ml
Solution B	4,000 ml.

Solution A:

Sodium phosphate (Na_2HPO_4)	47 gm
Formalin solution, 10%, to make	5,000 ml.

Solution B:

Potassium phosphate (K_2HPO_4)	45 gm
Formalin solution, 10%, to make	5,000 ml.

Solutions A and B must be stored in separate containers.

Mounting in Semisolid Material. Mounting in gelatin is an old although not widely used method.[17] An excellent semisolid embedding material is Schwerigal (S. Schwerin, Geiststr. 7, Göttingen, Germany[3]). The specimens float in the solidified mass, and no special mounting board or suspension is needed. If the jars are airtight and correctly sealed and if they can be stored and displayed under minimal exposure to daylight and at constant temperature, they seem to remain unchanged for many years.

    1. The fresh organs must be thoroughly fixed in fresh formalin solution, diluted to exactly 5%. Some organs will need special treatment such as the filling of cysts or cavities. Lungs are injected, after 3 days of formalin fixation, with a preparation consisting of:

Distilled water	1,000 ml
Schwerigal powder	80 gm
Colorostat*	2 gm
Softener*	1.5 ml
Hardener*	24 ml.

    2. Trim and rinse in running water for 10 to 20 hours. Immerse in 20 to 30% pyridine solution until colors begin to reappear. This generally will be the case after 1 to 2 minutes, and after 5 minutes with old specimens. Rinse and embed immediately.

    3. Fifty grams of Schwerigal powder is soaked in 1,000 ml of cold water for about 10 minutes. The mixture is then heated in a water bath to exactly 40 C. After the Schwerigal is completely dissolved the following, in this order, are stirred into the solution: 4 gm of Colorostat, 3 ml of softener, and 30 ml of hardener. This mixture is poured into carefully cleaned, degreased, dry glass jars. Until solidification, the specimens are suspended by long, thin, stainless steel needles. Air bubbles are removed with a glass rod. Foam is taken off the surface and embedding material is added until the jar is filled to the brim. Solidification can be accelerated by keeping the jar in a container which can be filled with cold water after the specimen has been suspended and air bubbles have been removed.

    4. The jar is sealed after about 18 hours at room temperature. The rim of the jar must be free from embedding material and should be cleaned with acetone. The lid should protrude somewhat. The glass is

---

* Also available from Schwerin.

sealed with UHU-plus (Medipharm, Franz Reinschmidt, Bahnhofstr. 12, Pforzheim, Germany). Keep the lid fixed in position during the hardening period of 12 hours. The surplus glue is removed and the glass is cleaned with acetone. A tape is adjusted around the jar, about 10 to 15 mm beneath the lid, and the space between the edge of the lid and the tape is filled with Metallon KP (Medipharm). The sealing material is again covered with black tape which should also overlie the periphery of the surface of the lid.

Mounting in Solid Plastic. If successful, embedding of specimens in solid blocks of plastic compounds yields excellent museum preparations. Numerous products are on the market, such as Metacrylates (Polysciences, Inc., Rydai, Penna., USA) and Polypal BC (Bolleter & Co. AG, Kanzleistr. 200, Zürich, Switzerland) or Vestopal W (Martin Jaeger, Vésenaz/Gèneve, Switzerland or Chemische Werke Hüls AG, Recklinghausen, Germany).

Unfortunately, the embedding procedures are complicated. The specimens must be carefully dehydrated, a procedure which will distort most autopsy tissues. Cracks, incomplete hardening, or clouding of the polymer may occur, and specimens may shrink or become spongy in appearance. Artifacts may also be created by the heat of the exothermic polymerization of the monomer. Best results are usually achieved with specimens such as bullets, concrements, or casts. The instructions of the suppliers must be followed strictly, and one must heed the warnings as to the danger of explosions and the need to protect eyes and hands. Specimens embedded in solid blocks are difficult or impossible to retrieve for further study. An exemption is the method of Segarra[16] which uses a clear silicone potting compound.

Labels. Labels to identify and describe museum specimens can be glued to the jar or inserted between an outer and an inner plastic bag. Labels on the outside of a container can accidentally be torn off, and an identifying tag should always be attached to the actual specimen inside the jar. Identifying tags or labels which are enclosed with the specimen must be made of a material capable of resisting the chemical action of the mounting fluid. Good labels for museum specimens can be prepared with engraving panels—for instance, with a black face and a white core.[8]

OTHER METHODS

Injection and Corrosion Techniques. Blood vessels, airways, hollow viscera, and cavities can be injected with a great variety of materials. If injection is combined with corrosion, excellent casts may be prepared but little or no material will be available for histologic study. The reader is referred to the descriptions of techniques for various organs and organ systems in chapters 3 through 7.

Barium Sulfate Mixtures. These are probably the most widely used radiopaque media for vascular injection. Commercially available preparations such as Barosperse (Mallinckrodt Chemical Works), Micropaque (Picker X-ray Corporation), and Chromopaque (Mallinckrodt) are preferred. The barium sulfate usually is diluted with 10% formalin solution. In most instances, 5% gelatin is added to cause the mass to solidify after injection. The viscosity of the solution can be decreased by decreasing the amount of gelatin added or by adding more saline. Vessels as small as 30 to 60 μ in luminal width will be filled. The actual viscosity of the medium within the specimen depends on many variables, including the speed of injection and the temperature of the injected tissues. Therefore, each laboratory will have to standardize its own techniques. The injection often is done by quite elaborate methods but, in my experience, injection by hand with a large glass syringe will give excellent results for routine examination and most qualitative studies.

We have used barium sulfate-gelatin mixtures to inject most organ-related vascular systems, the vessels of the lower extremities (see chapter 3), the aorta and its branches, and the inferior vena cava system.

Staining of the injection mass may be required — for example, for differential display of the right and left coronary artery systems. Barium sulfate with various pigment colors is commercially available (Chromopaque). We have occasionally stained gelatin mixtures with carmine, Berlin Blue, Naphthol Green, or Acridine Yellow.

Media Containing Heavy Metals. Like barium sulfate mixtures, these media are also usually prepared with gelatin. Metal salts such as lead carbonate and mercuric sulfide are used.[12] Schlesinger's[15] lead agar mass is a medium of this type widely used in the past.

Clinical Contrast Media. These media are expensive and, when pure, are lost for histologic identification during processing. However, they are readily available in most hospitals and can be recommended to pathologists who do injection work only on occasion. Hypaque (Winthrop Laboratories, New York, N.Y.) is an aqueous injection medium available as 50% and 75% suspensions. Both yield excellent roentgenograms. The contrast medium can be stained with pigment colors. Ethiodol (E. Fougera & Co., Inc., Hicksville, N.Y.) is an oily contrast medium which I have used extensively for postmortem lymphangiography (see chapter 3). A few drops of green oil paint mix readily with the medium and facilitate dissection. Some green pigment can then usually be identified histologically.

India Ink. This is used primarily for microscopic study of the microvasculature. The black pigment stands out readily and will withstand histologic processing.[11] India ink can be mixed with gelatin and water. Thick sections usually are studied. If these are to be studied microradiographically, a radiopaque mass such as diluted Chromopaque neutral medium is required (see chapter 3).

Plastics. Excellent casts of vessels and cavities can be prepared with colored vinyl plastic mixtures.[10] Some of these have also been made radiopaque. Most authors use Vinylite in acetone, with added kieselguhr to prevent shrinkage of the plastic material. The tissues usually are macerated with 35% hydrochloric acid. The use of these plastics has been described in chapters 3, 4, and 5 for coronary arteries, pulmonary vessels, hepatic vessels, bile ducts, and the renal vasculature.

A detailed discussion of casting with synthetic resins can be found in the textbook by Tompsett.[19] The use of Neoprene latex is also described there. This substance is preferred when the injected tissue is to be preserved. Its use for the demonstration of pulmonary vessels and airways is described in chapter 4 and for the hepatic vascular and biliary systems, in chapter 5.

Metal Casts. These are made of alloys with very low melting points such as Wood's metal. Bronchograms or casts of hydronephroses or cystic tumors can easily be prepared with this method. For tissue maceration, antiformin is suggested (see chapter 7).

Clearing Techniques. Clearing techniques are used to demonstrate bones or injected blood vessels without destroying the outline of the surrounding tissue. The smell of oil of wintergreen and the danger of skin irritation make this type of work unpleasant. The glue used for sealing the jars must be specially prepared to resist the chemical action of the mounting fluid. Only glassware can be used; most plastics will dissolve. The following methods yield instructive specimens.

Method of Spalteholz (After Edwards and Edwards[2] and Pulvertaft[13]).
1. Fix in 10% formalin-saline solution.
2. Bleach in 50% hydrogen peroxide, neutral or slightly alkaline.
3. Wash in tap water.
4. Dehydrate in sequential changes of 50, 60, 70, 80, and 95% ethyl alcohol and two changes of absolute ethyl alcohol. Two weeks are required for each change. During the second change of absolute alcohol, anhydrous copper sulfate is placed on the bottom of the container and covered by five layers of filter paper.
5. Soak in two changes of benzene. Two weeks are required for each change.
6. Soak in two changes of benzyl benzoate. Two weeks are required for each change.
7. Mount in a mixture consisting of equal parts of benzyl benzoate and oil of wintergreen. Use a glass jar.
8. Seal with the following mixture:

Powdered arabic gum	50 gm
Sugar	50 gm
Sodium silicate	2 gm
Formalin, 40%	1 ml.

Abbreviated Method of Spalteholz. This method, which we have used, is considerably less time-consuming than the original one and also yields good results.
1. Fix in 10% formalin or Kaiserling I solution.
2. Wash in tap water.
3. Dehydrate in changes of 80 and 95% ethyl alcohol for 24 hours at each change and in absolute ethyl alcohol for 48 hours.
4. Soak in benzene for 24 hours.
5. Mount in a glass jar with oil of wintergreen.
6. Seal with the following mixture:

Cabinetmakers' glue sticks	80 gm
Powdered arabic gum	20 gm
Glycerine	10 gm
Tap water	150 ml

Acetic acid	5 ml
Thymol crystals	0.05 gm.

Fixation and Clearing of Intact Fetus With Staining of Skeletal Structures.
Embryos and fetuses can be fixed intact in 5% formalin solution. After the
sixth month, the fetus should also be perfused through umbilical vessels.
The fetus is mounted in 10% formalin solution containing 3 gm of sodium
bisulfite per 1,000 gm of specimen.[2]

Clearing of the intact fetus with staining of skeletal structures can be
accomplished with the following solutions:

Ethyl alcohol, 95%	2 weeks
Rinse in tap water	
Potassium carbonate, 1%	4 weeks
Potassium hydroxide, 1%	10 days.

Prior to alcohol fixation, an abdominal incision should be made to facilitate
penetration. Formalin-fixed specimens are also suitable, but immersion in
potassium hydroxide must be prolonged to 4 to 6 weeks. If the tissue
requires hardening, the specimen should be immersed for 12 to 24 hours
in a solution of equal parts of glycerine, water, and 95% ethyl alcohol and
then returned into the clearing solution. During the last few days of
clearing, 0.5% potassium hydroxide solution can be used. Wash in running
water for 24 hours. Transfer the specimen into staining solution:

Alizarin solution*	30 minutes to 6 hours
Rinse in tap water	30 minutes
Decolorizing solution †	7 to 14 days.

Mount and dehydrate in alcohol-glycerine-water solutions. Eliminate water
stepwise until specimen can be mounted in a solution of equal parts of
alcohol and glycerine. Seal in glycerine and alcohol.

Williams described a modification of the alizarin method of Dawson
(see Edwards and Edwards[2]). Staining solutions with toluidine blue and
alizarin red S are used. This will permit differentiation between bone and
cartilage.

Staining of Skeletal Structures in Cleared Specimens. This method[2] has
already been described for fetuses. The dehydrated tissue is placed into an
alizarin solution (solution III, see below). The specimen is then dehydrated
again in ethyl alcohol of increasing concentrations and mounted in a mixture of oil of wintergreen and benzyl benzoate, 5:3 (w/w).

Solution I:

To 95% ethyl alcohol, add acetic acid until the smell of acetic acid
becomes obvious. Add crystalline alizarin until the solution is saturated.

Solution II:

Same as solution I only that alizarin cyanine is added instead of crystalline alizarin.

---

* Alizarin solution: alizarin red S, 1% aqueous solution, 1 liter; potassium hydroxide, 1%,
1 ml.
† Decolorizing solution: potassium hydroxide, 10 gm (or 5 gm if specimen is small);
glycerine, 200 ml; distilled water, 800 ml.

Solution III:

Solution I	9 parts
Solution II	1 part
Ethyl alcohol, 70%	190 parts.

Infiltration Techniques. Infiltration of organs with paraffin, beeswax, diglycol stearate, calcium chloride, gelatin, nitrocellulose products, glycerine compounds, or resins permits permanent preservation of dry specimens.[6] Some of these methods can be strongly recommended although they are time-consuming. Paraffin infiltration of the heart is described in detail in chapter 3 and may serve as an example of the infiltration technique.

Mummification Techniques. Mummification of organs is the simplest and oldest preservation technique. Mummification of whole bodies is described by Evans.[4] Shrinkage and loss of material for histologic study are the main disadvantages of organ mummification. This type of dry preservation is described for lungs in chapter 4 and for the intestine in chapter 5.

Organ Models. Organ models are of great didactic value primarily for the presentation of normal anatomic structures. The preparation of models made of resin has been thoroughly described by Tompsett.[19] He prefers Marco resin. Many other materials have been used for the preparation of models, such as blotting paper, cardboard, balsa wood,[1] beeswax, plaster of Paris, rolled sheet aluminum,[18] and acryl plates. Jørgensen[5] has reviewed the available methods.

The preparation of a paraffin model showing an enlarged version of a small portion of a cirrhotic liver is described in chapter 5 and may serve as an example of the general technical principles.

REFERENCES

1. Cummins H: Serial reconstruction with sheets of balsa wood: a teaching model of a 10 mm. pig embryo. J Tech Methods *22*:81–84, 1942
2. Edwards JJ, Edwards MJ: Medical Museum Technology. London, Oxford University Press, 1959
3. Ertelt M: Anweisung zur Einbettungstechnik mit "Schwerigal" nach den neuesten Erfahrungen. Präparator *11*:2–12, 1965
4. Evans WED: The Chemistry of Death. Springfield, Illinois, Charles C Thomas, Publisher, 1963
5. Jørgensen M: Three-dimensional reconstruction in histology: a short survey of available methods and description of a new technique. Acta Pathol Microbiol Scand [A] *79*:298–302, 1971
6. Kramer FM: Dry preservation of museum specimens: a review, with introduction of simplified technique. J Tech Methods *18*:42–50, 1938
7. Kramer FM: Review of the use of plastics in museum work. J Tech Methods *20*:14–26, 1940
8. Ladd R, Thompson JR: Permanent labels for museum specimens. J Tech Methods *21*:41–42, 1941
9. Lundquist LR, Robertson HE: Technic of mounting specimens in a partial vacuum without fluid. J Tech Methods *12*:32–35, 1929
10. Mann JD, Wakim KG, Baggenstoss AH: Alterations in the vasculature of the diseased liver. Gastroenterology *25*:540–546, 1953
11. Mitra SK: The terminal distribution of the hepatic artery with special reference to arterioportal anastomosis. J Anat *100*:651–663, 1966

12. Prinzmetal M, Kayland S, Margoles C, Tragerman IJ: A quantitative method for determining collateral coronary circulation: preliminary report on normal human hearts. J Mount Sinai Hosp NY *8*:933–945, 1942
13. Pulvertaft RJV: Museum techniques: a review. J Clin Pathol *3*:1–23, 1950
14. Schalm OW, Benguerel LA: The use of channel iron for the construction of low-cost museum jars. J Tech Methods *20*:35–37, 1940
15. Schlesinger MJ: An injection plus dissection study of coronary artery occlusions and anastomoses. Am Heart J *15*:528–568, 1938
16. Segarra JA: A new embedding procedure for the preservation of pathologic specimens, using clear silicone potting compounds. Am J Clin Pathol *40*:655–658, 1963
17. Shore THG: A method of mounting flat pathological and other specimens in gelatin. J Path Bact *24*:140–144, 1921
18. Thiessen NW: A method for making durable reconstruction models. J Tech Methods *21*:50–54, 1941
19. Tompsett DH: Anatomical Techniques. Edinburgh, E. & S. Livingstone, Ltd., 1956

CHAPTER 12

AUTOPSY PROTOCOLS, DEATH CERTIFICATES, AND INTERVIEWS

AUTOPSY DIAGNOSES

Autopsy diagnosis represents an interpretation of objective, primarily morphologic, findings. For the next of kin, attending physicians, insurance companies, and public health authorities, these diagnosis sheets are important documents, but they may become meaningless in the future. Interpretations change, names of syndromes and diseases change, and so do autopsy diagnoses. This is one of the reasons why protocols should include objective descriptions.

Autopsy diagnoses can be reported and listed (1) in order of causal relationships and relative importance (for example, chronic alcoholism; alcoholic liver cirrhosis; ruptured esophageal varices; gastrointestinal hemorrhage) or (2) in a standard sequence to facilitate anatomic orientation, statistical analysis, and coding (for example, cardiovascular system, respiratory system, digestive system, etc.). The former method will appeal more to the clinician and in fact conveys more interpretative information, while the latter method of reporting will be preferred by statisticians and by those charged with coding.

The preliminary diagnosis forms which we fill out in the autopsy room contain (1) name, age, weight, length, and clinic number and autopsy number of the patient, (2) date and time of death, (3) date and time of autopsy, (4) names of resident and staff pathologists, (5) preliminary autopsy diagnosis, primarily in the order of causal relationships, (6) directions as to which organs and lesions to photograph, to prepare for organ review, or to save permanently, and (7) directions for histologic sectioning and staining. Space for items 6 and 7 is provided on the back of the preliminary diagnosis form.

AUTOPSY PROTOCOLS

Purpose and Principles of Preparation.   The autopsy protocol represents a permanent record of objective, primarily morphologic, findings, with little interpretation. Its content should not be affected by the advance of science. Organs and lesions are described by (1) location and relationship to other organs and structures, (2) size, (3) weight, (4) shape, (5) color, (6) consistency, (7) odor, and (8) other special features,[4] such as texture of cut surfaces. Thus, the protocol describes the characteristics, extent, and severity of a lesion or condition interpreted in the diagnosis.

Numerous forms must be filled out for each autopsy, such as diagnosis sheets, protocol forms, weight sheets, and requests for histologic, microbiologic, or chemical studies. In order to save time in identifying each form, we have designed each sheet with a free space in the upper right hand corner. The clerk then uses carbon paper and types the identifying data only once. The free space on each form shows the name, clinic and autopsy numbers, age, and sex of the patient, date and time of death, and initials of the pathologist in charge. This method reduces typing and copying errors considerably.

There is no ideal format for protocols because the requirements which have to be satisfied are to some extent mutually exclusive. Autopsy protocols should contain complete, detailed, yet concise and well-organized descriptions of all normal and abnormal findings. The descriptions should be easily retrievable. Narrative or diagrammatic parts of the protocol must be typewritten, proofread, and signed. Autopsy protocols should require little time to complete by pathologists and secretaries. Protocol forms should be self-explanatory so that the resident pathologist is in some way guided by the protocol. And, finally, protocol forms should be inexpensive.

Each institution has to compromise between the limitations of available manpower and time and the need for optimal protocols for training, research, and record-keeping. This is probably one of the reasons why an "International Autopsy Protocol Form" is not yet available. Such a form, adapted for computer use, should be developed by the World Health Organization. The advantages of internationally uniform recording are obvious, and, because of the great demand, the printing costs would be low.

Autopsy protocol writing is an art. Descriptions should be brief yet complete. There should be no interpretations and no descriptions of the mechanics of dissection ("The left atrium of the heart is opened, and the mitral valve is found to be . . ."). The statement that a nodule is yellow will not become more informative by adding "in color."

Sizes should be stated in centimeters, and comparisons with fruits or other objects should be avoided.[9] Weights should be stated in grams and kilograms and volumes, in liters and milliliters.

Narrative Protocols.   This time-honored type of protocol is inexpensive and may be most instructive. The protocols of Virchow[18] are classic examples.

The narrative protocol permits detailed descriptions of complicated findings and, at the same time, utmost brevity in describing the normal.

There are no space limitations, and yet no space is wasted by printed provisions for abnormalities which do not apply. Unfortunately, good narrative protocols can be expected only from experienced pathologists whose style is lucid and whose descriptions are fitting. An established narrative pattern must be maintained. Those not fluent in the language in which it is written may have difficulties with this type of protocol.

Protocols Based on Sentence Completion and Multiple-Choice Selection. These protocols can be completed with ease and speed. Even the inexperienced can be expected to provide the most important information in most instances. However, the space limitations often make addenda on separate sheets necessary, and at the same time much paper is wasted by printed provisions for abnormalities which do not apply.

Pictorial Protocols. Narrative protocols with hand drawings, or sentence completion and multiple-choice selection protocols with diagrammatic outlines, also belong in this category but do not primarily rely on pictorial recording. In most instances the outlines of organs and organ systems are printed on the protocol forms. Some pathologists also use rubber stamps or photographs for this purpose. Coding is a special problem in protocols which are primarily pictorial.

We have tried various types of protocols and seem to have the best results with a combination of written descriptions and schematic drawings. For several years we have been using a commercially available form, the "Pictorial Necropsy Report System" (Washington Associates, Inc., 5850 Leesburg Pike, Falls Church, Virginia 22041). A special feature is use of adhesive-backed paste-on drawings. All drawings are printed into the original protocol form. The completed protocol with gross and microscopic descriptions is typed on blank paper and only those paste-on drawings which have been used to illustrate an autopsy finding are glued into the final copy (Fig. 12–1). This system saves time. The original protocol is filled out by the pathologist in the autopsy room and is completed after the histologic slides have been reviewed. The final copy is typed only once. No rough draft has to be edited. The saving of physician's and secretary's time and the quality of the final copy seem to make worthwhile the expense of forms and paste-on pictures. For neuropathologic records we use our own drawings, supplemented by a narrative protocol.

THE DEATH CERTIFICATE

Death certificates are required by law. They are needed for burial permits, life insurance claims, settlement of estates, and claims for survivorship benefits.[7] The death certificate requirement also serves crime detection. The public interest in medical certification of the cause of death reflects the demand for reliable morbidity data[14] which are rarely available in any other way. Death certificates help to locate cases for clinical investigators and aid in follow-back studies.[12]

The determination of the cause of death may be an extremely difficult task and philosophically may be impossible.[8] Certain rules and regulations

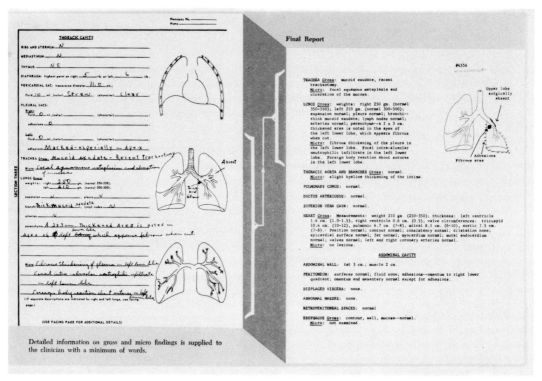

Figure 12–1. Pictorial autopsy report system. Left page shows pictorial report form which is filled out after completion of autopsy and microscopic examination. Schematic drawings are printed on this form. Right page shows the final report form which partly corresponds to the left page; the drawing on this page was prepared from an adhesive-backed paste-on with the part corresponding to the resected portion of the left lung cut away. (From Pictorial Necropsy Report System [copyright], Washington Associates, Inc. By permission.)

must be observed to secure reasonable and comparable data. The mechanisms causing a death may be so complex that the provisions of the death certificate are insufficient for adequate documentation, in proper relationship, of the events that led to death. Nevertheless, the law must be satisfied. Many civil and criminal court proceedings revolve around the "cause of death." The physician, the biostatistician, and the judge each accept as correct a different cause of death in a given case. This led Orth[8] to define three types of causes of death: scientific, statistical, and legal.

The death certificates in the United States are based on the "International Form of Medical Certificate of Cause of Death," designed by the 6th Decennial International Revision Conference, Paris, France, 1948. The conference suggested tabulating the "underlying causes" of death, defined as "(A) The disease or injury which initiated the train of morbid events leading directly to death" or "(B) The circumstances of the accident or violence which produced the fatal injury."

Death Certification Procedures. Instructions for physicians on the use of the "International Form of Medical Certificate of Cause of Death" have been published by the World Health Organization.[6] Guidelines for correct certification are given and suggestions are made how to avoid indefinite or inadequate terms and redundant or misplaced entries.

The proper use of United States death certificates is described in a Public Health Service publication.[17] Every physician in the United States who is charged with certifying deaths should have this booklet on hand.

The United States Standard Certificate of Death. Figure 12–2 illustrates a properly completed form. Instructions for the completion of each entry are given in the Public Health Service publication.[17]

The United States Standard Certificate of Fetal Death. Figure 12–3 illustrates a properly completed form. Instructions for the completion of each entry are given in the Public Health Service publication.[17]

Death Certificates in Medicolegal Cases. A United States Standard Certificate of Death is filled out. A form for medical examiners or coroners and a combined form for physicians, medical examiners, or coroners are available. Figure 12–4 shows an example of a properly completed combined form. The coroner or medical examiner is charged with filling out and signing the death certificate, or the appropriate section of it, in deaths due to violence (homicide, suicide, or accident) and in other cases if so defined

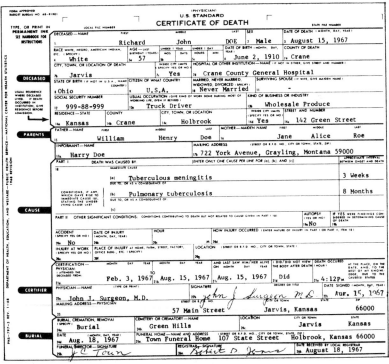

Figure 12–2. United States Standard Certificate of Death, physician form. (From US National Center for Health Statistics, Public Health Service: Physicians' Handbook on Medical Certification: Death, Fetal Death, Birth. [Publication No. 593-B.] Washington DC, US Government Printing Office, 1967. By permission.)

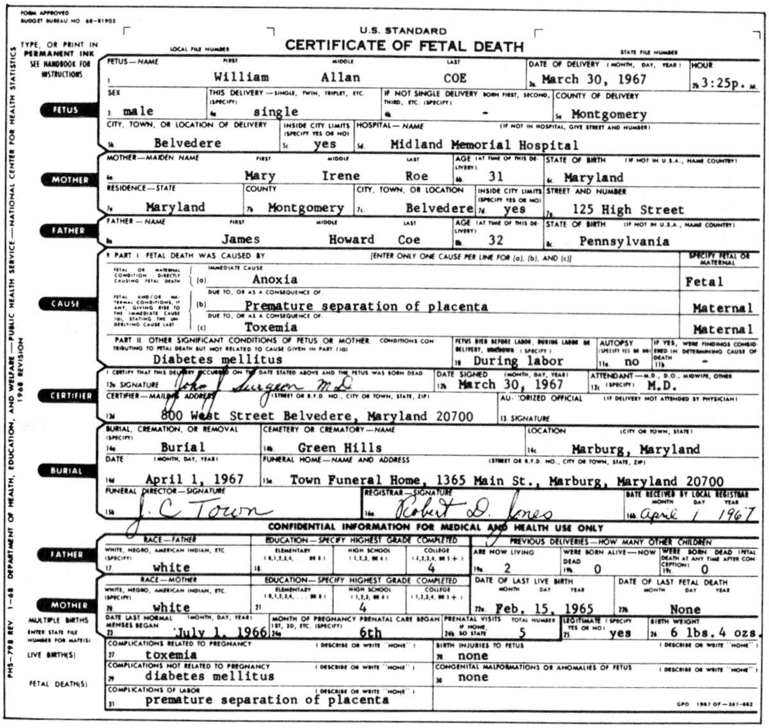

U.S. STANDARD CERTIFICATE OF FETAL DEATH

FETUS—NAME: William Allan COE
DATE OF DELIVERY: March 30, 1967 HOUR: 3:25 p.m.
SEX: male THIS DELIVERY: single
COUNTY OF DELIVERY: Montgomery
CITY, TOWN, OR LOCATION OF DELIVERY: Belvedere INSIDE CITY LIMITS: yes HOSPITAL—NAME: Midland Memorial Hospital
MOTHER—MAIDEN NAME: Mary Irene Roe AGE: 31 STATE OF BIRTH: Maryland
RESIDENCE—STATE: Maryland COUNTY: Montgomery CITY, TOWN, OR LOCATION: Belvedere INSIDE CITY LIMITS: yes STREET AND NUMBER: 125 High Street
FATHER—NAME: James Howard Coe AGE: 32 STATE OF BIRTH: Pennsylvania

PART I FETAL DEATH WAS CAUSED BY:
 (a) IMMEDIATE CAUSE: Anoxia — Fetal
 (b) DUE TO, OR AS A CONSEQUENCE OF: Premature separation of placenta — Maternal
 (c) DUE TO, OR AS A CONSEQUENCE OF: Toxemia — Maternal
PART II OTHER SIGNIFICANT CONDITIONS OF FETUS OR MOTHER: Diabetes mellitus
FETUS DIED BEFORE LABOR, DURING LABOR: During labor
AUTOPSY: no
DATE SIGNED: March 30, 1967
ATTENDANT: M.D.
CERTIFIER—MAILING ADDRESS: 800 West Street Belvedere, Maryland 20700

BURIAL, CREMATION, OR REMOVAL: Burial
CEMETERY OR CREMATORY—NAME: Green Hills LOCATION: Marburg, Maryland
DATE: April 1, 1967 FUNERAL HOME—NAME AND ADDRESS: Town Funeral Home, 1365 Main St., Marburg, Maryland 20700
FUNERAL DIRECTOR—SIGNATURE: J. C. Town
REGISTRAR—SIGNATURE: Robert D. Jones
DATE RECEIVED BY LOCAL REGISTRAR: April 1, 1967

CONFIDENTIAL INFORMATION FOR MEDICAL AND HEALTH USE ONLY

RACE—FATHER: white
RACE—MOTHER: white EDUCATION—COLLEGE: 4
PREVIOUS DELIVERIES—ARE NOW LIVING: 2 DEAD: 0 WERE BORN ALIVE—NOW DEAD: 0 WERE BORN DEAD: 0
DATE OF LAST LIVE BIRTH: Feb. 15, 1965
DATE OF LAST FETAL DEATH: None
DATE LAST NORMAL MENSES BEGAN: July 1, 1966
MONTH OF PREGNANCY PRENATAL CARE BEGAN: 6th
PRENATAL VISITS TOTAL NUMBER: 5
LEGITIMATE: yes
BIRTH WEIGHT: 6 lbs. 4 ozs.
COMPLICATIONS RELATED TO PREGNANCY: toxemia
COMPLICATIONS NOT RELATED TO PREGNANCY: diabetes mellitus
COMPLICATIONS OF LABOR: premature separation of placenta
BIRTH INJURIES TO FETUS: none
CONGENITAL MALFORMATIONS OR ANOMALIES OF FETUS: none

Figure 12–3. United States Standard Certificate of Fetal Death. (From US National Center for Health Statistics, Public Health Service: Physicians' Handbook on Medical Certification: Death, Fetal Death, Birth. [Publication No. 593-B.] Washington DC, US Government Printing Office, 1967. By permission.)

by state law. Pathologists must be familiar with the appropriate laws in the states where they practice. The correct use of medicolegal death certificates is described in a special publication of the Public Health Service.[16]

Proper Completion of Death Certificates. The Public Health Service has published the following general instructions for completing death certificates:[17]

(A) Use the current form designated by the state. (B) Type all entries whenever possible. Do not use worn typewriter ribbons. If a typewriter is not used, print legibly in dark, unfading ink. Black ink gives the best copies. (C) Complete all items or attach a note explaining any omissions. (D) Do not make alterations or erasures. (E) All signatures must be written. Rubber stamp or other facsimile signatures are not acceptable. (F) Do not submit carbon copies, reproductions or duplicates for filing. The registrar will accept originals only. (G) Avoid abbreviations. (H) Spell entries correctly. Verify names which sound the same, but have different spellings (Smith vs. Smyth, Gail vs. Gayle, Wolf vs. Wolfe, etc.). (I) Refer problems not covered in specific instructions to the state vital statistics office, or local registrar.

Classification and Nomenclature.   Entries should be based on "International Classification of Diseases, Adapted."[15] Another valuable source is the American Medical Association's *Standard Nomenclature of Diseases and Operations.*[13] (See also page 286).

Delayed Certification.   Occasionally, the cause of death can only be established after further, and often time-consuming, microbiologic, chemical, or other studies. The legal requirements in such cases vary somewhat throughout the United States, but the statement on the death certificate "Pending further investigations" will be accepted in most if not all places. Local laws, customs, or arrangements determine how long a delay will be acceptable. The following guidelines were recommended by the Public Health Service for delay of a definitive statement as to the cause of death:[16]

(1) The term "pending" is intended to apply only to cases in which there is a reasonable expectation that an autopsy, other diagnostic procedure, or investigation may significantly change the diagnosis.

(2) Certifications of cause of death should not be deferred merely because "all details" of a case are not available. Thus, for example, if it is clear that a patient died of "cancer of the stomach," reporting of the

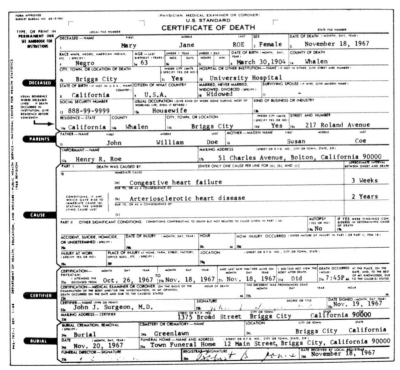

Figure 12–4. Death certificate for medicolegal cases; combined form for physician, medical examiner, or coroner. (From US National Center for Health Statistics, Public Health Service: Physicians' Handbook on Medical Certification: Death, Fetal Death, Birth. [Publication No. 593-B.] Washington DC, US Government Printing Office, 1967. By permission.)

cause should not be deferred while a determination of the histologic type is being carried out. Similarly, if a death is from "influenza," there is no justification for delaying the certification because a virological test is being carried out.

(3) In cases where death is known to be from an injury, but the circumstances surrounding the death are not yet established, the injury should be reported immediately. The circumstances of the injury should be noted as "deferred," and a supplemental report filed.

(4) Lastly, the term "pending" is not intended to apply to cases in which the cause of death is in doubt, but for which no further diagnostic procedures can be carried out. In this case, the "probable" cause should be entered on the basis of the facts available and the certification made in accordance with the best judgment of the certifier.

Daylight Saving Time. "Daylight Saving Time" has to be recorded on death certificates during the entire period in which daylight saving time is in effect.

What Happens to the Death Certificate?   After the physician has completed and signed the death certificate, he turns the document over to the funeral director or local registrar. Figure 12–5 shows the way data on the death certificates are passed on and how they are used.

Certification Problems.   All problems not answered by the *Physicians' Handbook on Medical Certification*[17] or the *Medical Examiners' and Coroners' Handbook on Death and Fetal Death Registration*[16] should be referred to the vital statistics office of the state or to the local registrar. Angrist[1] suggested that, in these instances, one should send to the responsible authorities the incomplete death certificate with the separate autopsy diagnosis and appropriate comments. In this way, correct completion of the death certificate is ensured. In the future, use of "multiple cause syndromes" would be valuable, particularly in the aged.[5]

Incorrect certification of cause of death is frequent. In about 10% of all cases, qualified physicians state the cause of death incorrectly, even when laboratory aids are available.[1] A reevaluation of death certificates from hospital records, autopsy findings, interviews with physicians, and other information was undertaken in 12 cities to determine the reasons for variations in reported mortality from different diseases in different localities.[10] In this study Sox and Holota[11] found that in San Francisco the percentage changes from original to final assignment of cause of death were +129% for alcoholism, +320% for alcoholic hepatic cirrhosis, +44% for syphilis, +18% for homicide, and +8% for suicide. Other causes of death decreased, such as respiratory diseases, diseases of blood and blood-forming organs, and cardiovascular and renal diseases. In a similar study, total coronary death was found to be over-reported in 39% of men and 59% of women; sudden death due to coronary disease was under-reported by 11% in men and 25% in women.[3]

Causes of death also change with time. Progress—atomic bombs, new drugs, insecticides, space travel—continuously provides new ways to die. While new causes of death emerge, others vanish. "Fever" is no longer ac-

RESPONSIBLE PERSON OR AGENCY	BIRTH CERTIFICATE	DEATH CERTIFICATE	FETAL DEATH CERTIFICATE (Stillbirth)
Physician, Other Professional Attendant, or Hospital Authority	1. Completes entire certificate in consultation with parent(s). Physician's signature required. 2. Files certificate with local office of district in which birth occurred.	1. Completes medical certification and signs certificate. 2. Returns certificate to funeral director.	1. Completes or reviews medical items on certificate. 2. Certifies to the cause of fetal death and signs certificate. 3. Returns certificate to funeral director. 4. In absence of funeral director, files certificate.
Funeral Director		1. Obtains personal facts about deceased. 2. Takes certificate to physician for medical certification. 3. Delivers completed certificate to local office of district where death occurred and obtains burial permit.	1. Obtains the facts about fetal death. 2. Takes certificate to physician for entry of causes of fetal death. 3. Delivers completed certificate to local office of district where delivery occurred and obtains burial permit.
Local Office (may be Local Registrar or City or County Health Department)	1. Verifies completeness and accuracy of certificate. 2. Makes copy, ledger entry, or index for local use. 3. Sends certificates to State Registrar.	1. Verifies completeness and accuracy of certificate. 2. Makes copy, ledger entry, or index for local use. 3. Issues burial permit to funeral director and verifies return of permit from cemetery attendant. 4. Sends certificates to State Registrar.	
	City and county health departments use certificates in allocating medical and nursing services, followups on infectious diseases, planning programs, measuring effectiveness of services, and conducting research studies.		
State Registrar, Bureau of Vital Statistics	1. Queries incomplete or inconsistent information. 2. Maintains files for permanent reference and as the source of certified copies. 3. Develops vital statistics for use in planning, evaluating, and administering State and local health activities and for research studies. 4. Compiles health related statistics for State and civil divisions of State for use of the health department and other agencies and groups interested in the fields of medical science, public health, demography, and social welfare. 5. Prepares copies of birth, death, and fetal death certificates or records for transmission to the National Center for Health Statistics.		
Public Health Service National Center for Health Statistics	1. Prepares and publishes national statistics of births, deaths, and fetal deaths; and constructs the official U.S. life tables and related actuarial tables. 2. Conducts health and social-research studies based on vital records and on sampling surveys linked to records. 3. Conducts research and methodological studies in vital statistics methods including the technical, administrative, and legal aspects of vital records registration and administration. 4. Maintains a continuing technical assistance program to improve the quality and usefulness of vital statistics.		

Figure 12-5. The Vital Statistics Registration System in the United States. (From US National Center for Health Statistics, Public Health Service: Physicians' Handbook on Medical Certification: Death, Fetal Death, Birth. [Publication No. 593-B.] Washington DC, US Government Printing Office, 1967. By permission.)

cepted as a sufficient explanation of death. "Bronchopneumonia" is accepted, but "*Staphylococcus aureus* bronchopneumonia" is preferred. This state of affairs led Bohrod,[2] aptly and somewhat cynically, to state: "The cause of death is a statement made by a pathologist to a clinician or a law enforcement agent which makes the latter say 'Well, I am not surprised that the patient died.'" An equally timeless definition of when death has occurred is the following: "A person is dead when a physician says so"—that is, when he pronounces a patient dead and signs the death certificate.

INTERVIEW WITH NEXT OF KIN

In most institutions the attending physician will explain the cause of death to the family of the deceased. However, after autopsy permission had been granted, the next of kin may want detailed information about the autopsy findings. In this instance the attending physician should discuss the matter with the pathologist and either convey the preliminary autopsy findings to the family himself or schedule an interview with the pathologist. Letters describing the autopsy findings are often delayed, and as a rule they are a poor alternative for an interview—letters cannot respond to unexpected problems and questions, and their preparation may be just as time-consuming as an interview. The granting of permission for an autopsy is a favor, and failure to inform the family speedily about the autopsy findings understandably causes anger and frustration.

Pathologists who elect not to conduct interviews should try hard to convey the preliminary autopsy diagnosis to the attending physician in the shortest possible time; the attending physician then has to talk or write to the relatives of the deceased and to the referring physician. Undue delay may cause embarrassment for the attending physician, strained relationships for the pathologist, and, ultimately, a decline of the autopsy service.

At this institution, through our clinical colleagues we offer, on request, an interview to the next of kin. The appointment usually is scheduled for 3 to 4 hours after the autopsy. Each hospital has a "Quiet Room," close to the religious center and chapel, for relatives of the deceased who wish privacy. The Death Record Book is kept in this room. This is a proper place for the attending physician to ask for permission to perform an autopsy and for the pathologist to explain the findings to the family.

Relatives may come to the interview frightened, upset, guilt-ridden, and with an attitude of hostility. After the interview the pathologist may have the satisfaction of seeing the family members leave calmly, composed, and often comforted and with a positive attitude toward their doctors. He who has explained to a terrified mother what we know about crib death, thus relieving her guilt feelings, knows what an interview can do. In the interview room, pathology and psychology are equally important so that most of us will feel not properly equipped for this task. I have found, however, that it does not take much more than tact, compassion, and understanding to adjust to the emotional needs of the bereaved family members. A proper attitude toward the next of kin is part of good patient care. Besides, such consideration will be noticed in the community and will decrease the reluctance of many people to grant autopsy permission.

Another important and often overlooked aspect of the interview with the next of kin is its role as a source of additional data. A patient with hepatic cirrhosis may have denied chronic alcoholism but at the time of the interview his family may readily volunteer the information. An unexpected amoebic abscess of the liver will prompt diligent inquiry about former residencies. A suicide may come to light.

An interview may serve to relieve feelings of hostility against the attending physicians, surgeons, or paramedical personnel. Many lawsuits originate from misunderstanding, misinformation, and lack of communication. The pathologist, at the time of the interview, may be the first one to sense such feelings. He may be able to provide the needed explanations, to correct misconceptions, or to realize the need for an interview of the next of kin with the attending physician.

Seven Rules for Conducting Interviews. 1. Before you go to an interview, read the hospital chart carefully, familiarize yourself with the history of the deceased, and discuss the case with the attending physician.

2. Do not wear a white gown or other hospital attire. Your attitude should be unhurried and adapted to the emotional needs of the family.

3. At the time of the interview introduce yourself, present a card with your name and address, and ask for the names of the persons present and their kinship to the deceased. Failing to do this, a pathologist may find himself inadvertently talking to newspaper reporters, private investigators, or curious neighbors. The possible legal consequences are obvious.

4. Report your findings in appropriate lay terms, adjusted to the intellectual level of the family members. Omit insignificant findings. Be sure that your report is understood, and encourage the family to ask questions. The risk of the same fatal disease afflicting other members of the family often needs to be discussed, and in some cases detailed genetic counseling may be in order.

5. Occasionally, the emotional shock to the next of kin may make an interview futile. In such a case it is better to postpone the interview or, if agreeable to the family, talk to their closest friend or clergyman. If the results of histologic, microbiologic, or chemical studies must be awaited, explain this to the next of kin and give a date when a final report can be expected. Point out that the attending and referring physicians also will receive such a report. Allow ample time for your work-up. It is easier to explain the difficulties of laboratory procedures and to point out to the next of kin that they may have to wait for 6 weeks than to promise an earlier date which cannot be kept.

6. Express your appreciation for the permission to perform an autopsy and point out that others may be helped with the insights which were gained from performing the autopsy.

7. After the interview, dictate and sign a report of what was said. This should also include the time and place of the interview, the names and addresses of the persons present, and their kinship to the deceased. Bring to the attention of the attending physician all grievances or other important points that might have come up during the interview.

REFERENCES

1. Angrist A: Certified cause of death: analysis and recommendations. JAMA *166*:2148–2153, 1958
2. Bohrod MG: The meaning of "cause of death." J Forensic Sci *8*:15–21, 1963
3. Gearing FR, Bergner L, Schweitzer MD: Death certificate data held often error-prone. Medical Tribune December 19, 1966

4. Gould SE: Descriptions of pathologic findings: with particular reference to myocardial infarcts. *In* Methods and Achievements in Experimental Pathology. Volume 1: An Introduction to Experimental Pathology. Edited by E Bajusz, G Jasmin. Chicago, Year Book Medical Publishers, Inc., 1966, pp 21–32

5. Heasman MA, Lipworth L: Accuracy of certification of cause of death. London, Her Majesty's Stationery Office, 1966

6. Medical Certification of Cause of Death: Instructions for Physicians on Use of International Form of Medical Certificate of Cause of Death. WHO Bull, Suppl 3, 1952

7. Moriyama IM: The importance of recording detailed birth and death certificates. Sandoz Panorama 7:21–25, 1969

8. Orth J: Was ist Todesursache? Berl Klin Wochenschr 45:485–490, 1908

9. Prichard RW: Descriptions in pathology: avoiding pathological descriptions. Arch Pathol 59:612–617, 1955

10. Puffer RR, Griffith GW: Patterns of Urban Mortality: Report of the Inter-American Investigation of Mortality. (Publication No. 151.) Washington DC, Pan American Health Organization, World Health Organization, 1967

11. Sox ED, Holota M: Underlying causes of death, cardiovascular disease: San Francisco experience in the Pan American Health Organization International Mortality Study. Read at the Annual Meeting of the American Public Health Association, San Francisco, 1966

12. Spiegelman M, Bellows MT, Erhardt CL, Keehn RJ, Moriyama IM, Parkhurst E, Sellers HH: Problems in the medical certification of causes of death. Am J Public Health 48:71–80, 1958

13. Thompson ET, Hayden AC: Standard Nomenclature of Diseases and Operations. Fifth edition. New York, McGraw-Hill Book Company, Inc., 1961

14. Treloar AE: The enigma of cause of death. JAMA 162:1376–1379, 1956

15. US National Center for Health Statistics, Public Health Service: Eighth Revision of the International Classification of Diseases. Volume 1: Tabular list, 1967; volume 2: Alphabetical index, 1968. Washington DC, US Government Printing Office

16. US National Center for Health Statistics, Public Health Service: Medical Examiners' and Coroners' Handbook on Death and Fetal Death Registration. (Publication No. 593-D.) Washington DC, US Government Printing Office, 1967

17. US National Center for Health Statistics, Public Health Service: Physicians' Handbook on Medical Certification: Death, Fetal Death, Birth. (Publication No. 593-B.) Washington DC, US Government Printing Office, 1967

18. Virchow R: Post-mortem Examinations With Especial Reference to Medico-legal Practice. Fourth German edition. (English translation by TP Smith.) Philadelphia, P. Blakiston, Son & Co., 1885

ORGANIZATION OF THE AUTOPSY SERVICE AND TISSUE REGISTRY AND METHODS OF DATA RETRIEVAL

With R. Thierbach and Robert C. Bahn

MAINTENANCE OF AUTOPSY FACILITIES

Maintenance and cleaning of autopsy facilities is well described in the handbook by Emery and Marshall.[16]

Dressings, cotton wool swabs, hair, and other loose cadaver material should be incinerated without delay. Protective garments and towels are first washed in cold water to remove blood, then soaked in a detergent for several hours, and finally autoclaved or sent to the laundry. Contaminated items are placed in a separate bag which is labeled with a warning tag and sent to the laundry for appropriate further treatment. Heavy rubber autopsy gloves are washed with detergent, autoclaved, and checked for leaks before they are used again. We also use surgical gloves which are discarded when they wear out. Plastic or rubber aprons are washed. Metal instruments are washed to remove all particulate matter and then are soaked in a detergent—for example, a 1:40 Lysol solution or Haemo-sol, 15 gm per 3.8 liters of water. Metal instruments also can be autoclaved. Plastic syringes and needles are discarded. Glass syringes are autoclaved. Sponges should be washed and soaked in detergent. We do not recommend the use of sponges.

275

The walls and floors of the autopsy facilities are washed regularly with soft brushes and antiseptic solution. We use Wescodyne (95 ml in 20 liters of water). The autopsy table is rinsed with water and cleanser after each autopsy. Lysol is used after heavily contaminated cases.

AUTOPSY ROOM ACCIDENTS AND INFECTIONS

Autopsy room infections and first aid are well discussed in Emery and Marshall's handbook,[16] and this should be required reading for autopsy technicians. Some chapters of this book also will be of great benefit to pathologists.

Bacterial autopsy room infections were a serious problem, but in this century this has changed dramatically. In fact, I am not aware of any recent reports of fatal bacterial infections from autopsies. The reasons are manifold. The number of highly infectious autopsy cases is smaller, and treatment with antibiotics is most effective. Whether better protective autopsy techniques play a role is difficult to decide.

Tuberculosis may still be significant as an autopsy room infection, but this is difficult to trace in a specific case. Skin inoculation (cutaneous tuberculosis or "prosector's wart") still occurs occasionally.[28]

Viral infections represent a great possible danger for pathologists and autopsy technicians, particularly infections with the hepatitis virus. I do not know of systematic studies of viral hepatitis from autopsy infections. A few years ago a fatal smallpox infection occurred in a pathologist who had done an autopsy on an unsuspected case.[16]

Wounds and injuries do occur in the autopsy room but seem rarely to be of significance. All such accidents must be reported for possible workman's compensation. Because of the limited exposure, autopsy or pathology department injuries have not been listed separately in the tables of the US Bureau of Labor Statistics.[8]

All persons with puncture wounds or more than superficial cuts which occurred in the autopsy area are sent to the emergency room for proper surgical treatment. If there is a risk of hepatitis virus infection, γ-globulin is administered.

HANDLING OF SPECIMENS AND DOCUMENTS

Our organization of the autopsy and related services and the tissue registry is schematically represented in Table 13–1. The pathologist selects the gross specimens for preliminary storage. On the back of the preliminary autopsy diagnosis he enters instructions for further processing of the specimen, including requests for refrigeration, fixation, preparation for organ review, photography, roentgenography, gross staining procedures, or immediate storage. Xerox copies of the preliminary autopsy diagnosis and of the instructions for technicians are prepared immediately after the

TABLE 13-1.   ORGANIZATION OF THE AUTOPSY SERVICE

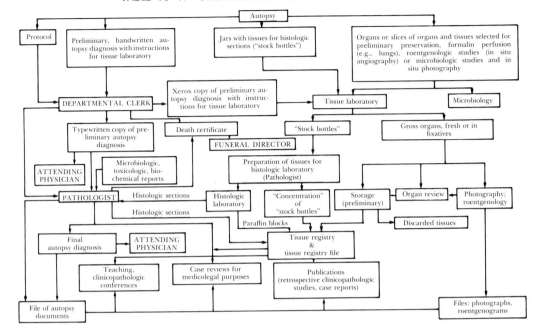

original form has been completed. Material for deep freezing and for microbiologic or chemical studies is sent directly from the autopsy room.

When a gross specimen is to be saved it is immediately identified with a plastic tag which shows the autopsy number and, for paired organs, the side (one punched-out notch for right and two notches for left). After the autopsy tissue laboratory has received a Xerox copy of the preliminary autopsy diagnosis with the instructions for the technicians, the gross specimens are processed accordingly. As a rule, gross specimens are stored for some time in the autopsy tissue laboratory in stainless steel tanks (Fig. 13-1).

After the organ review conference and selection of additional histologic material, some of the gross specimens and tissues are discarded. The remaining specimens are entered into the record book of the autopsy tissue laboratory. On completion of the final autopsy diagnosis, the gross specimens are sent to the tissue registry for permanent storage.

Specimens for microscopic examination are kept in 10% formalin solution in "stock bottles." These stock bottles contain fragments of all organs, tissues, and lesions. Gallbladders are stored separately. The case number is carried on a plastic tag inside the jar and on a label on the outside. Tissues requiring special identification or fixatives are kept in separate jars. After material for histologic study has been selected, the remaining tissues in the stock bottle are trimmed and transferred to jars with fresh formalin solution. These "concentrated stock bottles" are saved permanently in the tissue registry.

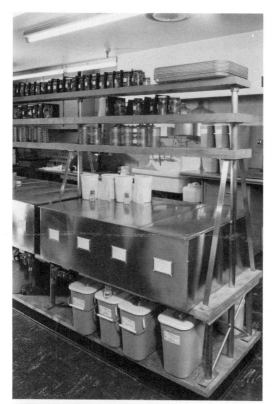

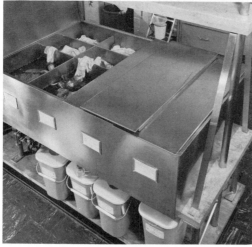

Figure 13-1. *Upper,* **Storage in autopsy tissue laboratory.** Racks hold stainless steel tanks for temporary storage of autopsy tissues and shelves with "concentrated stock bottles." Steel containers with perforated walls are used for washing tissues. Lowest shelf shows plastic containers for storing brains. White plastic containers in center are preliminary stock bottles used in autopsy room. *Lower,* **Stainless steel tanks with autopsy tissues** in formalin solution. Each tank has removable dividers so that up to 16 compartments can be built. We have six such tanks in operation. Towels soaked with formalin solution are used to improve fixation of floating tissues.

If a pathologist desires to review an old specimen, he sends a request card to the autopsy tissue laboratory where the record books are kept. If the requested specimen is listed in the record books as being stored in the tissue registry, the request is passed on by phone (if large numbers of specimens are requested for study a list is prepared for the tissue registry). In either case the master index cards in the tissue registry file are checked, as well as the separate files for autopsy or surgical specimens; in this way the crock or jar in which the requested specimens are stored is located. When this material arrives in the autopsy tissue laboratory, the request card is returned to the pathologist to notify him that the specimens are available for study. After the review is completed, the pathologist initials the request card, indicating that the material can be returned to storage. The same procedure is used for surgical specimens or stock bottles with tissue fragments for histologic study.

THE TISSUE REGISTRY

A well-organized tissue registry is the most valuable source of material for service and research work in anatomic and surgical pathology.

The tissue registry of the Mayo Clinic saves or keeps on file: (1) all histologic slides (an estimated 2 to 3 million) prepared in the pathologic anatomic and surgical pathologic laboratories (also more than $1\frac{1}{4}$ million paraffin blocks which are stored separately), (2) all surgical and anatomic pathologic gross specimens, and (3) the concentrated stock bottles with the autopsy tissue samples

Histologic slides and paraffin blocks are saved permanently. Concentrated stock bottles with tissues for histologic study are saved permanently or for 25 years. Gross specimens are saved for at least 20 years. After 20 years, a pathologist reviews the autopsy diagnoses and tissue registry file cards and selects the specimens which are to be saved permanently; the rest are then discarded.

Tissue Registry File. In order to make a tissue registry operational, fairly elaborate records must be maintained (Fig. 13–2). We keep (1) "master index cards" of all autopsies which show the clinic and autopsy numbers, name of patient, date of death, and types of specimens saved and (2) "surgical index cards" which show the clinic number and name of the patient and the type of surgical specimen saved. Also identified on the master and surgical index cards are the code numbers of the crocks and muslin sacks in which the specimens are stored. When applicable, master index cards and surgical index cards are cross indexed.

Storage Material. Glass jars are used when tissues are preserved in alcohol, xylol, carbolic acid, or oil of wintergreen. For storage in formalin solution, the glass containers are being replaced by plastic jars. Concentrated stock bottles, small surgical specimens, and bottles with gallbladders are filed on shelves in the tissue registry storage area, according to autopsy or case number and year.

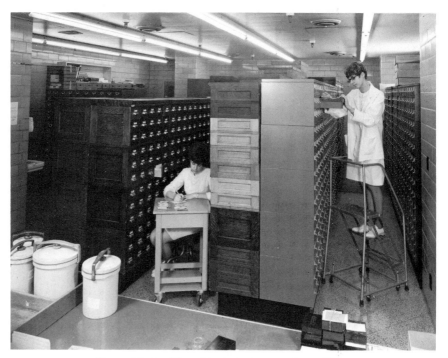

Figure 13–2. **File cabinets** in tissue registry office.

Plastic bags* are now popular for storage in tissue registries. Mylar plastic roll stock yields larger plastic bags when sealed on both ends. For the sealing of plastic bags we use the Clamco heat sealer (CLAMCO Heat Sealing & Packaging Co., Cleveland Detroit Corporation, Cleveland, O.) (Fig. 13–3).

Comparison of a large number of commercially available plastic films revealed that fluorohalocarbon film (Aclar 22A and 33C; General Chemical Division, Allied Chemical Corporation, Film Department, P.O. Box 70, Morristown, N.J.), particularly when included in a laminated film, gave the best results.[10] Bags were prepared from these films by using a Vertrod Model 24 PC impulse sealer (Vertrod Corp., Brooklyn, N.Y.). Fluorohalocarbon was found to be almost completely transparent and superior in terms of impermeability to fixation fluids. Simple polyethylene bags and bags of laminates containing polyethylene were most durable. Simple fluorohalocarbon film must be sealed with a thermal impulse sealing device in which the sealed area cools under pressure; the seal may rupture when under stress. When fluorohalocarbon was one of the layers in laminated plastic films of high tensile strength, the bags combined durability with a high degree of impermeability. These laminated films can be sealed with a simple heating device if polyethylene is the inner layer of the film.

---

* Plastic bags 15 by 17.8 or 26.7 cm are available through J. R. Blade Co., 2666 Shaker Road, Cleveland Heights, O.

Organs or organ fragments which are sealed in plastic bags for storage are either individually labeled and wrapped in gauze or they are sealed without wrapping. The plastic bags are identified by the autopsy number.

Plastic bags are also useful for disposal of autopsy tissues. The specimens are placed in the bag with some formalin solution and cotton, and the bag is placed in the abdominal or chest cavity of the cadaver.[18]

The tagged gross autopsy or surgical specimens are placed in muslin bags. The autopsy number is also shown on a tag on the outside of each bag. Surgical specimens are identified by type of lesion, site of lesion, and date. Several small bags are put into a large bag which is submerged in a 75.5-liter (20-gallon) crock (Fig. 13–4). Some crocks now being sold permit formalin solutions to leak. An alternative is 75.5-liter (20-gallon) Brute containers which are made of white plastic (Rubbermaid Commercial Products Inc., Winchester, Va. 22601). All autopsy, crock, and sac numbers are pounded onto red plastic tags which are tied to the outside of the large bags.

Brains are stored separately but in a similar manner.

All stored material is identified by rigid plastic tags, which can be cut from larger sheets (Standard Pyroxoloid Corp., Nile St. Plant, Leominster, Mass.), or by Scotch Brand labeling tape marked with a Dymo-Mite Tapewriter (Dymo Products, Berkeley, Calif.). The autopsy number and year are imprinted onto the tag with a bench press (Model 131, Numberall Stamp & Tool Co., Inc., 379 Huguenot Ave., Staten Island, N.Y.). Labels also can be prepared from old roentgenograms. The emulsion is removed with hot water. The films are then dipped in glacial acetic acid for 10 sec-

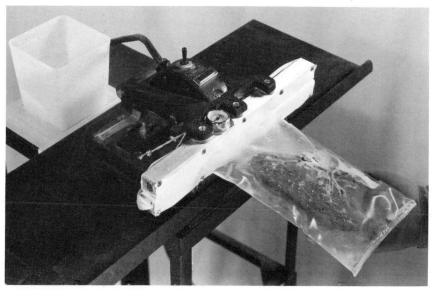

Figure 13–3. Heat-sealing for storage of slice of lung in plastic bag containing formalin solution.

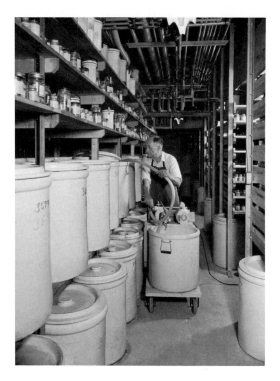

Figure 13–4. Tissue registry storage area. For refilling of crocks, an electric pump and a crock with formalin solution, on a cart, is used. The pump can also be used to remove formalin solution from the crocks. The crocks are identified by code numbers. The containers on the upper shelves are used for storage of surgical specimens.

onds and are made opalescent in a solution of 5 gm of sodium carbonate in 3.8 liters of water.[34]

Plastic bags can be identified by writing on filter paper with a lead pencil and sealing this tag into the seam of the plastic bag; in this case we include an identifying plastic tag with the specimen.

Tissue Registry Storage Area. The space requirements are exemplified by the following data from our facilities. By the end of 1971 the Mayo Clinic tissue registry was storing about 94,000 autopsy specimens and 687,680 surgical specimens. There were 23,100 concentrated stock bottles. Gross specimens were stored in 3,500 large (75.5-liter) crocks or plastic containers, and in 379,857 jars. The total storage space covered 1,681 square meters (18,075 square feet).

One 75.5-liter crock occupies a space of about 56 by 51 by 51 cm and holds about 18 brains or tissues from 18 autopsies. The stock bottles occupy a space of about 15 by 8 by 8 cm each.

From the average autopsy case we save four gross specimens, one stock bottle, and an occasional glass bottle with a specimen requiring special identification or special preservation fluid. Hearts and brains are permanently saved from all autopsies. Slices of formalin-perfused lungs are sealed into plastic bags (Fig. 13–3) and stored on shelves or in containers.

Personnel Requirements. At the present time there are nine employees working in the tissue registry of the Mayo Clinic. Their duties include preparation and updating of files, retrieval of cards for requested tissues or slides, filing of slides, concentration of tissues in crocks, arranging of bottles on shelves, refilling crocks to replace evaporated formalin solution, retrieval and returning of tissues used for studies, disposal of tissues at the end of the 20-year storage period, and transportation of tissues and slides. The cost of running a tissue registry of this type is considerable. However, less elaborate systems quickly prove useless because slide and tissue retrieval becomes too cumbersome, if not impossible.

METHODS OF DATA RETRIEVAL

By R. Thierbach, Robert C. Bahn, and Jurgen Ludwig

Most autopsy records are relatively voluminous. They usually are numbered consecutively and filed by year. If no further provisions are made, information retrieval is possible only by manually searching each individual record. Although this approach is probably the most flexible and adaptable to individual objectives, with moderate or large amounts of stored material, manual information retrieval becomes too laborious and time-consuming. Alternative methods of information processing are required.

There is no single ideal method for all purposes. The pathologist usually evolves an information retrieval system which functions in an optimal manner for himself and his institution. In this evolution, compromises are made between the desired precision, speed, versatility, completeness, and reliability of the system on the one hand and the restrictions of resources such as funds, personnel, and equipment on the other.

Planning of Data Processing. The development or modernization of an autopsy data-processing system requires a decision as to how much can be invested in terms of time, personnel, and funds to maintain files capable of supporting the realistic responsibilities and objectives of an individual laboratory. An honest appraisal of these responsibilities and objectives and an accounting of available resources are essential for the proper design of a retrieval system.

The various members of the staff responsible for anatomic pathology, surgical pathology, diagnostic cytology, the museum, teaching, and research often desire to use the same data-processing system rather than different ones. Cooperation with other pathology departments has been found useful.[48] The importance of autopsy data for clinicians and for public health work makes it imperative that the information be made part of an integrated data-processing system, either within the clinic and medical center or as part of the medical record linkage of larger territories.[51] One should remember, however, that a comprehensive retrieval system invariably involves personal compromises. This also can lead to increased rather than decreased costs accompanied by decreased accessibility, increased complexity of rules for accessing files, and prolongation of the time between the request and the receipt of the desired information.

How elaborate the data-processing system will be depends on whether all or only a portion of relevant autopsy data is to be retrievable. Most general pathologists are principally interested in a basic documentation.[23,24] Such documentation would provide a continuous processing system which stores a large amount of predominantly morphologic data not geared to any specific medical discipline. The objectives of such a system would be to provide a means of statistical surveillance of the work load and to provide a means of identifying the existence of other records, protocols, photographs, references, or diagrams which would contain information germane to the specific question.

The Nature of the Data.   The pathologist's contribution to autopsy data usually is expressed in natural language and consists of gross and microscopic descriptions of organs and tissues accompanied by summarizing diagnostic statements. Photographs and diagrams at times play important roles. An important additional part of the data arises from the patient's medical record and consists of clinical data as well as the results of microbiologic, serologic, chemical, and other laboratory tests. The traditional autopsy record is therefore principally a collection of narrative supplemented by photographs, diagrams, graphs, and limited amounts of numerical data.

With the exception of drawings, diagrams, and graphs, which contain analog data, the greatest portion of the autopsy data are recorded in digital representation—that is, the record consists of numerical characters, alphabetic characters, and special characters organized as prose which is intended to be read and interpreted by a trained human being. The essence of any retrieval system is the development of a scheme which in some way relates these complex concepts to a logically organized number system. Later sections of this chapter will illustrate (1) the process of selection of concepts by means of a logically organized number system, (2) the use of various procedures whereby these numbers can be sequentially or spatially ordered, and (3) methods which utilize the foregoing organization of information for the retrieval of desired data.

The following data for basic documentation of autopsy pathology can be expressed numerically by conventions which can easily be defined by the individual responsible for file maintenance.

1. Demographic patient data. Sex; race; dates of birth and death; age; first, middle and last names; mailing address; occupation.

2. Clinical data. Person or department requesting the autopsy; duration of final admission; number (if any) of biopsy or cytology examinations; diagnoses (causes of death and other).

3. Autopsy data. Autopsy number and date; prosector; weights and measurements of body and organs; diagnoses (causes of death and other).

Demographic data can be extended to include items such as place of birth, birth order, and marriage status; these may be part of an identification number. Clinical data can be extended to include place of death and clinic number. The diagnoses may also include clinical symptoms, laboratory findings, and the mode of dying. Statements as to the completeness of

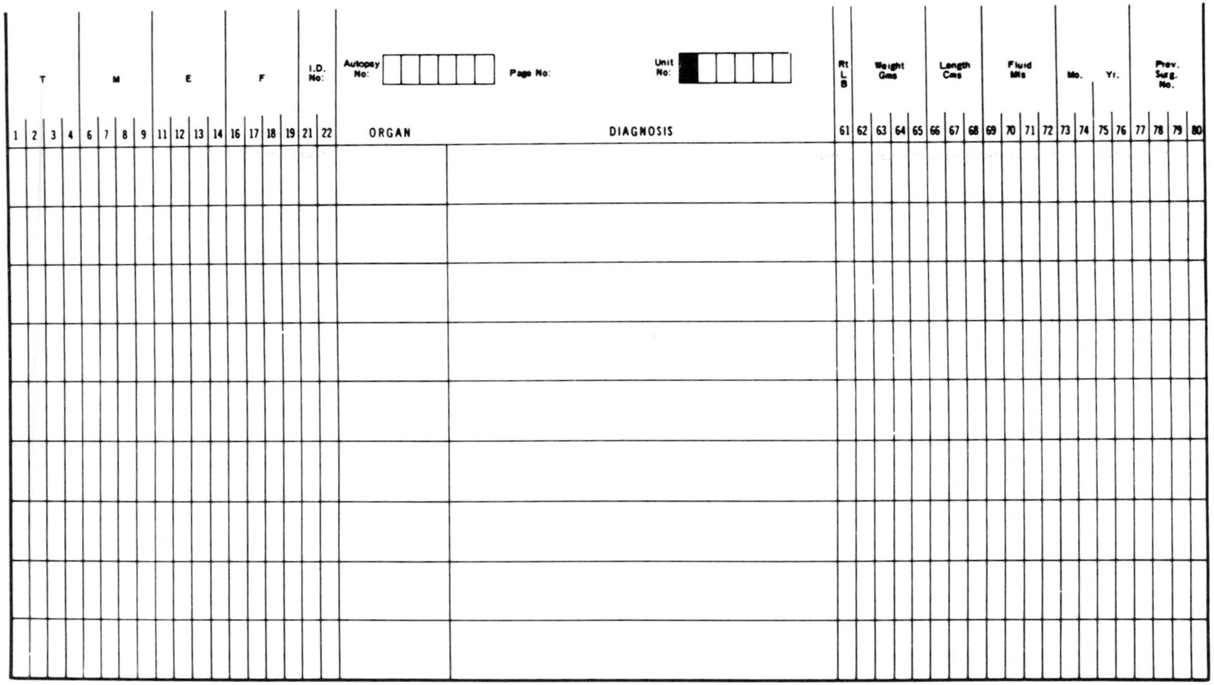

Figure 13–5. Work sheet for autopsy data. Center space is for entries in natural language. Spaces to right are for primary numerical data; spaces to the left are for SNOP code numbers. Form contains 80 columns to correspond with punch cards which are prepared from this form. (From Crocker DW: Preparation of anatomic pathology data for automation. In Pathology Annual 1969. Edited by SC Sommers. New York, Appleton-Century-Crofts, Inc., 1969. By permission.)

the autopsy or special postmortem studies may facilitate data retrieval. The institution must be identified if the data are to be linked with those of other institutions. The minimal requirements for any basic documentation are autopsy number, sex, age, and principal autopsy diagnoses (causes of death).

Coding. Coding can mean (1) the transformation of data from natural language into an abbreviated form, as exemplified by the use of code numbers in place of verbal diagnoses, and (2) the manner of data storage in a data carrier—for instance, the site and type of entry in a work sheet or punched card (Fig 13–5). In this chapter, both senses of coding are used.

It is imperative for those who provide data for coding to base these on a common nomenclature, common definitions, and a common (systematic) classification of diseases and lesions. Of great practical use for this purpose are the following publications:

1. *Systematized Nomenclature of Pathology (SNOP 1965)*.[13] Nomenclature and classification according to topography, morphology, etiology, and function. No terminology.

2. *Manual of Tumor Nomenclature and Coding (MTNC 1968)*.[32] Nomenclature and classification according to topography and morphology or histology. No terminology.

3. *Illustrated Tumor Nomenclature (ITN 1969)*.[19] Nomenclature in six languages; illustration of histologic appearances. Mixed topographic and histologic classification.

4. *International Histological Classification of Tumours (IHCT 1969)*.[30] Histologic classification in each issue, topographic classification of the whole series. Nomenclature and terminology with illustrations.

5. *Standard Nomenclature of Diseases and Operations (SNDO 1961)*.[49] Nomenclature. Topographic and etiologic classification. No terminology.

6. *Current Medical Terminology (CMT 1966)*.[17] Nomenclature and terminology. No classification.

7. *International Classification of Diseases (ICD 1967 and 1969)*,[21] *International Classification of Diseases (ICDA 1967 and 1968)*,[50] and *Hospital Adaptation of ICDA (H-ICDA 1968)*.[12] Mixed topographic, morphologic, etiologic, and nosologic-functional classification. No nomenclature. No terminology.

MTNC is cross-referenced with *ICD* and *SNOP; ITN* is cross-referenced with *ICD*. With the exception of *IHCT*, all of these listings contain code numbers 0 to 9. *SNOP* and *SNDO* also contain the symbols X and Y. A magnetic tape is being prepared which will permit matching the *CMT* code with the *ICD, SNDO,* and *SNOP* codes.[1]

It should be noted that, since there is not perfect correspondence between codes, some information can be expected to be lost in "translation." Because all the coding systems are not equivalent, the selection of the particular code which will be used primarily will depend upon the specific objectives of the retrieval system as well as the availability of data-processing facilities.

Manual coding is cumbersome, time-consuming, and error-prone. It represents a bottleneck of data processing.[39,40] This difficulty can be circumvented by a computer which will automatically produce the stored code numbers. Coded data are preferred because they need less space than data in natural language. For instance, a diagnosis consisting of several words can be expressed by a 4-digit number. Although a computer may not be available in many institutions, coding is still necessary to impose a defined logical organization upon the data as well as to save space on the postprimary data carriers. If a numerical code is used, it is obvious that numerical data such as autopsy numbers, age of patients, and measurements do not need to be transformed. Other nondiagnostic data such as sex, residence, or occupation often can be expressed by a simple code — for instance, male = 1; female = 2.

A manual code should be simple and easy to read; a mixed alphanumeric code may serve this purpose well. Three to four numeric digits are used in the ICD,[21] four in CMT,[17] maximal 2 times 4 in SNDO[49] (and in addition a 1-digit malignancy code for neoplasms), 2 times 4 in MTNC,[32] and maximal 4 times 4 in SNOP.[13]

Spaces for code numbers can be provided on a separate code form or punch card form or on the primary data carriers. If data are worked on outside the institution — for instance, when key punching work is done commercially — the codes must be made separable from the text in natural language in order to prevent disclosure of confidential information. A perforated line in the data carrier will permit easy separation of the portion with the code numbers.

Primary Data Carriers. The objective of an information system is to select and abstract, from a large body of data, pertinent items which are then organized in a manner which facilitates examination of a given body of knowledge. The autopsy record arises from certain source documents such as the death certificate and related data sheets, hospital charts or the clinician's report of death, work sheets arising from the gross and microscopic examinations of tissues and organs (Fig. 13–5), and summarizing diagnostic statements relating to the previous categories of data (Fig. 13–6).

Once a decision is made concerning the selection of data, the design of primary and postprimary data carriers should be considered. The primary data carriers are those documents which carry the information which has been abstracted from the primary source documents. The primary data carriers are usually paper documents which can be quite generalized in that their form could be considered independent of the final retrieval method. In contrast, the postprimary data carriers are usually cards, paper tapes, or magnetic tapes which arise from the primary data carriers. Their form is completely specified by the retrieval method.

The primary data carriers are usually completed by the process of human data selection, editing, abstraction, and recording. These intellectually complex tasks should be carried out by a trained individual.

Transfer of data from the primary to the postprimary carrier is much more mechanical. The transfer is usually done by an individual familiar with the general technical aspects of the retrieval system. In some cases, such as keypunching of cards, this individual may be completely unfamiliar with the implications of the information being transferred.

All forms serving as primary data carriers should have a common

PETER BENT BRIGHAM HOSPITAL
PATHOLOGY DEPARTMENT

| UNIT NUMBER | 7 2 2 7 1 | AUTOPSY NUMBER | A 6 8 0 0 4 |

AGE 0 5 9 SEX M RACE 1 (1=WHITE 2=NEGRO 3=OTHER) SERVICE 1 (1=MEDICAL 2=SURGICAL 3=NEUROLOGY) OCCUPATION

NAME

Prosector:
Final review by:

DURATION OF FINAL ADMISSION	DEATH DATE	MO	DAY	YR	HOUR	AUTOPSY DATE	MO	DAY	YR	HOUR
10 days		0 1	0 2	6 8	8:25 P.M.		0 1	0 3	6 8	11:00 A.M.

76 COMPLETENESS OF AUTOPSY	77 MEDICOLEGAL EXAMINER	78 SPECIAL OR NEW CLINICAL STUDY	79 SPECIAL POST-MORTEM STUDIES	80 SUGGESTED USE
1. COMPLETE 2. NO BRAIN 3. RESTRICTED 4. SELECTED ORGANS 5. FETUS 6. OTHER (SPECIFY DETAILS)	0. NOT REPORTED 1. DECLINED 2. ACCEPTED, NATURAL DEATH 3. ACCIDENTAL DEATH 4. SUICIDE OR HOMICIDE 5. CERTIFICATION PENDING OR COURT CASE 6. OTHER (SPECIFY DETAILS)	0. NONE 1. LABORATORY DX 2. RADIOLOGIC 3. MEDICAL THERAPY 4. SURGICAL THERAPY 5. COMBINATIONS 6. OTHER (LIST SPECIAL STUDIES)	0. ROUTINE 1. SPINAL CORD OR ORGANS OF SENSES 2. BONES AND JOINTS 3. OTHER SPECIAL DISSECTIONS 4. X-RAYS (INC. ANGIOGRAMS) 5. MICROBIOLOGY AND SEROLOGY 6. VIROLOGY 7. HORMONE ASSAYS 8. TOXICOLOGY 9. OTHER (LIST ALL SPECIAL STUDIES)	0. ROUTINE 1. CLINICAL-PATH. CONFERENCE 2. NEUROLOGICAL TEACHING 3. OTHER CLINICAL CONFERENCES 4. PATHOLOGY DEMONSTRATION 5. DIAGNOSTIC REVIEW 6. OTHER (SPECIFY)

DIAGNOSTIC SUMMARY

Code	Site	Diagnosis
7100 3558 0000 0000 01	KIDNEY:	POLYCYSTIC DISEASE, BILATERAL
5600 3557 0000 0000 01	LIVER:	POLYCYSTIC DISEASE
3200 7200 0000 0000 02	HEART:	BIVENTRICULAR HYPERTROPHY
2800 3840 0000 0000 03	LUNG:	PULMONARY EDEMA
2700 3831 0000 0000 03	PLEURA:	BILATERAL SEROUS EFFUSIONS
0200 3851 0000 0000 04	SKIN:	Petechiae, general
0200 3853 0000 0000 05	SKIN:	Purpura, left arm
0200 5400 1101 0000 06	SKIN:	Necrosis skin of R. foot, pseudomonas
0X00 0000 1601 9013 07 1101	BLOOD:	Sepsis, Staph. coagulase positive (clinical culture) Pseudomonas aeruginosa (postmortem culture)
3100 4050 0000 0000 08	PERICARDIUM:	Fibrinous pericarditis
6000 3850 0000 0000 09	PHARYNX:	Submucosal hemorrhage, extensive
6000 3840 0000 0000 10	PHARYNX:	Edema
5600 5731 0000 0000 11	LIVER:	Hemosiderosis, extensive (spleen and bone marrow moderate)
7100 4202 0000 0000 12	KIDNEY:	Chronic active pyelonephritis
7700 4200 0000 0000 13	PROSTATE:	Chronic active prostatitis

Figure 13–6. Autopsy face sheet with blocked entries for key punching. The diagnoses are listed by site and process. Major diagnoses are capitalized. Numbers to the left represent SNOP codes. (From Crocker DW: Preparation of anatomic pathology data for automation. In Pathology Annual 1969. Edited by SC Sommers. New York, Appleton-Century-Crofts, Inc., 1969. By permission.)

design to permit easy orientation so that entries can be made in a logical order, either in writing or by appropriate marks in spaces. Properly arranged questions in the primary data carriers are most likely to provide complete information and will minimize the time required for coding. In some instances the possible answers can be printed into the forms so that the appropriate spaces need only to be marked with a graphite pencil. This method has found some clinical use[15] and may be applicable, for instance, to sentence-completion protocols (see chapter 12).

Recording and proper arrangement of data which identify autopsy cases or which give weights and measurements offer little difficulty. Much more complicated is the preparation for encoding of autopsy diagnoses, particularly when they represent a mixture of objective and interpreted findings phrased and arranged in speculative combinations or in accordance with presumptions of importance.[41] Because autopsy diagnoses of this type convey more information they are preferred by most clinicians. This is difficult to reconcile with the standard arrangement of diagnoses (Fig. 13–7), which is preferred for data recording. A compromise can be made by subclassifying diagnoses—for instance, as "causes of death" and "others."

Postprimary Data Carriers and Data Storage. Primary data carriers are not amenable to handling, merging, sorting, computing, and other procedures. Moreover, for efficient data storage—that is, the retention of data for subsequent reference—a postprimary data carrier must be used, such as file cards (Fig. 13–8), punch cards (Figs. 13–9 and 13–10), paper tape, or magnetic tape. Cards can be kept in files and can be written on but require large amounts of file space, while tapes have great data storage capacity,

```
                                          Autopsy No.:
                                          Date:

Name:
Demographic Data:
                        Principal Diagnoses
               Recent thrombus of left coronary artery
               Recent infarct of myocardium
               Bronchopneumonia of right lung
                    Diagnoses by Anatomic Systems
Cardiovascular
   Recent thrombus of left coronary artery
   Recent infarct of myocardium
   Acute fibrinous epicarditis
Respiratory
   Bronchopneumonia, lower lobe of right lung
   Acute fibrinous pleuritis, right lung
Digestive
   Acute passive hyperemia of liver
Genitourinary
   Arteriolar nephrosclerosis
Hematopoietic
   Passive hyperemia of spleen
Endocrine
   No pathologic diagnosis
Musculoskeletal
   No pathologic diagnosis
Craniospinal
   Permission for examination not granted
Integumentary
   Scars of the skin
     (Tissue diagnoses expressed as process-site
conjunctions, one per line, according to
anatomic systems. In some instances a
diagnostic word includes both process and
site, eg, nephrosclerosis and epicarditis.)
```

Figure 13–7. Autopsy diagnosis in topographic order with separate listing of principal diagnosis. (From Smith JC: Intermediate data retrieval system for the anatomic pathologist. Arch Pathol 87:432–438, 1969. By permission of the American Medical Association.)

T-63 Stomach		Peptic Ulcer	M-4003
5-62-6			
A-62-315			
5-62-429			
5-62-536			
5-62-647			
A-62-693			
5-62-704			
5-62-743			

Figure 13–8. File card for "Peptic ulcer of stomach" with SNOP code numbers. Some autopsy and surgical pathology case numbers are entered. (From Committee on Nomenclature and Classification of Disease: Systematized Nomenclature of Pathology [SNOP]. Chicago, College of American Pathologists, 1965. By permission.)

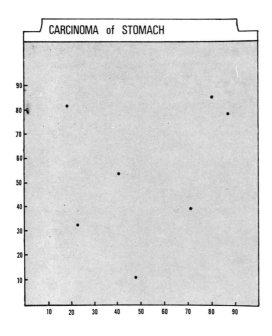

Figure 13–9. Light-transmitting card for "Carcinoma of stomach." Holes indicate cases which fall under this diagnosis. (From Smith JC: Intermediate data retrieval system for the anatomic pathologist. Arch Pathol 87:432–438, 1969. By permission of the American Medical Association.)

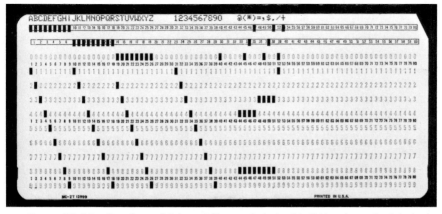

Figure 13–10. Punch card (about 2/3 actual size) with IBM code and alphabetic, numeric, and special characters on upper margin.

require relatively less physical space for their storage, and provide for speedy retrieval.

Transfer of data from primary to postprimary carriers can be achieved by the following methods.

1. Data are transferred by a separate procedure—for instance, by preparing a punch card or by writing the autopsy number on a file card which lists all cases falling under a specific diagnosis heading (Fig. 13–8). Punch cards may be prepared directly or a form is prepared which is later used for the actual punching.

2. Data are transferred concomitantly with the typing of the final autopsy diagnosis—for instance, by using a tape-typewriter. The paper or magnetic tape so prepared can in turn be used for the preparation of punch cards.

3. Data are transferred automatically—for instance, onto punch cards—from special forms by using an optical character reader.[46]

The quality and quantity of data on the postprimary carriers determine to what extent the original documents can be retrieved later.[5]

Retrieval Systems. Modern data-processing and retrieval techniques in anatomic and surgical pathology have come into wide use only during the last 15 years. Manual-mechanical, electromechanical, and electronic systems are available. They are characterized, in the order listed, by increasing capacity and cost.

Manual-Mechanical Systems. For institutions where data accumulate relatively slowly, manual-mechanical systems can still be recommended. Among the disadvantages are the large number of cards (one card per case or per card heading must be kept on file) and the necessity to count manually the retrieved data.

Typewriters can be used to prepare cards, and simple machines are available for sorting and punching. Data are put on cards made of cardboard or plastic. The cards may come with or without punched holes.

1. Simple file cards. The autopsy numbers are merely entered onto the file card which has the appropriate heading, such as "Peptic ulcer of stomach" (Fig. 13–8) or "Peptic ulcer of stomach, male, 50–59." There is no necessity for coding. Cards are stored in the alphabetic order of the headings or by code number if numbers are used. Manual retrieval is required but can be aided by use of card riders or cards of various colors. The system is easily extendable by introducing cards with new headings.

2. Pin-sort cards. Autopsy data can be entered in natural language. Round holes are punched, usually along lines parallel with the periphery of the card. The holes which are to be marked are either connected with the free edge of the card with a special punch so as to create a notch[25] or they are connected in pairs by a punching machine so as to create slots.[35] The limited storage capacity of these cards requires transformation of data into code. Data are retrieved by sorting the cards with metal needles. The cards which are searched for fall out or protrude from the stack. The operation may be aided by special vibrating halters. The cards do not have to be in a special order. Pin-sort card systems permit little extension for the incorporation of new data which had not originally been provided for.

3. Light-transmitting cards. As in the case of simple file cards, one card per title is used. Light-transmitting cards (Fig. 13–9) have a grid of numbered lines (not shown in the illustration). The capacity of the system depends on how close together the lines of the grid are in the various types of cards.[11,20,40,52] Instead of writing down an autopsy number, a hole is made into the grid at the appropriate intersection of vertical and horizontal coordinates. This requires precisely working punching machines because the site of the hole which permits light transmission characterizes the cases in question. If combined data are requested, several cards can be placed on top of each other (optical coincidence system). To make diagnoses retrievable by site and process, a dual-deck card system is recommended.[40,41]

Electromechanical Systems.   The data carrier is a punch card (Fig. 13–10). The data are usually coded and transferred to the card with a numerical or alpha-numeric punching apparatus; a similar apparatus checks the punched holes for errors.[9] Mixing and duplicating of cards can also be achieved electromechanically. For data retrieval, sorting machines are used which are equipped with mechanical counters or with devices to print data on the punch card or to tabulate them on strips of paper, together with the results of simple calculations. The cards do not need to be stored in a specific order. Electromechanical systems can be adapted to continuous data storage in pathology departments.[47,48] However, disadvantages, such as the time required for coding and the limited capacity of the punch cards, make electronic systems clearly superior. This should be considered when plans are made for data processing with machines.

Electronic (or Combined Electromechanical-Electronic) Systems.   Computers of various sizes and complexity can be used for data processing.[9,38,45] Basically, they consist of a central unit and peripheral units for input and output. Data input can be accomplished with punch cards, paper or magnetic tapes, data-reading devices, or alpha-numeric typing. The processing of data in the computer requires a set of directions for processing which are stored within the computer;[45] this set of instructions is called the computer program.

Computers can also process uncoded data such as natural language, provided a properly programmed system is available. Data can be retrieved as print-outs on paper or punch cards, as an optical display, or by other means.[38,45]

Techniques for transition from electromechanical to electronic systems are available.[14,22-24] Experience in converting conventional to electronic systems has been reported by Becker and associates.[6,7] The exclusive use of computers of various sizes has been discussed by numerous authors.[4,5,26,27,29,31,33,36,37,42-44]

Automatic data processing becomes a necessity whenever a large number of clinical data are to be correlated with autopsy data or when correlations with other files are desired — for instance, with sociologic data.[2,3,39]

Comment. Some applications of these data-retrieval systems to pathology have only been suggested, others have actually been tried, and still others may already have been dropped. While the methods have often been described in detail, reports on results are scanty and even fewer economic evaluations are available.[38] Added to these uncertainties are the compromises which must usually be made when a pathologist is to decide on a system. In the planning stage of complicated systems, advice is needed from specialists in data processing and from pathologists experienced in this field. This notwithstanding, the output quality of any processing system will not be greater than the quality of the collected data. In addition, one should always keep in mind that data retrieval is no end in itself. It serves only as a first step to operations such as statistical analysis and interpretation.

REFERENCES

1. Alexander MK: Data processing in histopathology. J Clin Pathol 22(Suppl 3):74–76, 1969
2. Angrist A: Fitting the old-fashioned autopsy into the modern medical scene. Am J Clin Pathol 45:202–207, 1966
3. Angrist A: Breaking the postmortem barrier. Bull NY Acad Med 44:830–842, 1968
4. Bahn RC, Schmit RW, Lutz TD: Potential uses of a digital computer in the Section of Experimental and Anatomic Pathology. Mayo Clin Proc 39:830–834, 1964
5. Bahn RC, Schmit RW, Young GG: An information-retrieval system for research associated with the postmortem examination. Mayo Clin Proc 39:835–840, 1964
6. Becker H: Aufbau und Auswertungen einer pathologisch-anatomischen Diagnosenkartei durch Computer-Einsatz. Methods Inf Med 5:105–113, 1966
7. Becker H, Breitenlohner H, Lang C, Schwarz F: Computer in der Pathologie: Methodik und Erfahrungen nach Auswertung von 27000 Sektionsprotokollen. Methods Inf Med 8:60–67, 1969
8. Bresnahan MF: Personal communication
9. Brooks FP Jr, Iverson KE: Automatic Data Processing. New York, John Wiley & Sons, Inc., 1969
10. Cantway D, Fitch FW: Plastic films for storage of pathology tissue storage specimens. Arch Pathol 81:448–452, 1966
11. Carpenter HM: A system for storage and retrieval of data from autopsies. Am J Clin Pathol 38:449–467, 1962

12. Commission on Professional Hospital Activities: Hospital Adaptation of ICDA (H-ICDA). Vol 1, Tabular List. Vol 2, Alphabetic Index. Ann Arbor, Michigan, 1968

13. Committee on Nomenclature and Classification of Disease: Systematized Nomenclature of Pathology (SNOP). Chicago, College of American Pathologists, 1965

14. Crocker DW: Preparation of anatomic pathology data for automation. *In* Pathology Annual 1969. Edited by SC Sommers. New York, Appleton-Century-Crofts, Inc., 1969, pp 31–41

15. Ehlers CT, Wick DP: Datenverarbeitung im Krankenhauswesen. II. Erfassung und Bewertung medizinischer Daten mit dem Markierungsleser. IBM Nachr *17*:533–539, 1967

16. Emery JL, Marshall AG: Handbook for Mortuary Technicians. Oxford, Blackwell Scientific Publications, 1965

17. Gordon BL, Hussey HH: Current Medical Terminology (CMT). Third edition. Chicago, American Medical Association, 1966

18. Gordon H: Method for storing wet histologic accessions and disposing of autopsy material. Lab Invest *2*:152–153, 1953

19. Hamperl H, Ackerman LV: Illustrated Tumor Nomenclature. Second revised edition. Berlin, Springer Verlag, Inc., 1969

20. Hienz HA: Statistische Erfassung der Sektionsbefunde mit Hilfe einer Sichtlochkartei. Frankfurt Z Pathol *69*:342–356, 1958

21. International Classification of Diseases: Manual of the International Statistical Classification of Diseases, Injuries, and Causes of Death. Eighth revision. Vol 1, Tabular List, 1967. Vol 2, Alphabetical Index, 1969. Geneva, World Health Organization.

22. Jacob W: Über ein neues Prinzip der halbautomatischen Verschlüsselung in der medizinischen Dokumentation – das sog. "over-cross" Verfahren – und seine Anwendung in der pathologischen Anatomie. Frankfurt Z Pathol *74*:700–715, 1965

23. Jacob W: Basis-Dokumentation in der Pathologie. Methods Inf Med *6*:166–173, 1967

24. Jacob W: Moderne Dokumentationsmethoden im Routinebetrieb eines pathologischen Instituts. *In* Automatisierung des klinischen Laboratoriums. Edited by G Griesser, G Wagner. Stuttgart, Schattauer Verlag, 1968, pp 77–87

25. Jansen HH: Hat sich die Randlochkartei bei der Erfassung und Auswertung des Sektionsgutes wirklich bewahrt? Verh Dtsch Ges Pathol *41*:210–213, 1957

26. Lamson BG, Dimsdale B: A natural language information retrieval system. Proc Inst Electric Electron Engineers *54*:1636–1640, 1966

27. Lamson BG, Glinski BC, Hawthorne GS, Soutter JC, Russell WS: Storage and Retrieval of Uncoded Tissue Pathology Diagnoses in the Original English Free-Text Form. Poughkeepsie, New York, Proceedings of the 7th IBM Medical Symposium, 1965, pp 411–426

28. Minkowitz S, Brandt LJ, Rapp Y, Radlauer CB: "Prosector's wart" (cutaneous tuberculosis) in a medical student. Am J Clin Pathol *51*:260–263, 1969

29. Myers J, Gelblat M, Enterline HT: Automatic encoding of pathology data: computer-readable surgical pathology data as a by-product of typed pathology reports. Arch Pathol *89*:73–78, 1970

30. Notes: International histological classification of tumours. Methods Inf Med *8*:104–105, 1969

31. Paplanus SH, Shepard RH, Zvargulis JE: A computer-based system for autopsy diagnosis storage and retrieval without numerical coding. Lab Invest *20*:139–146, 1969

32. Percy CL, Berg JW, Thomas LB: Manual of Tumor Nomenclature and Coding. New York, American Cancer Society, 1968

33. Pratt AW, Thomas LB: An information processing system for pathology data. *In* Pathology Annual. Edited by SC Sommers. New York, Appleton-Century-Crofts, Inc., 1966, pp 1–21

34. Pulvertaft RJV: Museum techniques: a review. J Clin Pathol *3*:1–23, 1950

35. Ross W: Dokumentation und Auswertung von Sektionsbefunden mittels Schlitzlochkartei. Virchows Arch Pathol Anat *333*:466–478, 1960

36. Röttger P, Reul H, Klein I, Sunkel H: Die vollautomatische Dokumentation und statistische Auswertung pathologisch-anatomischer Befundberichte. Methods Inf Med *8*:19–26, 1969

37. Röttger P, Reul H, Sunkel H, Klein I: Neue Auswertungsmöglichkeiten pathologisch-anatomischer Befundberichte: Klartextanalyse durch Elektronenrechner. Methods Inf Med *9*:35–44, 1970

38. Sharpe WF: The Economics of Computers. New York, Columbia University Press, 1969

39. Smith JC: Anatomic pathology and data processing (editorial). Arch Pathol *81*:279–280, 1966

40. Smith JC: Intermediate data retrieval system for the anatomic pathologist. Arch Pathol *87*:432–438, 1969
41. Smith JC: Basis of data control for anatomical pathology. J Clin Pathol *22*(Suppl 3):77–81, 1969
42. Smith JC, Melton J: Automated retrieval of autopsy diagnoses by computer technique. Methods Inf Med *2*:85–90, 1963
43. Smith JC, Melton J: Manipulation of autopsy diagnoses by computer technique. JAMA *188*:958–962, 1964
44. Smith JC, Melton J: Data Control for Anatomic Pathology. Institute of Pathology, Western Reserve University, Cleveland, 1965
45. Spencer DD: Fundamentals of Digital Computers. Indianapolis, Indiana, Howard W. Sams & Co., Inc., 1969
46. Stulle P: Mehrfunktionsbelegleser IBM 1287 – Der Beginn eines neuen Abschnitts der Datenerfassung. IBM Nachr *16*:335–343, 1966
47. Thierbach R: Die Erschließung der Informationen im pathologisch-anatomischen Sektionsgut: Studie zur Dokumentation medizinischer Daten unter Verwendung konventioneller Lochkartenmaschinen und der Internationalen Krankheitsklassifikation der Weltgesundheitsorganisation. Med Habil-Schr (Thesis), Halle (Saale), 1967
48. Thierbach R, Zschoch H: Erfahrungen aus der Dokumentation von Autopsiedaten in 2 Pathologischen Instituten. Zentralbl Allg Pathol *114*:251–272, 1971
49. Thompson ET, Hayden AC: Standard Nomenclature of Diseases and Operations. Fifth edition. New York, McGraw-Hill Book Company, Inc., 1961
50. US National Center for Health Statistics: Eighth Revision of the International Classification of Diseases. Vol 1, Tabular list, 1967. Vol 2, Alphabetical index, 1968. Washington DC, US Government Printing Office
51. Wagner G, Newcombe HB: Record linkage: its methodology and application in medical data processing; a bibliography. Methods Inf Med *9*:121–138, 1970
52. Ziegler HK: Erfahrungen mit der Sichtlochkartei im Rahmen eines Pathologischen Institutes. Dok Med Biol *3*:57–59, 1959

CHAPTER 14

MEDICOLEGAL CONSIDERATIONS

With Gregg Orwoll

In this chapter only some general legal principles pertaining to autopsies are discussed. Each pathologist should familiarize himself with the laws of his state which govern the performance of all autopsies.

MEDICOLEGAL SAFEGUARDS PRIOR TO PERFORMANCE OF AUTOPSY

Prior to performing an autopsy, the pathologist should do the following. These three steps should be taken by the pathologist personally and should not be delegated to technicians or other personnel.

1. Identify the body of the deceased (name tag, clinic number, etc.) to ascertain that the body is in fact the one for which an autopsy permission has been granted. The pathologist who performs an unauthorized autopsy in the mistaken belief that authorization has been obtained could be found to be liable unless he is able to show that his actions have not resulted from his negligence.[10]

2. Consider whether the case falls under the jurisdiction of the official who is in charge of ordering medicolegal autopsies and, if it does, consult with the appropriate official to discuss how the case should be handled.

3. Scrutinize the autopsy authorization form to ascertain that it is properly completed and signed (if written authorization is used) and to learn about any restrictions which may have been imposed. Details of these restrictions should be told immediately to technicians and assistants who may help in performing the autopsy. If a *signed* authorization form is not

297

used for this purpose, a form which contains all pertinent information should, nevertheless, be used to avoid errors and misunderstandings.

MEDICOLEGAL AUTOPSIES

Authorization. In most states, medicolegal autopsies may be authorized by one or more of the following: coroners or county physicians (also deputy coroners, coroners' physicians, coroners' juries, and ex officio coroners such as justices of the peace or district, deputy, and county magistrates), medical examiners, attorneys general (or county, district, state, and prosecuting attorneys), and judges (superior court, circuit court, district court, or county court judges). In a few instances, medicolegal autopsies may be authorized by other officials, such as the county sheriff or the county manager.

Medicolegal autopsies may be performed without the consent or even against the expressed will of the surviving spouse or next of kin.

Who May Perform Autopsy. In most states, medicolegal autopsies may be performed by medical examiners and their deputies, coroners (if they are physicians), and coroners' physicians, county physicians, and their deputies or other designated physicians who may be referred to in the statute as "qualified physicians and surgeons," or whose required qualifications may have been specified as "competent pathologists or toxicologists."

When May Medicolegal Autopsy Be Performed. In most instances, statutes authorize medicolegal autopsies when death has resulted from violence (apparent homicide, suicide, or accident) or from unlawful or criminal means. Some state laws also include deaths in penal institutions, deaths due to self-induced abortions, deaths involving a possible threat to public health, or when cremation is intended.

Statutes in some states also authorize autopsies when the death took place without an eyewitness, when the decedent was not attended by a physician at the time of death, when death was sudden and unexplained, or when the death was of unknown cause. In most states, however, death also must have occurred in an unusual manner or under circumstances giving rise to a suspicion that death was by unlawful or criminal means before a medicolegal autopsy will be warranted.[18]

The burden of proving that a medicolegal autopsy was unjustified is on the claimant.[10] A presumption exists that the public official acted in good faith.

Source Material. The laws governing medicolegal autopsies vary greatly from state to state. An excellent compilation of the medicolegal autopsy laws of the 50 states and the District of Columbia has been published by the Armed Forces Institute of Pathology.[19] This booklet lists separately, for each state, the persons who may authorize and perform medicolegal autopsies, the circumstances under which medicolegal autopsies may be authorized, and references to the statutes which contain these provisions. A somewhat similar compilation was prepared earlier by Regan.[13]

AUTHORIZATION OF AUTOPSIES BY STATUTE

In most states the directors or administrators of hospitals, prisons, or other public institutions may give permission for autopsies on bodies which have to be buried at public expense and when no persons are known who would legally be entitled to take custody of the body for burial.[7] Autopsies may be done on such bodies or they may be surrendered to established medical or dental schools for scientific studies. In all these instances, reasonable efforts must be made over a specified period to communicate with relatives or friends who might want to assume custody of the body and the costs of burial.

Authorization by statute may be contested unless the procedures outlined in the statute are followed carefully. Some state workmen's compensation laws provide statutory immunity for autopsies performed by order of the Industrial Commission. However, unless so provided by statute, courts generally have held that the economic interest of the insurance carrier involved in a workmen's compensation claim is not a sufficient interest to override the refusal of the next of kin to grant an autopsy permission.[10]

AUTOPSIES AUTHORIZED BY RELATIVES, FRIENDS, OR THE DECEASED

Autopsies may not be performed without a proper authorization. The right to grant, restrict, or withhold authorization for an autopsy usually rests with the surviving spouse or the next of kin. Although the dead human body is not property in the commercial sense and may not be bargained for, bartered, or sold,[2,17] there is a right, protected by law, to possess the body for the purpose of burying it. Figure 14–1 shows a proper authorization form.

Persons Who May Authorize Autopsy. An autopsy permission may be granted by one of the following persons.[9]

1. The deceased. In some but not all states, the deceased, prior to his death, may authorize in writing an autopsy on himself.[2,8,9] It seems wise, however, to secure also the consent of the person(s) who would otherwise be entitled to give permission for an autopsy.

2. Surviving spouse. The widow's or widower's wishes in regard to the autopsy clearly override those of the next of kin, with a possible exception in some cases in which the man and wife were separated.[7,9,18]

3. Children of the deceased, if they are of age.

4. Grandchildren of the deceased, if they are of age.

5. Parents.

6. Brothers and sisters.

7. Cousins, nieces, nephews, grandparents, uncles, and aunts (local law should be consulted with regard to right to consent and priority).

8. Friends or any person of legal age who assumes responsibility for

AUTHORIZATION FOR AUTOPSY

A.M.
Date_____ Time_____P.M.

I (We) request and authorize the physicians and surgeons in attendance at the _____ Hospital to perform a complete autopsy on the remains of _____ and I (we) authorize the removal and retention or use for diagnostic, scientific, or therapeutic purposes of such organs, tissues, and parts as such physicians and surgeons deem proper.

This authority is granted subject to the following restrictions:

_____

(If no restrictions, write "None.")
The following special examinations shall be made:

_____

I (We) wish the remains to be released to:

_____

(Name of undertaking establishment)   (City)   (State)

I (We) represent that I am (we are) the _____ of the

(relationship)

deceased and entitled by law to control the disposition of the remains.

Signed_____

Signed_____

Witnesses:

_____

Name of person obtaining Authorization:

_____

Figure 14–1. Example of proper autopsy authorization form. (From American Medical Association Law Department: Medicolegal Forms With Legal Analysis. Chicago, American Medical Association, 1961, pp 45–49. By permission.)

burial. In the case of a friend, an affidavit may be required stating the facts of the friendship and that the friend will assume the costs of burial.[7]

State statutes generally establish the order of priority among those authorized to make decisions concerning the remains. A decision made by the person(s) having the highest priority is binding and may not be over-ruled by a person with a lower priority. Under the laws of most states, a person with a lower priority may act if persons with higher priorities are not available.[9] Many states have statutes which state that the authorization for an autopsy is sufficient if given by the surviving spouse, children, parents, siblings, friends, or anybody who has assumed custody of the body.[2,9] Thus, one who has lived with and cared for the deceased in a friendly and intimate relationship may have a right to possess the body for burial which is superior to the right of kinsmen,[18] if no such relationship existed with the members of the family. Under some statutes, one of the persons involved may authorize the autopsy even though several persons have assumed custody of the body. A very recent Illinois lower court decision has cast doubt on the confidence with which one can act in reliance on authorization by fewer than all of those persons who might authorize the autopsy. In the case of *Sam Leno & Ralph Leno v. St. Joseph's Hospital* (Cook County Case #67L, 13251), the court declared unconstitutional the portion of an Illinois statute giving hospitals the right to perform an au-topsy with the permission of only one surviving relative. A motion leading to an appeal of the case has been made. When acting on the authority of one such individual, it would be wise to require this person to indicate that he has authority to act for all members of the group.

In general, it seems prudent not to perform an autopsy whenever the right of custody of the body seems questionable and there is a risk of litigation.

Authorization for an autopsy without specified restrictions is given with the understanding that the autopsy will be carried out in the usual manner—that is, the chest and abdominal cavities may be examined and the brain may be removed. For any procedures which require additional incisions, particularly of the face, neck, or hands, or which may interfere with proper reconstruction, such as total removal of the spinal column, it seems prudent to secure a special permission spelling out the nature of the intended procedure. This also holds true for removal of the eyes.

A good professional relationship with the funeral director is of great importance. Extended autopsy procedures should be discussed with him first and every effort should be made to avoid interfering with the embalming. Funeral directors who have a proper understanding and attitude toward the objectives of the autopsy may be expected to make their skills available when defects from extended autopsies must be reconstructed or when an occasional technical mishap must be repaired.

Restricted Authorization for Autopsy. Autopsies may be restricted as to place, manner, and extent.[10,12] Restrictions regarding place generally are intended to secure privacy. Even without this specification, the pathologist is well advised to admit to the autopsy room only physicians, autopsy technicians on duty, and funeral directors in charge of embalming the bodies. While it is customary to admit medical students as part of specific courses, the admission of nurses, physical therapists, law enforcement officers, or others for the purpose of general instruction in pathology should be discouraged. The relatives who authorize the autopsy probably do not anticipate the presence of persons not necessary for the conduct of the examination or handling of the body. A pathologist who admits mere spectators runs the risk of being found liable in an action for damages,[17] although it is likely that any such finding would result in a nominal damage award.

The extent of the autopsy may be restricted to the abdominal or chest cavity, to exploration through an operative incision, or in other ways. Even the usual autopsy procedures may be prohibited if the person authorizing the autopsy insists on such restrictions. He may, for instance, not allow temporary removal of organs from the body for histologic examination or other purposes. Whether the examination should be conducted at all under such conditions should be carefully considered by the pathologist.

Unauthorized Autopsies. The performance of an unauthorized autopsy may be construed as a mutilation of the body of the deceased. The same holds true when restrictions on the extent of the autopsy have been disregarded. The survivors may claim that this has caused them "mental anguish."[10] Damages are collectible without proof of physical injury to the claimant. The proper party claimant, and the person to recover for the mutilation of the dead body, generally would be the one who had the right to custody of the body and who therefore had the right to restrict or withhold authorization for the autopsy.

Many insurance policies providing indemnity for accidental death contain clauses which give the insurer the right to demand an autopsy.[10,13,18]

However, the economic interest of the insurance carrier does not override the right of the surviving spouse and of the next of kin to control the disposition of the body.[10]

Retention of Organs and Tissues for Study. Temporary removal of organs and tissues for histologic study is accepted as a normal part of the autopsy.[10] Permanent retention of entire organs may not be contemplated by the next of kin, and consequently, one should be satisfied that the authorization which has been obtained is broad enough to permit such retention.

Donation of Body, Organs, and Tissues. A number of states have enacted laws permitting the donation of dead bodies or parts of them. Suggested provisions for inclusion in a will are available.[8] Figure 14–2

AUTHORIZATION TO USE EYES (DONOR)

Date_____ Time_____ A.M.
P.M.

I authorize, at the time of my death, the removal of both or either of my eyes for donation to any eye bank serving the area in which my death occurs and for such purpose as the eye bank may see fit.

Signed_____

(Donor)

Witness_____

AUTHORIZATION TO USE EYES (NEXT OF KIN)

Date_____ Time_____ A.M.
P.M.

I authorize any member of the medical staff of the _____ Hospital to remove both or either of the eyes of _____, the deceased, for donation to any eye bank serving the area and for such purpose as the eye bank may see fit.

Signed_____

(next of kin)

_____
(relationship to deceased)

Witness_____

AUTHORIZATION TO RETAIN AND DISPOSE OF BODY

Date_____ Time_____ A.M.
P.M.

We request and authorize the release of the body of baby _____ to the Pathology Staff of the laboratory at _____ Hospital, for scientific purposes and study with privilege of ultimate disposal.

Signed_____
(Mother)

Signed_____
(Father)

Witnesses:

_____

_____

Figure 14–2. Samples of authorization forms. (From American Medical Association Law Department: Medicolegal Forms With Legal Analysis. Chicago, American Medical Association, 1961, pp 45–49. By permission.)

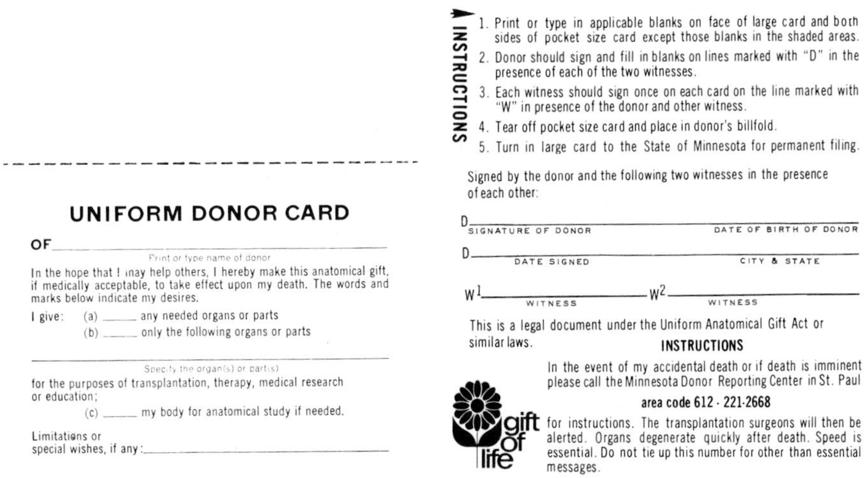

INSTRUCTIONS

1. Print or type in applicable blanks on face of large card and both sides of pocket size card except those blanks in the shaded areas.
2. Donor should sign and fill in blanks on lines marked with "D" in the presence of each of the two witnesses.
3. Each witness should sign once on each card on the line marked with "W" in presence of the donor and other witness.
4. Tear off pocket size card and place in donor's billfold.
5. Turn in large card to the State of Minnesota for permanent filing.

Signed by the donor and the following two witnesses in the presence of each other:

UNIFORM DONOR CARD

OF_____
Print or type name of donor

In the hope that I may help others, I hereby make this anatomical gift, if medically acceptable, to take effect upon my death. The words and marks below indicate my desires.

I give: (a) _____ any needed organs or parts
(b) _____ only the following organs or parts

_____
Specify the organ(s) or part(s)

for the purposes of transplantation, therapy, medical research or education;

(c) _____ my body for anatomical study if needed.

Limitations or special wishes, if any :_____

D_____
SIGNATURE OF DONOR   DATE OF BIRTH OF DONOR

D_____
DATE SIGNED   CITY & STATE

W1_____ W2_____
WITNESS   WITNESS

This is a legal document under the Uniform Anatomical Gift Act or similar laws.

INSTRUCTIONS

In the event of my accidental death or if death is imminent please call the Minnesota Donor Reporting Center in St. Paul

area code 612 - 221-2668

for instructions. The transplantation surgeons will then be alerted. Organs degenerate quickly after death. Speed is essential. Do not tie up this number for other than essential messages.

gift of life

Figure 14–3. **Donor card** in use under Uniform Anatomical Gift Act in Minnesota. Cards bearing substantially similar language are in use in most states which have adopted the Act.

shows authorization forms for the use of the eyes and for the retention and disposition of the body of a baby. In the many states which now have adopted the Uniform Anatomical Gift Act, a small card (Fig. 14–3) signed by the deceased and two witnesses is a legal document providing for the donation of organs for transplantation purposes or for the donation of the body for anatomic study, or both. The card also has a space in which limitations of its provisions or special wishes may be entered.

The subject of organ transplantation has been reviewed by Dukeminier and Sanders,[3] and many of their thoughts and suggestions are implemented in the Uniform Anatomical Gift Act. Background information concerning the Uniform Anatomical Gift Act is outlined in a publication of the National Research Council[11] and in two other articles.[14,15]

DEATH CERTIFICATES AND AUTOPSY PROTOCOLS—ADMISSIBILITY AS EVIDENCE

The death certificate is a public record and is admissible in court as prima facie evidence of the facts recorded.[1] Autopsy protocols and diagnoses usually are admitted into evidence by laws pertaining to the admissibility of hospital records or by specific provisions of the law covering autopsy reports and death certificates. Direct testimony of the pathologist usually is required but he will be allowed to use the autopsy documents while testifying.[1,16] In most jurisdictions, information gained at autopsy is not privileged because a dead body is not considered a patient. However, a physician who discloses autopsy findings must be careful not to reveal facts he learned during the patient's life while he had a professional relationship with him.[1,13a]

Autopsy diagnoses or opinions concerning autopsy findings frequently are sought by private insurance carriers. Generally it is a good practice not to disclose such information without an authorization signed by the person who had custody of the body and who gave permission for the autopsy.

The foremost reason for surviving spouses or the next of kin to authorize autopsies is their desire to have the findings explained to them, either in an interview or in writing. In either case, care must be taken that the findings are disclosed primarily to the person who had custody of the body and that others are informed through or in the presence of this person. It is recommended that autopsy findings not be discussed on the telephone and that interviews be held only with the closest relatives. Occasionally, when the consent of those who have custody of the body has been obtained, an interview may be held with a clergyman or friend. Letters with autopsy findings should be addressed to the surviving spouse or the next of kin who had custody of the body.

The findings of medicolegal autopsies also often are explained to the relatives, but this should not be done without previously discussing the matter with the official who has ordered the medicolegal autopsy. Interviews after medicolegal autopsies obviously should not be held if there is a pending criminal investigation, but they are justified in some instances, such as in cases of crib death.

TRANSPORTATION OF BODIES

The autopsy pathologist should become familiar with the laws of the state in which he practices, the regulations issued by the appropriate state health agency, and the local rules concerning the transportation of bodies within his area or from his location to other states by various means of conveyance. Minnesota regulations are fairly typical as they pertain to such transportation. In Minnesota, regulations specify that the remains of the dead must be prepared for transportation by an embalmer.[4] Transportation permits must be issued for each body by local or state registrars. The signatures of the embalmer, the registrar, and the person in charge of the conveyance are required on the transportation permit. Transportation and burial permits are delivered with the body to the person in charge of the cemetery or to the health officer in cities that have local ordinances requiring burial permits by this official.

When bodies are transported in caskets, an outside container is required unless transportation is by automobile. In this instance, only the casket or an ambulance cot is needed. The body must be properly dressed and covered with clean sheets, or it must be encased in a zipper pouch or bag. When the patient died with a communicable disease, thorough embalming of the body by specified techniques is prescribed. There are also regulations governing the types of caskets and containers which must be used. Transportation by airplane within the state requires thorough embalming and a casket but no outside container. For transportation outside the state by airplane, an outside container is required.

The following letter must be written in triplicate for each body sent to a foreign country. One copy stays with the funeral director, one copy is kept by the airline, and one copy remains with the body:

To Whom It May Concern:

    This is to certify that the death of _____

of _____, _____, _____, who died at _____

Hospital, _____,* Minnesota, on _____, was due

to a non-communicable cause. The cause of death was _____

_____; due to _____

Sincerely yours,

 * City or town   _____, M.D.

There are numerous regulations concerning embalming, caskets, and containers, depending on how long the remains will be in transit. For shipment of disinterred bodies, approval of the health authorities is required.

Cremation of the body is considered a final disposal. For the transportation, interment, or other disposal of ashes of a cremated body, no additional permit is required and there are no regulations as to the type of container to be used for preservation or transportation.

EMBALMING

In the United States, embalming is a widely practiced procedure. Some exceptions should be noted. As an example, embalming and application of cosmetics both are in direct violation of the religious beliefs of orthodox Jews.[9] For the transportation of bodies, embalming usually is required by state law. In Minnesota, embalming is not required if a person dead of a noncommunicable disease is buried within 72 hours after death.

EXHUMATION

Exhumation—that is, disinterment of bodies—is carried out on rare occasions for the investigation of homicides, suspected homicides disguised as suicides, and suspected homicidal poisoning, for death as result of criminal abortion, for the comparison of an exhumed body with the body of another person thought to have been deceased, to identify war and accident victims, to settle accidental-death, double-indemnity insurance, and workmen's compensation claims, to settle liability claims for malpractice, negligence, or torts, or to search for a lost foreign object.[5,6] It follows that autopsies on exhumed bodies may be done both in criminal and in civil court cases.

State laws define who may authorize disinterment and under what circumstances it may be done. In most instances, a court order is required.

The procedural steps, either in civil or criminal cases, are as follows.[6]

1. Application is made to a court, setting forth good and substantial reasons for a disinterment—namely, that the cause of justice requires it.

2. A copy of the court order is sent to the cemetery, the pathologist, the undertaker, and such other selected persons as may be necessary under the circumstances, such as a dentist, a fingerprint expert, or a photographer.

3. Notice is given to the interested parties of the time and the place of the disinterment.

4. An autopsy is done and the body is reburied.

5. The results of the autopsy and exhumation procedure are fully reported to the court.

The principal participants in the exhumation procedure are the next of kin, the petitioner and his attorney, the court having jurisdiction, the coroner or medical examiner of the place where the body is located, the funeral director and cemetery authority, a pathologist, a dentist, a court reporter, a photographer, and a fingerprint expert. Of course, not all these persons will be required in all cases.

REFERENCES

1. Chayet NL: Autopsy protocols—confidentiality and admissibility. N Engl J Med *271*:728–729, 1964
2. Chayet NL: Consent for autopsy. N Engl J Med *274*:268–269, 1966
3. Dukeminier J Jr, Sanders D: Organ transplantation: a proposal for routine salvaging of cadaver organs. N Engl J Med *279*:413–419, 1968
4. Fitzgibbons JP: Personal communication
5. Gonzales TA, Vance M, Helpern M, Umberger CJ: Legal Medicine: Pathology and Toxicology. Second edition. New York, Appleton-Century-Crofts, Inc., 1954, pp 95–99
6. Hall GE: To exhume or not to exhume. JAMA *198*:301–302, 1966
7. Hayt E, Landau B: Autopsy laws in American hospitals. Acta Med Leg Soc (Liege) *19*:127–131, 1966
8. Heise HA, Fisher RS, Groeschel AH, Sadusk JF, Torrens JK: Disposition of dead bodies. JAMA *183*:606–610, 1963
9. Hershey N: Who may authorize an autopsy? Am J Nurs *63*:103–105, 1963
10. Holder AR: Unauthorized autopsies. JAMA *214*:967–968, 1970
11. National Research Council Division of Medical Sciences: Medical-Legal Aspects of Tissue Transplantation. (A Report to the Committee on Tissue Transplantation From the Ad Hoc Committee on Medical-Legal Problems.) Washington DC, Government Printing Office, 1968
12. O'Hern VM: Authorization for autopsies. JAMA *203*:199–200, 1968
13. Regan LJ: Legal authorization for autopsy. Ann West Med Surg *5*:287–311, 1951
13a. Rose EF: Pathology reports and autopsy protocols: confidentiality, privilege, and accessibility. Am J Clin Path *57*:144–155, 1972
14. Sadler AM Jr, Sadler BL, Schreiner GE: A uniform card for organ and tissue donation. Mod Med *37*:20–23, 1969
15. Sadler AM Jr, Sadler BL, Stason EB, Stickel DL: Transplantation—a case for consent. N Engl J Med *280*:862–867, 1969
16. Sagall EL, Reed BC: Documentary evidence: autopsy reports. *In* The Heart and the Law: A Practical Guide to Medicolegal Cardiology. New York, The Macmillan Company, 1968, pp 256–262
17. Schultz OT: The law of the dead human body. Arch Pathol *9*:1220–1241, 1930
18. Stump A, Emswiller B: The law pertaining to autopsies. J Indiana State Med Assoc *49*:761–765, 1956
19. Wecht CH, Turshen EA, Rule WR: The Medico-legal Autopsy Laws of the Fifty States and the District of Columbia. Washington DC, American Registry of Pathology, Armed Forces Institute of Pathology, 1966

CHAPTER 15

AUTOPSIES — PAST, PRESENT, AND FUTURE

The psychoanalyst knows everything and
does nothing.
The surgeon knows nothing and does
everything.
The dermatologist knows nothing and does
nothing.
The pathologist knows everything but
always a day too late.

PAST AND PRESENT FUNCTIONS OF THE AUTOPSY

More than 100 years ago, John H. Bennett stated: "It is daily becoming more and more apparent that the results of post-mortem examination have ceased to furnish us with facts sufficiently novel and important enough to advance the study of pathology."[22] The spirit of this statement is still with us. The scene in many institutions is symbolic. The autopsies are done by an ill-tempered first-year resident, unattended and unsupervised, in a dreary room in the basement of the hospital. The procedure is kept alive for little more than to fulfill the quota required for teaching institutions.[10]

Autopsies are time-consuming and often repetitious or, worse yet, unrewarding. There is little, if any, financial support. In 1969, the cost of an autopsy at the Mayo Clinic was about $300. The ailing autopsy has caused much concern. Outstanding pathologists have come to the defense of the autopsy in leading journals, some stressing its time-honored merits and most demanding new approaches.[2,5,9,12,13,17,20,21,24,31] What are the functions of the autopsy today? What is its potential?

The Educational Functions of the Autopsy. For pathologists at any level

307

of experience the educational value of the autopsy is self-evident.[8] However, for many clinicians this remains to be debated. The autopsy ranks low
on the list of their educational priorities. Organ reviews become rare, and
Clinicopathologic Conferences, if they are held, remain the only meeting
ground between autopsy pathologist and clinician. There are many reasons
for this alienation, among them unattractive morgue facilities often at a
considerable distance from the wards and, above all, the lack of skill in the
demonstrations of cases. Robertson[26] said it best: "To watch an interne
or a staff physician thumb over a voluminous collection of clinical notes
and then listen to him attempting to read all sorts of findings, most of them
irrelevant and immaterial, is not only time consuming, but it is likely to
'kill' the meeting almost before it starts."

The history should be presented briefly and clearly. For the listeners,
most laboratory data become interesting only after they know about the
pathologic findings. The display of specimens must be attractive and informative. Someone has to be in charge to keep to the time schedule and to
moderate a pertinent discussion. For the student, only a close liaison
between pathologist and clinician can make the autopsy truly rewarding.[25]
There is no reason why, on occasion, organs should not be shown first or a
brief "Reversed Clinicopathologic Conference" be attempted. Ritual is secondary when education is the concern.

Another aspect of the educational function of the autopsy is the use of
the cadaver in training in surgery.[6] Students can learn basic techniques and
experienced surgeons may need cadavers to work out new approaches.

The Autopsy in Research.   The foundations of modern medicine are
based on the results of research in autopsy pathology. Our classifications of
diseases are still based primarily on anatomic findings. Autopsy research
has fallen far behind other disciplines. Yet, major contributions have been
made in recent years. Corrective surgery of congenital heart diseases developed from the combined efforts of surgeons, physiologists, and autopsy
pathologists. Hypertensive pulmonary vascular disease and its prognostic
significance in heart surgery was first evaluated on autopsy material.
Bronchitis and emphysema have been reevaluated and reclassified[23] based
on modern autopsy research. Autopsies must still be used to determine
the relevance in man of experiments performed on nonhuman animals.[5]
This is another, often overlooked, research function. At the same time,
important stimulation for experimental study may come from autopsy
observations.

The Autopsy as a Control Function for Clinicians and Clinical Research.
Prutting[21] quoted a review of 1,000 autopsies which showed that the antemortem diagnosis was correct in only 55.4% of the cases. In other autopsy series, pulmonary embolism was diagnosed in less than 50% and gastrointestinal hemorrhages, in only 67%.[21] In a study of 9,501 cases by
Heasman and Lipworth,[14] "disagreement of fact" (underlying cause of
death given by one of the certifying physicians and not by the other, as
compared with "disagreement of wording") was found in 25% of the
deaths. One should admit, however, that these data appear overly pes-

simistic. Thus, "disagreement of fact" does not necessarily mean diagnostic error on the part of the clinician who may be in a better position to judge the sequence of events and the significance of anatomic findings. Such disagreement rarely reflects a clinical diagnostic error being responsible for the patient's demise. Nevertheless, autopsies often refute, clarify, modify, or elaborate on clinical, surgical, biopsy, roentgenologic, and laboratory diagnoses.

Finally, autopsies are an important tool for the detection of iatrogenic diseases. Phenacetin papillitis, potassium ulcers of the intestine, and steroid-induced osteoporosis are pertinent examples. Surgical techniques and other procedures also must be controlled by autopsies. For instance, there may be ulcerations from indwelling catheters, heart valve prostheses may be displaced or infected, bile peritonitis may have developed after a needle biopsy of a liver, or a fatal hemorrhage may have occurred after a needle biopsy of the kidney.

The Autopsy in Medical Statistics, Epidemiology, and Population Genetics. It was only about 1912 that autopsies were recognized, in the United States, as important for these disciplines of medicine.[30] The collection and analysis of death certificates provides information on incidence, trends, geographic distribution, and population selectivity of disease. Autopsy diagnoses undoubtedly improve the reliability of death certificates. In studies such as those currently under way in Olmsted County, Minnesota, on the incidence, trends, and survivorship of several hundred diseases and syndromes and in chronic disease epidemiology studies, an extraordinary level of accuracy in the diagnosis of all cases is essential if the rates, trends, or correlations with risk factors are to be meaningful. Thus, the complete detection of suspected and unsuspected lesions is a prerequisite of successful research in such population-based programs. There can be no meaningful selection of cases, and an autopsy rate of 100% must remain the goal. The incidence of congenital malformations recorded in autopsied infants was approximately twice that recorded for nonautopsied premature infants.[17]

The Autopsy in Public Health. This particular function of the autopsy is closely related to that of surveillance and accuracy of reporting. However, there are rare instances in which autopsies may play a much more immediate role in the early diagnosis, treatment, and prevention of diseases. For instance, an asymptomatic reactivated caseating tuberculous hilar lymphadenitis with perforation of caseous material into the bronchus, detected at autopsy in an old woman, requires an immediate thorough examination of all persons with whom the deceased had had contact.

The Autopsy as a Medicolegal Procedure. A sizable proportion of all autopsies are performed for medicolegal purposes. Criminal investigation has been discussed in chapter 2. More important for physicians is the function of the autopsy as protection against false accusations of malpractice. Certainly, an autopsy may also support the claim of the damaged party. Important for the public is the role of the autopsy diagnosis in insurance claims. Without an autopsy, double-indemnity or workmen's compensation benefits may be in jeopardy.[29]

The Autopsy in Tissue Transplantation.   The following organs and tissues have been utilized for homografting[3]: heart, heart valves, arteries, blood, lungs, kidneys, liver, pancreas, cornea, bone, cartilage, dura, fascia, and skin. While the removal of organs is an operating-room procedure, heart valves, arteries, bone, cartilage, dura, fascia, and skin often are provided by autopsy pathologists. Aortic valve homografts are already used to an extent such that the demand occasionally exceeds the supply. Homografts of this type appear very promising. Freeze-dried dura mater functioned successfully in 98% of 175 patients in a 15-year period.[1] Legal problems are still a major obstacle.[11]

The Autopsy and the Recovery of Prosthetic Material.   We routinely recover, at autopsy, Küntscher nails, Vitallium screws, and other prosthetic material. Heart valve prostheses are also removed.

Autopsy Tissues for Pharmacologic Extraction and Tissue Culture Work. The most widely used procedure is the extraction of pituitary growth hormones. We send all grossly normal pituitary glands to the National Pituitary Foundation except when the nature of the case requires histologic study of the gland.

Kidney and lung tissues from autopsies of premature infants have been used as growth media for virologic studies.[19]

AUTOPSY PATHOLOGY IN THE FUTURE

One can safely predict that none of today's autopsy functions will be given up but that many will be extended and, hopefully, improved. Three examples may emphasize this prediction.

1. The demand for transplantable tissues will continue to increase, and the procurement of material such as aortic valve homografts for tissue banks may become a major autopsy function in the future. Cadaver blood or blood components may come into use although this so far has appeared impractical in the western hemisphere.

2. Pollution control may require federally or internationally supervised screening programs for the detection, in autopsy tissues, of substances such as mercury or pesticides.

3. Autopsy research and the role of autopsies in epidemiology are two areas which are most deserving of extension and improvement. Many rare cases of great scientific value are lost for research purposes because at the time of the autopsy the pathologist knows little more than the name of the condition he is dealing with, or he is not aware of ongoing studies and optimal techniques required for proper preservation and documentation. For the same reason, in-depth statistical or related studies are severely hampered. Computers are ideally suited to provide necessary information if fed with key words giving age, sex, clinical or pathologic diagnosis, and cause(s) of death. The computer would then identify the interested researchers, the nature of the studies in question, and the procedures and techniques required to supply the material and data of interest. This would

permit prospective studies on a much larger scale than now is possible. Even in the absence of ongoing research, optimal techniques and documentation or preservation methods could be made instantly available.

Wherever future autopsy services proliferate, problems of autopsy rates, manpower, and finance will become major concerns.

Autopsy Rates.   A meaningful selection of cases for autopsy, either by pathologists or by an autopsy committee, is nearly impossible. We should try to influence our clinical colleagues to increase their efforts in acquiring autopsy permission. The knowledge of the potential services will greatly affect their attitude. We also have to pay more attention to relationships with funeral directors,[27] a field greatly neglected in the past. It is my experience that funeral directors will cooperate gladly once an understanding of the mutual problems has been achieved by sensible discussion. Education of the public and actions in the state legislatures may be needed to ensure autopsy rates which satisfy public and scientific interests.

The attitude toward the body in the autopsy room may also be a detrimental factor.[27,28] Appropriate decorum should be as much a part of the autopsy as it is part of the examination of the patient during life. Lack of care by the technicians in handling the remains may impress students or attending physicians as showing lack of respect. Experiences of this kind have done much harm. Laymen such as police officers or paramedical personnel such as nurses are more likely to be shocked rather than to be instructed by autopsies. Therefore, at the Mayo Clinic, we admit to the autopsy room only physicians, the small crew of trained autopsy technicians, funeral directors, and crime investigators.

Manpower.   There is a shortage of autopsy pathologists, which is most likely to persist. The training of competent autopsy technicians appears to be the best answer.[3,4] A model for such training has been developed in Great Britain where an apprentice-type teaching of future autopsy technicians is supplemented by instruction in anatomy, physiology, microbiology, disinfection, and law.[15] Completion of such training is recognized by the award of a certificate or diploma. Adequate remuneration will make such programs attractive. Certified autopsy technicians will be able to perform all autopsy procedures, in most cases requiring the physician pathologist only to make the gross and microscopic diagnoses. In the United States, the experience with licensed morticians acting not only as autopsy technicians but also as "pathology assistants" in a much wider sense has been good.[7] At the end of their training, such assistants who are also licensed morticians will be charged with unifying and simplifying all procedures that precede, accompany, and follow the autopsy.

In the University Hospitals of Cleveland,[7] a mortician is on duty 24 hours a day. His previous training in the psychology of bereavement makes him ideally suited to deal with the family of the deceased. He becomes the link among clinicians, pathologists, administrative personnel, nurses, and funeral directors. He ensures that all necessary information is gathered and all forms are properly filled out. Then, and always in the presence of a physician pathologist, he assumes his functions as a professional prosector.

The physician pathologist, at the same time, studies the clinical history, dissects specimens of special interest, points out sites he wants to examine histologically, and orders special procedures that might be indicated. The mortician is charged with most activities related to the autopsy, except that the embalming is left to the funeral directors so as not to interfere with their financial interests. The impartial assignment of funeral directors, usually on a rotating basis, is one of the most sensitive areas in programs of this type.

None of these solutions seems ideal, but little can be done to increase the number of autopsy pathologists. For the young physician, the teaching pathologist or preceptor represents the most important factor affecting the choice of pathology as a career.[16] Here lies our challenge. Unfortunately, for the certified pathologist, autopsies are likely to rank behind clinical and surgical pathology which are more attractive financially and behind experimental research which conveys more status.

Financing. If one considers that the average cost for one autopsy is about $300 and that larger institutions perform between 500 and 2,000 autopsies per year, the financial burden from autopsy services is truly severe. Use of sophisticated techniques will push the cost even higher. Certified autopsy technicians may help to achieve cost reduction. Certain autopsy procedures may have to be curtailed to save money. For instance, there is no reason why some routine autopsies should not be limited to gross examination,[18] possibly aided by the preparation of frozen sections. To limit the number of autopsies or to study only special cases[13] appears to be an unacceptable solution.

Angrist[2] has suggested supporting autopsies financially from general study grants, specific training grants, fees, health and hospital insurance, and social security death benefit allowances.

REFERENCES

1. Abbott WA, Dupree EL Jr: The procurement, storage, and transplantation of lyophilized human cadaver dura mater. Surg Gynecol Obstet *130*:112–118, 1970
2. Angrist A: What remedies for the ailing autopsy? JAMA 193:806–808, 1965
3. Angrist A: Progress and paradox in pathology and medicine. Pharos *32*:48–53 (Apr.) 1969
4. Bloodworth JMB Jr: Non-physician prosectors. Bull Path 7:16, 1966
5. Bohrod MG: Uses of the autopsy. JAMA *193*:810–812, 1965
6. Butterworth RF: Missed opportunities in the post-mortem room. Med J Aust 2:805–806, 1955
7. Carter JR, Martin DL: A pathology assistant program: the role of licensed morticians. Am J Clin Pathol *53*:26–31, 1970
8. Corrigan GE: Decline of the autopsy. N Engl J Med *282*:633, 1970
9. Davidson CS: The autopsy in the age of molecular biology. JAMA *193*:813–814, 1965
10. Editorial: Of autopsies. JAMA *191*:1078–1079, 1965
11. Ersek RA, Cutting E, Chou S, Tierney JR, Najarian JS, Lillehei RC: Procurement of transplantable tissues. Minn Med *52*:183–193, 1969
12. Gall EA: Case for necropsy in medicine: photobrief by Ohio pathologist. Hosp Tribune, Dec. 2, 1968, pp 12–13
13. Hazard JB: The autopsy. JAMA 193:805–806, 1965
14. Heasman MA, Lipworth L: Accuracy of Certification of Cause of Death. London, Her Majesty's Stationery Office, 1966

15. Heggie JF: Training of post-mortem room technicians. J Clin Pathol *20*:793–794, 1967
16. Hotchkiss SM: Survey of American Pathologists. Baltimore, Williams & Wilkins Company, 1966
17. Kane SH: Significance of autopsies in premature infants. JAMA 187:865, 1964
18. Madden SC: How many autopsies? JAMA *193*:812–813, 1965
19. Marymont JH Jr: Hospital virologic cultures employ necropsy tissues. (Presented at the meeting of the American Society of Clinical Pathologists, Miami Beach.) Antibiotic News, November, 1968, p 5
20. McManus JFA: The autopsy as research. JAMA *193*:808–810, 1965
21. Prutting J: Lack of correlation between antemortem and postmortem diagnoses. NY State J Med *67*:2081–2084, 1967
22. Rather LJ: Rudolf Virchow's views on pathology, pathological anatomy, and cellular pathology. Arch Pathol *82*:197–204, 1966
23. Reid L: The Pathology of Emphysema. Chicago, Year Book Medical Publishers, Inc., 1967, p 309
24. Robertson HE: Our responsibility to our deaths. South Med J *18*:125–127, 1925
25. Robertson HE: The isolation problem in the teaching of pathology. J Assoc Am Med Coll *6*:209–216, 1931
26. Robertson HE: The clinical pathological conference. Surg Gynecol Obstet *55*:785–786, 1932
27. Robertson HE: Postmortem examinations in the practice of medicine. Wis Med J *35*:370–373, 1936
28. Robertson HE: Postmortem examinations. Minn Med *27*:548–550, 1944
29. Sagall EL, Reed BC: The hypothetical question. Med Sci *18*:74–79, 1967
30. Stenn F: The achievement of the committee on necropsies of the Institute of Medicine of Chicago. Bull Am Coll Pathol *22*:87–94, 1968
31. Wilson RR: In defense of the autopsy. JAMA *196*:1011–1012, 1966

APPENDIX

NORMAL WEIGHTS AND MEASUREMENTS

CONVERSION FACTORS

To convert from	To	Multiply by
Metric to English		
Centimeters (cm)	Inches (US) (in.)	0.394
Centimeters (cm)	Feet (US) (ft)	0.033
Square meters (m²)	Square feet (US) (ft²)	10.753
Grams (gm)	Ounces (avoirdupois) (oz)	0.035
Grams (gm)	Pounds (avoirdupois) (lb)	0.002
Kilograms (kg)	Ounces (avoirdupois) (oz)	35.274
Kilograms (kg)	Pounds (avoirdupois) (lb)	2.205
Milliliters (ml)*	Ounces (US fluid) (fl oz)	0.034
Liters (liters)	Quarts (US liquid) (qt)	1.057
Liters (liters)	Gallons (US) (gal)	0.264
English to metric		
Inches (US) (in.)	Centimeters (cm)	2.540
Feet (US) (ft)	Centimeters (cm)	30.480
Square feet (US) (ft²)	Square meters (m²)	0.093
Ounces (avoirdupois) (oz)	Grams (gm)	28.350
Pounds (avoirdupois) (lb)	Grams (gm)	453.592
Pounds (avoirdupois) (lb)	Kilograms (kg)	0.454
Ounces (US fluid) (fl oz)	Milliliters (ml)	29.574
Pints (US liquid) (pt)	Milliliters (ml)	473.179
Quarts (US liquid) (qt)	Liters (liters)	0.946
Gallons (US) (gal)	Liters (liters)	3.785
Temperature conversion		

To convert °C to °F: $°F = (1.8 \times °C) + 32$

To convert °F to °C: $°C = \dfrac{(°F - 32)}{1.8}$

---

* For most purposes, cubic centimeter (cc) is the same as milliliter (ml).

FETUSES AND NEWBORNS

Body Length

LENGTH (cm) OF FETUS IN RELATION TO AGE (MONTH)*

Lunar month	Crown-rump length		Crown-heel length	
	Streeter	Scammon and Calkins	Dietrich	Scammon and Calkins
Second	2.3	. . .	3.0	. . .
Third	7.4	5.1	9.8	7.0
Fourth	11.6	10.7	18.0	15.5
Fifth	16.4	15.5	25.0	22.7
Sixth	20.8	19.7	31.5	29.2
Seventh	24.7	23.6	37.1	35.0
Eighth	28.3	27.1	42.5	40.4
Ninth	32.1	30.5	47.0	45.4
Tenth	36.2	33.6	50.0	50.2

* From Potter EL: Pathology of the Fetus and Infant. Second edition. Chicago, Year Book Medical Publishers, Inc., 1961. By permission.

Body Weight

WEIGHT OF FETUS (gm) IN RELATION TO AGE (MONTH)*

Lunar month	Streeter	Scammon and Calkins
Second	1.1	3.5
Third	14.2	14.3
Fourth	108.0	86.8
Fifth	316.0	260.9
Sixth	630.0	551.6
Seventh	1,045.0	971.4
Eighth	1,680.0	1,519.0
Ninth	2,378.0	2,196.1
Tenth	3,405.0	2,998.8

* From Potter EL: Pathology of the Fetus and Infant. Second edition. Chicago, Year Book Medical Publishers, Inc., 1961. By permission.

Organ Weight

ORGAN WEIGHT (gm) IN RELATION TO TOTAL BODY WEIGHT (gm)*

	Total body weight								
Organ	500–999	1,000–1,499	1,500–1,999	2,000–2,499	2,500–2,999	3,000–3,499	3,500–3,999	4,000–4,499	≧4,500
Thyroid	0.8	0.8	0.9	1.1	1.3	1.6	1.7	1.9	2.4
Thymus	2.1	4.3	6.6	8.2	9.3	11.0	12.6	14.3	17.3
Both lungs	18.2	27.1	37.9	43.6	48.9	54.9	58.0	65.8	74.0
Heart	5.8	9.4	12.7	15.5	19.0	21.2	23.4	28.0	36.0
Spleen	1.7	3.4	4.9	7.0	9.1	10.4	12.0	13.6	16.7
Pancreas	1.0	1.4	2.0	2.3	3.0	3.5	4.0	4.6	6.2
Both kidneys	7.1	12.2	16.2	19.9	23.0	25.3	28.5	31.0	33.2
Both adrenals	3.1	3.9	5.0	6.3	8.2	9.8	10.7	12.5	15.1
Brain	108.7	179.5	255.6	307.6	358.7	403.3	420.6	424.1	406.2
Liver	38.8	59.8	76.3	98.1	127.4	155.1	178.1	215.2	275.6

* From Potter EL: Pathology of the Fetus and Infant. Second edition. Chicago, Year Book Medical Publishers, Inc., 1961. By permission.

INFANTS AND CHILDREN

Adrenal Glands

ADRENAL GLANDS (COMBINED): 1 TO 12 MONTHS*

Age (mo)	Body length (cm)		Weight (gm), mean ± SE	
	Boys	Girls	Boys	Girls
1	51.4	51.9	5.1 ± 0.3	4.8 ± 0.4
2	54.0	54.0	5.0 ± 0.3	4.7 ± 0.2
3	57.7	57.0	5.0 ± 0.2	4.8 ± 0.3
4	60.4	59.0	4.9 ± 0.3	4.6 ± 0.4
5	62.0	62.2	5.3 ± 0.3	4.8 ± 0.6
6	64.2	63.0	5.2 ± 0.3	4.6 ± 0.4
7	66.7	65.4	5.5 ± 0.4	5.5 ± 0.5
8	68.2	66.5	5.4 ± 0.6	5.3 ± 0.6
9	69.4	68.3	5.4 ± 0.5	5.4 ± 0.5
10	69.7	67.5	5.7 ± 0.5	5.7 ± 0.5
11	70.5	70.5	6.1 ± 0.5	6.2 ± 0.6
12	73.8	71.5	6.3 ± 0.7	6.0 ± 0.4

* Data from Schulz DM, Giordano DA, Schulz DH: Weights of organs of fetuses and infants. Arch Pathol 74:244–250, 1962.

ADRENAL GLANDS: 1 TO 18.7 YEARS*

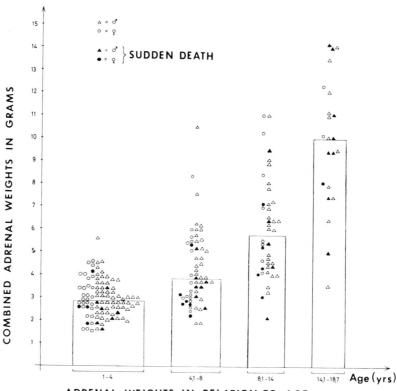

ADRENAL WEIGHTS IN RELATION TO AGE

The boxed-in areas designate the median values. The data are from the weights of 216 normal pairs of adrenal glands. The organs had been formalin-fixed, and it should be noted that the organs lose about 20% of their weight within 4 days after fixation in formalin solution. There was no sex difference.

* From Dhom G, Piroth M: Das Wachstum der Nebennierenrinde im Kindesalter. Verh Dtsch Ges Pathol 53:418–422, 1969. By permission of Gustav Fischer Verlag.

BODY WEIGHT, BODY LENGTH, AND HEAD CIRCUMFERENCE IN
RELATION TO AGE: BOYS, BIRTH TO 28 MONTHS*

INFANT BOYS

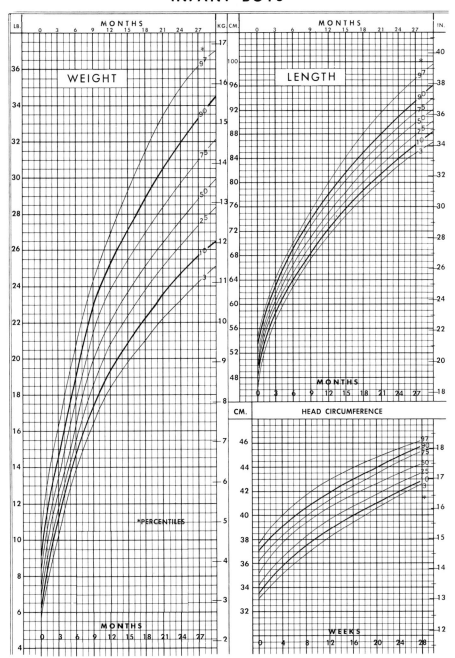

* From Stuart HC, et al: Anthropometric Charts of Infant Boys and Girls From Birth to 28 Months.
Harvard School of Public Health, Department of Maternal and Child Health. Boston: Children's Medical
Center (no date). By permission.

BODY WEIGHT, BODY LENGTH, AND HEAD CIRCUMFERENCE IN RELATION TO AGE: GIRLS, BIRTH TO 28 MONTHS*

INFANT GIRLS

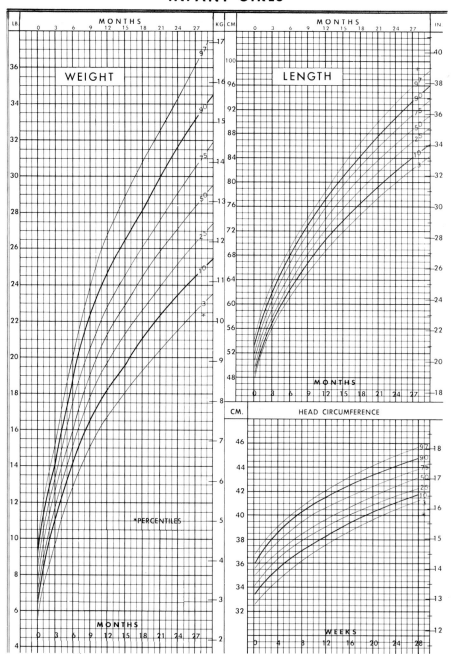

* From Stuart HC, et al: Anthropometric Charts of Infant Boys and Girls From Birth to 28 Months. Harvard School of Public Health, Department of Maternal and Child Health. Boston: Children's Medical Center (no date). By permission.

BODY WEIGHT AND LENGTH IN RELATION TO AGE:
BOYS, 2 TO 13 YEARS*

PERCENTILE CHART FOR MEASUREMENTS OF BOYS

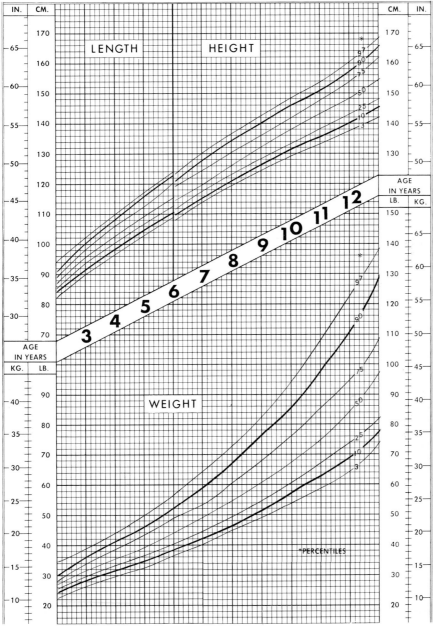

* From Stuart HC, et al: Anthropometric Charts for Boys and Girls From 2 Years to 13 Years. Harvard School of Public Health, Department of Maternal and Child Health, Boston: Children's Medical Center (no date). By permission.

BODY WEIGHT AND LENGTH IN RELATION TO AGE:
GIRLS, 2 TO 13 YEARS*

PERCENTILE CHART FOR MEASUREMENTS OF GIRLS

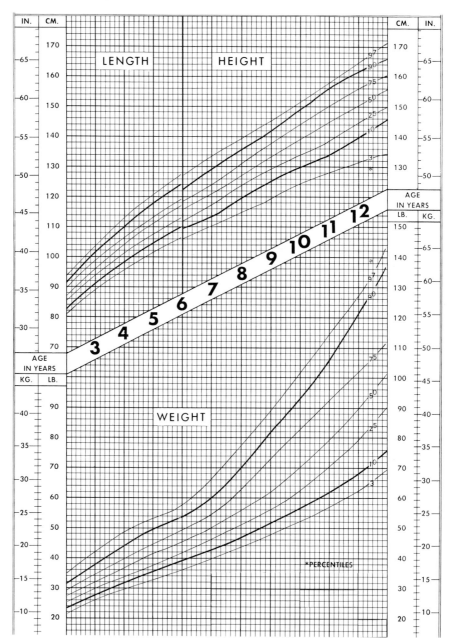

* From Stuart HC, et al: Anthropometric Charts for Boys and Girls From 2 Years to 13 Years. Harvard School of Public Health, Department of Maternal and Child Health. Boston: Children's Medical Center (no date). By permission.

BODY SURFACE AREA FROM HEIGHT AND WEIGHT*

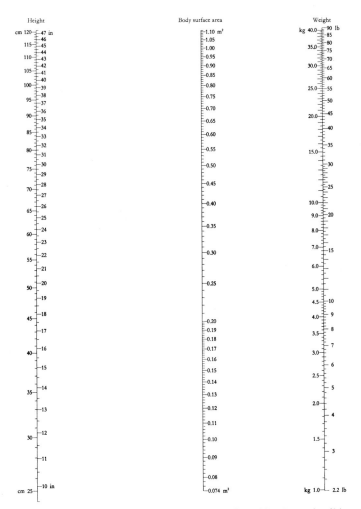

* From Diem K: Documenta Geigy: Scientific Tables. Seventh edition. Ardsley, New York, Geigy Pharmaceuticals, 1970, p. 538. By permission.

BODY SURFACE AREA: 1 TO 19 YEARS*
(Limits of hatched area indicate the 95th percentiles after
Heimendinger [1964])

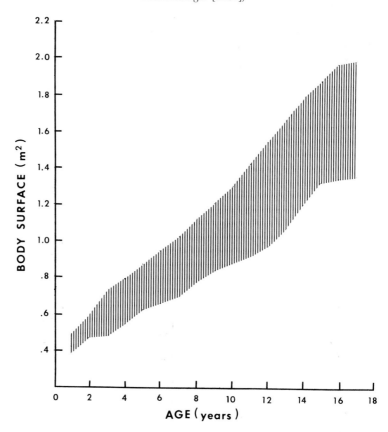

* Modified from Dhom G, Piroth M: Das Wachstum der Nebennierenrinde im Kindesalter. Verh Dtsch Ges Pathol 53:418–422, 1969.

Brain

BRAIN: 1 TO 12 YEARS*

Age	Body length (cm)	Brain weight (gm)
Birth–3 days	49	335
3–7 days	49	358
1–3 wk	52	382
3–5 wk	52	413
5–7 wk	53	422
7–9 wk	55	489
3 mo	56	516
4 mo	59	540
5 mo	61	644
6 mo	62	660
7 mo	65	691
8 mo	65	714
9 mo	67	750
10 mo	69	809
11 mo	70	852
12 mo	73	925
14 mo	74	944
16 mo	77	1,010
18 mo	78	1,042
20 mo	79	1,050
22 mo	82	1,059
24 mo	84	1,064
3 yr	88	1,141
4 yr	99	1,191
5 yr	106	1,237
6 yr	109	1,243
7 yr	113	1,263
8 yr	119	1,273
9 yr	125	1,275
10 yr	130	1,290
11 yr	135	1,320
12 yr	139	1,351

* Data from Sunderman FW, Boerner F: Normal Values in Clinical Medicine. Philadelphia, W. B. Saunders Company, 1949.

For brain weights listed separately for boys and girls, ages 1 to 12 months, see Kissane and Smith.[7] Minckler and Boyd[10] give detailed data and references on the physical growth of the central nervous system. On fixation with formalin solution by penetration there is a mean weight increase of 14.1% (range, 8.0 to 22.3%).[14]

Heart

HEART: BOYS, 1 MONTH TO 20 YEARS*

Age	Body Length (cm)	Weight (kg)	Heart weight (gm), mean ± SD
1 mo	51.4		23 ± 7
2 mo	54.0		27 ± 7
3 mo	57.7		30 ± 7
4 mo	60.4		31 ± 7
5 mo	62.0		35 ± 5
6 mo	64.2		40 ± 8
7 mo	66.7		43 ± 8
8 mo	68.2		44 ± 8
9 mo	69.4		45 ± 7
10 mo	69.7		46 ± 6
11 mo	70.5		48 ± 7
12 mo	73.8		50 ± 6
13–18 mo	78		54 ± 9
19–24 mo	84		60 ± 11
3 yr	90		72 ± 12
4 yr	101		88 ± 13
5 yr	109		94 ± 9
6 yr	114		105 ± 14
7 yr	121		110 ± 15
8 yr	127		119 ± 11
9 yr	132		138 ± 12
10 yr	138		150 ± 22
11 yr	144		154 ± 29
12 yr	149		169 ± 25
13 yr	155		212 ± 30
14 yr	159		219 ± 27
15 yr	163		224 ± 34
16 yr		43.81	253
17 yr		49.34	279
18 yr		42.40	217
19 yr		55.99	285
20 yr		51.99	282

* Data from Reiner L: Gross examination of the heart. *In* Pathology of the Heart and Blood Vessels. Third edition. Edited by SE Gould. Springfield, Illinois, Charles C Thomas, Publisher, 1968, pp 1111–1149.

HEART: GIRLS, 1 MONTH TO 20 YEARS*

Age	Body Length (cm)	Body Weight (kg)	Heart weight (gm), mean ± SD
1 mo	51.9		21 ± 5
2 mo	54.0		26 ± 6
3 mo	57.0		28 ± 4
4 mo	59.0		30 ± 6
5 mo	62.2		36 ± 5
6 mo	63.0		37 ± 7
7 mo	65.4		40 ± 9
8 mo	66.5		41 ± 7
9 mo	68.3		41 ± 5
10 mo	67.5		43 ± 7
11 mo	70.5		44 ± 8
12 mo	71.5		49 ± 6
13–18 mo	77		54 ± 12
19–24 mo	84		58 ± 11
3 yr	91		72 ± 10
4 yr	100		81 ± 12
5 yr	108		88 ± 7
6 yr	115		101 ± 16
7 yr	119		107 ± 19
8 yr	126		122 ± 19
9 yr	129		129 ± 19
10 yr	139		145 ± 25
11 yr	145		154 ± 23
12 yr	150		168 ± 36
13 yr	152		203 ± 32
14 yr	155		210 ± 35
15 yr	159		222 ± 33
16 yr		50.23	205
17 yr		47.66	220
18 yr		44.55	226
19 yr		47.83	255
20 yr		56.10	262

* Data from Reiner L: Gross examination of the heart. *In* Pathology of the Heart and Blood Vessels. Third edition. Edited by SE Gould. Springfield, Illinois, Charles C Thomas, Publisher, 1968, pp 1111–1149.

Heart weight tables have also been prepared or reproduced by Sunderman and Boerner,[15] Kissane and Smith,[7] and Eckner et al.[3] A table of the weights of the partitioned heart (right ventricle, left ventricle, and ventricular septum) from birth to 3 years of age has been published by Reiner.[12] The thickness of the ventricular walls, the valve circumferences, the length of ventricular inflow or outflow tracts, and the chamber perimeters or ventricular volumes in relation to body length and weight or age have been tabulated by Eckner et al.[3] This study was carried out on hearts after standard fixation by controlled pressure coronary perfusion. On fixation with formalin solution by penetration there is a mean weight loss of 5.8% (range, 0.9 to 19.2%).[14]

Kidneys

KIDNEYS: BIRTH TO 12 YEARS*

Age	Body length (cm)	Kidney weight (gm)	
		Right	Left
Birth–3 days	49	13	14
3–7 days	49	14	14
1–3 wk	52	15	15
3–5 wk	52	16	16
5–7 wk	53	19	18
7–9 wk	55	19	18
3 mo	56	20	19
4 mo	59	22	21
5 mo	61	25	25
6 mo	62	26	25
7 mo	65	30	30
8 mo	65	31	30
9 mo	67	31	30
10 mo	69	32	31
11 mo	70	34	33
12 mo	73	36	35
14 mo	74	36	35
16 mo	77	39	39
18 mo	78	40	43
20 mo	79	43	44
22 mo	82	44	44
24 mo	84	47	46
3 yr	88	48	49
4 yr	99	58	56
5 yr	106	65	64
6 yr	109	68	67
7 yr	113	69	70
8 yr	119	74	75
9 yr	125	82	83
10 yr	130	92	95
11 yr	135	94	95
12 yr	139	95	96

* Data from Sunderman FW, Boerner F: Normal Values in Clinical Medicine. Philadelphia, W. B. Saunders Company, 1949.

On fixation with formalin solution by penetration there is a mean weight loss of 3.3% (range, 0.2 to 6.0%).[14]

Liver

LIVER: BIRTH TO 12 YEARS*

Age	Body length (cm)	Liver weight (gm)
Birth–3 days	49	78
3–7 days	49	96
1–3 wk	52	123
3–5 wk	52	127
5–7 wk	53	133
7–9 wk	55	136
3 mo	56	140
4 mo	59	160
5 mo	61	188
6 mo	62	200
7 mo	65	227
8 mo	65	254
9 mo	67	260
10 mo	69	274
11 mo	70	277
12 mo	73	288
14 mo	74	304
16 mo	77	331
18 mo	78	345
20 mo	79	370
22 mo	82	380
24 mo	84	394
3 yr	88	418
4 yr	99	516
5 yr	106	596
6 yr	109	642
7 yr	113	680
8 yr	119	736
9 yr	125	756
10 yr	130	852
11 yr	135	909
12 yr	139	936

* Data from Sunderman FW, Boerner F: Normal Values in Clinical Medicine. Philadelphia, W. B. Saunders Company, 1949.

For liver weights listed separately for boys and girls, ages 1 to 12 months, see Kissane and Smith.[7]

On fixation with formalin solution by penetration there is a mean weight loss of 4% (range, 0.7 to 6.6%).[14]

Lungs

LUNGS: BIRTH TO 11 YEARS*

Age	Body length (cm)	Lung weight (gm)	
		Right	Left
Birth–3 days	49	21	18
3–7 days	49	24	22
1–3 wk	52	29	26
3–5 wk	52	31	27
5–7 wk	53	32	28
7–9 wk	55	32	29
3 mo	56	35	30
4 mo	59	37	33
5 mo	61	38	35
6 mo	62	42	39
7 mo	65	49	41
8 mo	65	52	45
9 mo	67	53	47
10 mo	69	54	51
11 mo	70	59	53
12 mo	73	64	57
14 mo	74	66	60
16 mo	77	72	64
18 mo	78	72	65
20 mo	79	83	74
22 mo	82	80	75
24 mo	84	88	76
3 yr	88	89	77
4 yr	99	90	85
5 yr	106	107	104
6 yr	109	121	122
7 yr	113	130	123
8 yr	119	150	140
9 yr	125	174	152
10 yr	130	177	166
11 yr	135	201	190

* Data from Sunderman FW, Boerner F: Normal Values in Clinical Medicine. Philadelphia, W. B. Saunders Company, 1949.

For lung weights listed separately for boys and girls, ages 1 to 12 months, see Kissane and Smith.[7]

Ovaries

OVARIES: BIRTH TO 16 YEARS*

Age (yr)	Weight (gm)	
	Right	Left
Birth	0.2	0.2
1	0.5	0.5
2	0.5	0.4
3	0.7	0.7
4	0.7	0.7
5	1.1	1.0
6	1.1	1.1
8	1.6	1.5
9	1.6	1.5
10	1.6	1.5
11	2.2	2.1
12	2.2	2.1
16	2.0	2.0

* Data from Sunderman FW, Boerner F: Normal Values in Clinical Medicine. Philadelphia, W. B. Saunders Company, 1949.

Pancreas

PANCREAS: 1 TO 12 MONTHS*

Age (mo)	Body length (cm)		Pancreas weight (gm), mean ± SE	
	Boys	Girls	Boys	Girls
1	51.4	51.9	6.2 ± 0.5	5.0 ± 0.4
2	54.0	54.0	7.2 ± 0.8	7.1 ± 0.6
3	57.7	57.0	7.7 ± 0.6	8.5 ± 0.6
4	60.4	59.0	11 ± 1	9.0 ± 0.7
5	62.0	62.2	11 ± 1	11 ± 1
6	64.2	63.0	11 ± 1	11 ± 1
7	66.7	65.4	12 ± 2	10 ± 1
8	68.2	66.5	13 ± 2	11 ± 1
9	69.4	68.3	16 ± 2	14 ± 2
10	69.7	67.5	14 ± 2	13 ± 2
11	70.5	70.5	16 ± 1	14 ± 2
12	73.8	71.5	14 ± 2	15 ± 3

* Data from Schulz DM, Giordano DA, Schulz DH: Weights of organs of fetuses and infants. Arch Pathol 74:244–250, 1962.

Pituitary Gland

The mean weight is 0.56 gm for both sexes, ages 10 to 20 years.[15]

Prostate

PROSTATE: BIRTH TO 25 YEARS*

Age (yr)	Prostate weight (gm)
Birth	0.9
1	1.2
3	1.1
5	1.2
8	1.3
10	1.4
11	2.3
12	2.8
13	3.7
14	3.5
15	5.1
16	6.1
17	11.4
21–25	17.9

* Data from Sunderman FW, Boerner F: Normal Values in Clinical Medicine. Philadelphia, W. B. Saunders Company, 1949.

Seminal Vesicles

SEMINAL VESICLES: BIRTH TO 15 YEARS*

Age (yr)	Vesicle weight (gm)
Birth	0.05
1	0.08
2	0.09
3	0.09
4	0.09
5	0.09
8	0.1
9	0.1
10	0.1
12	0.12
14	0.15
15	1.5

* Data from Sunderman FW, Boerner F: Normal Values in Clinical Medicine. Philadelphia, W. B. Saunders Company, 1949.

Spleen

SPLEEN: BIRTH TO 12 YEARS*

Age	Body length (cm)	Spleen weight (gm)
Birth–3 days	49	8
3–7 days	49	9
1–3 wk	52	10
3–5 wk	52	12
5–7 wk	53	13
7–9 wk	55	13
3 mo	56	14
4 mo	59	16
5 mo	61	16
6 mo	62	17
7 mo	65	19
8 mo	65	20
9 mo	67	20
10 mo	69	22
11 mo	70	25
12 mo	73	26
14 mo	74	26
16 mo	77	28
18 mo	78	30
20 mo	79	30
22 mo	82	33
24 mo	84	33
3 yr	88	37
4 yr	99	39
5 yr	106	47
6 yr	109	58
7 yr	113	66
8 yr	119	69
9 yr	125	73
10 yr	130	85
11 yr	135	87
12 yr	139	93

* Data from Sunderman FW, Boerner F: Normal Values in Clinical Medicine. Philadelphia, W. B. Saunders Company, 1949.

For spleen weights listed separately for boys and girls, ages 1 to 12 months, see Kissane and Smith.[7] On fixation with formalin solution by penetration there is a mean weight loss of 3.1% (range, 0.2 to 6.6%).[14]

Testes

TESTES: BIRTH TO 15 YEARS*

Age (yr)	Weight (gm) Right	Left	Size (cm)
			Newborn
Birth	0.2	0.2	1 × 0.5 × 0.4
1	0.7	0.7	
2	0.9	0.9	
3	0.9	0.9	
4	0.9	0.9	
5	0.9	0.9	
8	0.8	0.8	
9	0.8	0.8	
10	0.8	0.8	
11	1.2	1.3	Puberty
12	1.5	1.5	3 × 2 × 1.6
14	1.5	1.5	
15	6.8	6.8	

* Data from Sunderman FW, Boerner F: Normal Values in Clinical Medicine. Philadelphia, W. B. Saunders Company, 1949.

Thymus

THYMUS: 1 TO 12 MONTHS*

Age (mo)	Body length (cm) Boys	Girls	Thymus weight (gm), mean ± SE Boys	Girls
1	51.4	51.9	7.8 ± 0.9	6.6 ± 1.3
2	54.0	54.0	9.4 ± 0.8	5.8 ± 0.9
3	57.7	57.0	10 ± 1	9.7 ± 1.4
4	60.4	59.0	10 ± 1	9.0 ± 2.0
5	62.0	62.0	12 ± 1	13 ± 1
6	64.2	63.0	10 ± 1	10 ± 1
7	66.7	65.4	12 ± 2	10 ± 2
8	68.2	66.5	10 ± 2	8 ± 1
9	69.4	68.3	10 ± 1	9 ± 2
10	69.7	67.5	9 ± 1	12 ± 3
11	70.5	70.5	19 ± 2	15 ± 3
12	73.8	71.5	12 ± 1	11 ± 4

* Data from Schulz DM, Giordano DA, Schulz DH: Weights of organs of fetuses and infants. Arch Pathol *74*:244–250, 1962.

Sunderman and Boerner[15] report the following values for both sexes:

Age group	Mean weight (gm)	Weight range (gm)
Newborn	13.98	6.05–25.88
1 to 9 months	20.14	6.74–34.10
9 to 24 months	26.60	19.97–37.72
6 to 25 years	25	

Uterus

UTERUS: BIRTH TO 25 YEARS*

Age (yr)	Uterus weight (gm)
Birth	4.6
1	2.3
2	1.9
3	2.5
5	2.9
6	2.9
7	2.6
8	2.6
9	3.4
10	3.4
11	5.3
12	5.3
13	15.9
16	43.0
21–25	48.0

* Data from Sunderman FW, Boerner F: Normal Values in Clinical Medicine. Philadelphia, W. B. Saunders Company, 1949.

ADULTS

Adrenal Glands

ADRENAL GLANDS

	Mean weight (gm)	Weight range (gm)	Reference
Single gland	6		15
Single gland after complete stripping of fat tissue		3.5–4.5	11
Combined glands:			
Males	9.7		1
Females	8.3		1
Combined glands in relation to body length (cm):			
158–162 (N = 14)	10.0	7.0–13.2	15
170 (N = 16)	11.1	7.7–18.6	
174–176 (N = 12)	11.5	8.2–18.2	
178–182 (N = 9)	14.8	9.6–20.3	

Aorta

<table>
<tr><td colspan="3" align="center">AORTA</td></tr>
<tr><td></td><td align="center">**Mean**
circumference (cm)</td><td align="center">**Reference**</td></tr>
<tr><td>Ascending aorta</td><td align="center">8.5</td><td></td></tr>
<tr><td>Descending aorta
(thoracic)</td><td align="center">4.5–7.0</td><td align="center">4</td></tr>
<tr><td>Abdominal aorta</td><td align="center">3.5–4.5</td><td></td></tr>
</table>

Blood Volume

The mean total blood volume is 65 to 70 ml/kg body weight, with a normal range of 50 to 85 ml.[5]

Nomogram Relating Height and Weight to Blood Volume*

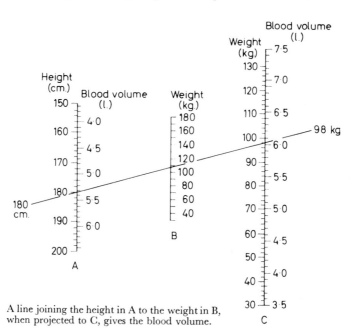

A line joining the height in A to the weight in B, when projected to C, gives the blood volume.

* From Furbank RA: Conversion data, normal values, nomograms and other standards. *In* Modern Trends in Forensic Medicine. Vol. 2. Edited by K Simpson. New York, Appleton-Century-Crofts, Inc., 1967, pp 344–364. By permission.

Body Dimensions

Nomogram for Determination of Body Surface
Area From Height and Weight*

Height		Body surface area	Weight	
cm.	in.	sq.m.	kg.	lb.
200	79	2·80	150	330
	78	2·70	145	320
195	76		140	310
190		2·60	135	300
	74	2·50	130	290
185	72	2·40	125	280
180	70	2·30	120	270
			115	260
175	68	2·20	110	250
170	66	2·10	105	240
165	64	2·00	100	230
		1·95	95	220
160	62	1·90	90	210
		1·85	85	200
155	60	1·80	80	190
150	58	1·75		180
		1·70	75	170
145	56	1·65	70	160
		1·60		150
140	54	1·55	65	140
135	52	1·50	60	130
		1·45		
130	50	1·40	55	120
125	48	1·35	50	110
		1·30		105
120	46	1·25	45	100
		1·20		95
115	44	1·15	40	90
110	42	1·10		85
		1·05	35	80
105	40	1·00		75
		0·95	30	70
100	39	0·90		66
		0·86		

*From Furbank RA: Conversion data, normal values, nomograms and other standards. *In* Modern Trends in Forensic Medicine. Vol 2. Edited by K Simpson. New York, Appleton-Century-Crofts, Inc., 1967, pp 344–364. By permission.

BODY WEIGHT AND LENGTH: 15 TO 30 YEARS*

In this table, three weights (without clothing) are given for each body length:
1. Weight for persons of average build = middle entry.
2. Weight for lightly built persons = top entry.
3. Weight for heavily built persons = bottom entry.

Women					Men				
Body length (cm)	**Weight (kg)**				**Body length (cm)**	**Weight (kg)**			
	15 yr	20 yr	25 yr	30 yr†		15 yr	20 yr	25 yr	30 yr†
	40.8	43.0	44.0	45.3		41.7	45.8	47.6	49.4
142.5	45.3	47.6	49.0	50.3	150	46.2	50.7	53.0	54.8
	51.2	53.0	55.3	56.6		51.6	57.1	59.3	61.6
	41.2	43.5	44.8	46.2		42.6	46.7	48.5	50.3
145	45.8	48.5	49.8	51.2	152.5	47.1	51.6	53.9	55.7
	51.6	53.9	56.2	57.5		53.0	58.0	60.7	62.5
	41.7	44.4	45.8	47.1		43.5	47.6	49.4	51.2
147.5	46.2	49.4	50.7	52.1	155	48.5	53.0	54.8	56.6
	52.1	55.7	57.1	58.4		54.4	59.3	61.6	63.4
	42.6	45.3	46.7	47.6		44.9	48.9	50.7	52.1
150	47.1	50.3	51.6	53.0	157.5	49.8	54.4	56.2	58.0
	53.0	56.6	58.0	59.8		56.2	61.2	63.0	65.2
	43.5	46.7	47.1	48.5		46.2	50.3	52.1	53.5
152.5	48.5	51.6	52.6	53.9	160	51.2	55.7	58.0	59.3
	54.4	58.0	59.3	60.7		57.5	62.5	65.2	66.6
	44.8	47.6	48.5	49.8		47.6	51.6	53.9	55.3
155	49.8	53.0	53.9	55.3	162.5	53.0	57.5	59.8	61.2
	55.3	59.8	60.7	62.1		59.3	64.8	67.0	68.9
	46.2	48.9	50.3	51.2		49.4	53.5	55.7	56.6
157.5	51.2	54.4	55.7	56.6	165	54.8	59.3	61.6	63.0
	57.5	61.2	62.5	63.9		61.6	66.6	69.3	70.7
	47.1	50.3	51.2	52.5		51.2	55.3	57.1	58.4
160	52.5	55.9	57.1	58.4	167.5	56.6	61.2	63.4	64.8
	59.3	62.5	64.3	65.7		63.4	68.9	71.1	72.9

* From Wissenschaftliche Tabellen. Basel, J. R. Geigy A. G., 1953, p. 199. By permission.
† Fourth decade weight should be maintained throughout life.

(Continued on next page.)

BODY WEIGHT AND LENGTH: 15 TO 30 YEARS* (Continued)

In this table, three weights (without clothing) are given for each body length:
1. Weight for persons of average build = middle entry.
2. Weight for lightly built persons = top entry.
3. Weight for heavily built persons = bottom entry.

Women					Men				
Body length (cm)	Weight (kg)				Body length (cm)	Weight (kg)			
	15 yr	20 yr	25 yr	30 yr†		15 yr	20 yr	25 yr	30 yr†
162.5	48.9	51.2	52.5	53.9	170	52.5	56.6	58.9	59.8
	54.4	57.1	58.4	59.8		58.4	63.0	65.2	66.6
	61.2	64.3	65.7	67.5		65.7	70.7	73.4	74.7
165	50.7	53.0	54.4	55.7	172.5	54.4	58.4	60.2	61.6
	56.2	58.9	60.2	61.6		60.2	64.8	67.0	68.4
	63.4	66.1	67.5	69.3		67.5	73.0	75.2	77.0
167.5	52.1	54.9	55.7	57.1	175	55.7	59.8	62.1	63.9
	58.0	60.7	62.1	63.4		62.1	66.6	68.9	70.7
	65.2	68.4	69.8	71.6		69.8	74.7	77.5	79.3
170	53.9	56.2	57.5	58.9	177.5	58.0	61.6	63.9	65.7
	59.8	62.5	63.9	65.2		64.3	68.4	71.1	72.9
	67.5	70.2	71.6	73.4		72.0	77.0	79.7	82.0
172.5	55.3	57.5	59.3	60.2	180	59.8	63.9	66.1	68.0
	61.6	63.9	65.7	67.0		66.6	70.7	73.4	75.7
	69.3	72.0	73.8	75.7		74.7	79.3	82.4	85.2
175	57.1	59.3	60.7	61.6	183	62.1	65.7	68.4	70.7
	63.4	65.7	67.5	68.4		68.9	72.9	76.1	78.4
	71.6	73.8	75.7	77.0		77.5	82.0	85.6	87.9
178	59.3	60.7	62.1	63.4	185.5	63.9	68.0	71.1	72.9
	65.7	67.5	68.9	70.2		71.1	75.2	78.8	81.1
	73.9	76.1	77.5	78.9		79.7	84.3	88.3	91.1
180	61.2	63.0	63.4	64.8	188	66.1	69.8	73.0	75.7
	68.0	69.8	70.7	72.0		73.4	77.5	81.1	83.8
	76.1	78.4	79.7	81.1		82.4	87.0	91.1	94.2

* From Wissenschaftliche Tabellen. Basel, J. R. Geigy A. G., 1953, p 199. By permission.
† Fourth decade weight should be maintained throughout life.

Bones

The weight of the bones is approximately 11.6% of the body weight.[5]

Brain

BRAIN: 17 TO 85 YEARS*

	Brain weight (gm)			
	Men		Women	
Age (yr)	Mean	Range	Mean	Range
17–19	1,340	1,170–1,527	1,242	1,120–1,420
20–29	1,396	1,158–1,620	1,234	1,057–1,565
30–39	1,365	1,075–1,685	1,233	1,038–1,440
40–49	1,366	1,069–1,605	1,240	995–1,543
50–59	1,375	1,113–1,665	1,200	820–1,447
60–69	1,323	1,018–1,610	1,178	920–1,372
70–85	1,279	1,039–1,485	1,121	832–1,370

* Data from Sunderman FW, Boerner F: Normal Values in Clinical Medicine. Philadelphia, W. B. Saunders Company, 1949.

The weight of the brain is approximately 1.4% of the body weight.[5] Various effects of fixation with formalin solution have been reported. On fixation by penetration there is a mean weight increase of 8.8% (range, 3.3 to 19.2%).[14] On fixation by perfusion with 1,000 ml of 10% formalin solution there is a mean weight increase of 5.7% (range, 0.7 to 31.8%).[8] On fixation by perfusion with 2,000 ml of 10% formalin solution the mean weight increase is 8.8% (range, 1.0 to 26.3%).[8]

Colon

The length is 150 to 170 cm.[15]

Duodenum

The length is 30 cm.[15]

Esophagus

The length is 25 cm.[15]

Fat Tissue

On fixation with formalin solution by penetration the mean weight increase is 2.2% (range, 0.1 to 4.8%).[14]

Heart

HEART WEIGHT IN RELATION TO BODY WEIGHT BY SEX*

Men				Women			
Body weight		Heart weight (gm)		Body weight		Heart weight (gm)	
Pounds	Kilograms	Mean	Range	Pounds	Kilograms	Mean	Range
105	47	205	165–241	90	40	162	135–193
110	50	215	173–253	95	43	171	143–204
115	52	225	181–264	100	45	180	150–215
120	54	235	190–276	105	47	189	158–226
125	56	245	198–287	110	50	198	165–237
130	58	255	206–299	115	52	207	172–248
135	60	265	213–310	120	54	215	180–259
140	63	274	221–322	125	56	225	188–268
145	65	284	229–333	130	58	234	195–277
150	68	294	237–345	135	60	244	203–286
155	70	304	245–356	140	63	253	211–295
160	72	313	253–368	145	65	262	219–304
165	74	323	261–370	150	68	272	225–313
170	77	333	268–371	155	70	282	233–322
175	79	343	280–372	160	72	288	240–330
180	81	353	288–373	165	74	297	247–337
185	83	363	296–382	170	77	306	255–343
190	86	373	304–392	175	79	315	283–350
195	88	382	312–402	180	81	324	301–356
200	90	392	320–412	185	83	333	309–361
				190	86	342	317–366
				195	88	351	325–371

Average weight of adult male heart: 294 gm

Average weight of adult female heart: 250 gm

* Data from Smith HL: The relation of the weight of the heart to the weight of the body and of the weight of the heart to age. Am Heart J 4:79–93, 1928.

The heart weight is approximately 0.45% of the body weight in men and 0.40% in women.[6] The value given by Furbank[5] for both sexes is 0.3%. Rössle and Roulet[13] prepared tables which show heart weights in relation to age, body weight, and sex. Tables relating heart weight to body length and sex have been prepared by Zeek.[18] The thickness of ventricular walls, the valve circumferences, the length of ventricular inflow or outflow tracts, and the chamber perimeters or ventricular volumes in relation to body length and weight or age have been tabulated by Eckner et al.[3] These studies were carried out on hearts fixed by controlled-pressure coronary perfusion.

The mural volume and weight of the heart after removal of the epicardial fat were studied by Hegglin. A table from Hegglin's work, reproduced by Reiner,[12] shows mean volumes, mean weights, and specific gravity of these hearts for both sexes from 20 to 89 years of age.

An elegant approach was described by Masshoff et al[9] who calculated the weight of the myocardial and fat tissue from the specific gravity of the heart:

$$\text{Specific gravity} = \frac{\text{total heart weight}}{\text{total heart volume}}.$$

The heart is weighed in isotonic saline for this determination. From the table below, one uses the specific gravity to find the factor which, when multiplied by heart weight, gives heart muscle mass. *Example:* A heart weighing 700 gm has a specific gravity of 1.032. The table shows a factor (X) of .798, or 79.8%. The muscle mass of this heart is 79.8% of 700 gm, or 558.6 gm.

FACTORS FOR CALCULATION OF MUSCLE CONTENT OF HEART FROM SPECIFIC GRAVITY*

Sp. grav.	X	Sp. grav.	X	Sp. grav.	X	Sp. grav.	X	Sp. grav.	X
1.055	1.000	1.032	0.798	1.009	0.569	0.986	0.395	0.963	0.193
1.054	0.991	1.031	0.789	1.008	0.588	0.985	0.386	0.962	0.184
1.053	0.982	1.030	0.781	1.007	0.579	0.984	0.377	0.961	0.175
1.052	0.974	1.029	0.772	1.006	0.570	0.983	0.368	0.960	0.167
1.051	0.965	1.028	0.763	1.005	0.561	0.982	0.360	0.959	0.158
1.050	0.956	1.027	0.754	1.004	0.553	0.981	0.351	0.958	0.149
1.049	0.947	1.026	0.746	1.003	0.544	0.980	0.342	0.957	0.140
1.048	0.939	1.025	0.737	1.002	0.535	0.979	0.333	0.956	0.132
1.047	0.930	1.024	0.728	1.001	0.526	0.978	0.325	0.955	0.123
1.046	0.921	1.023	0.719	1.000	0.518	0.977	0.316	0.954	0.114
1.045	0.912	1.022	0.711	0.999	0.509	0.976	0.307	0.953	0.105
1.044	0.904	1.021	0.702	0.998	0.500	0.975	0.298	0.952	0.096
1.043	0.895	1.020	0.693	0.997	0.491	0.974	0.289	0.951	0.088
1.042	0.886	1.019	0.684	0.996	0.482	0.973	0.281	0.950	0.079
1.041	0.877	1.018	0.675	0.995	0.474	0.972	0.272	0.949	0.070
1.040	0.868	1.017	0.667	0.994	0.465	0.971	0.263	0.948	0.061
1.039	0.860	1.016	0.658	0.993	0.456	0.970	0.254	0.947	0.053
1.038	0.851	1.015	0.649	0.992	0.447	0.969	0.246	0.946	0.044
1.037	0.842	1.014	0.640	0.991	0.439	0.968	0.237	0.945	0.035
1.036	0.833	1.013	0.632	0.990	0.430	0.967	0.228	0.944	0.026
1.035	0.825	1.012	0.623	0.989	0.421	0.966	0.219	0.943	0.018
1.034	0.816	1.011	0.614	0.988	0.412	0.965	0.211	0.942	0.009
1.033	0.807	1.010	0.605	0.987	0.404	0.964	0.202	0.941	0.000

* From Masshoff W, Scheidt D, Reimers HF: Quantitative Bestimmung des Fett- und Myokardgewebes im Leichenherzen. Virchows Arch [Pathol Anat] *342*:184–189, 1967. By permission of Springer-Verlag.

HEART MEASUREMENTS*

	Mean (cm)	Range (cm)
Thickness, left ventricular muscle	1.5	
Thickness, right ventricular muscle	0.5	
Thickness, atrial muscle	0.2	
Circumference, mitral valve	10	8–10.5
Circumference, aortic valve	7.5	6–7.5
Circumference, pulmonary valve	8.5	7–9
Circumference, tricuspid valve	12	10–12.5
Circumference, pulmonary artery	8.0	
Circumference, aorta	see under Aorta	

* Modified from Sunderman FW and Boerner F: Normal Values in Clinical Medicine. Philadelphia, W. B. Saunders Company, 1949.

On fixation with formalin solution by penetration there is a mean weight loss of 4.0% (range, 0.4 to 9.0%).[14] During storage of normal or hypertrophic unfixed hearts which were refrigerated 1 to 2 hours after the autopsy and kept at 6 C and a humidity of 96%, the mean weight loss was 2.6% of the original heart weight after 2 days and 6.2% after 5 days.[19]

Kidneys

The weight of the kidneys is approximately 0.3% of the body weight.[5] The mean combined weight in males is 313 gm (range, 230 to 440 gm). The mean combined weight in females is 288 gm (range, 240 to 350 gm).[15]

The mean size, for both sexes, of a normal adult kidney is 11 to 12 by 5 to 6 by 3 to 4 cm.

On fixation with formalin solution by penetration there may be a weight increase or a weight loss. The mean weight change is 1.9% (range, 0.1 to 6.4%).[14] During storage of unfixed kidneys which were refrigerated 1 to 2 hours after the autopsy and kept at 6 C and a humidity of 96%, the mean weight loss was 5.6% of the original fresh kidney weight after 2 days and 13.3% after 5 days.[19]

Liver

The weight of the normal liver has been reported[5] to be approximately 1.8% of the body weight. I have found the weight range of normal liver to be 1.9 to 3.1% of the total body weight. The data in the following table are based on a study of 318 autopsy cases (221 males and 97 females). These were mostly accident cases and were considered to be normal in respect to the liver and to the body weight.

NORMAL LIVER WEIGHTS

		Males		Females
Age (yr)	N	Liver weight (% of total body weight)*	N	Liver weight (% of total body weight)*
10–19	31	1.9–3.1	14	2.0–3.0
20–29	35	1.9–3.1	6	2.4–3.0
30–39	11	2.1–3.0	6	2.1–2.6
40–49	35	2.0–3.1	14	1.9–3.1
50–59	29	2.1–3.1	9	1.9–2.9
60–69	22	1.9–3.1	7	1.9–2.9
70–79	13	2.0–2.9	7	2.0–3.0
80–89	6	1.9–2.6	9	2.1–3.0

* Range shown represents values between 10th and 90th percentiles.

PERCENTILES OF WEIGHTS OF NORMAL LIVER*

Age (yr)	N	Max. weight (gm)	97.5	90	75	50	25	10	2.5	Min. weight (gm)
					Males					
20–29	38	2,500	2,480	2,300	2,000	1,820	1,640	1,420	1,300	1,235
30–39	54	2,515	2,520	2,310	2,030	1,830	1,670	1,490	1,370	1,327
40–49	58	2,900	2,600	2,290	2,030	1,840	1,670	1,510	1,350	1,470
50–59	39	3,020	2,570	2,190	2,000	1,840	1,640	1,510	1,350	1,200
60–69	37	2,400	2,420	2,070	1,890	1,740	1,580	1,420	1,320	1,300
70–79	13	2,263	2,140	1,860	1,640	1,380	1,180	1,020	900	900
					Females					
20–29	19	1,920	1,900	1,720	1,560	1,440	1,280	1,140	1,080	1,114
30–39	14	2,120	2,040	1,820	1,620	1,460	1,320	1,200	1,080	1,023
40–49	11	2,130	2,100	1,910	1,690	1,440	1,290	1,180	1,220	1,250
50–59	11	2,000	1,990	1,870	1,700	1,430	1,260	1,140	1,010	1,020
60–69	13	1,780	1,880	1,780	1,590	1,380	1,150	1,050	910	925
70–79	5	1,595	1,760	1,600	1,380	1,180	1,100	1,040	1,000	1,100

Percentiles of weight (gm) spans the columns 97.5, 90, 75, 50, 25, 10, 2.5.

* From Boyd E: Normal variability in weight of the adult human liver and spleen. Arch Pathol *16*:350–372, 1933. By permission of the American Medical Association.

On fixation with formalin solution by penetration there was a mean weight loss of 4.0% (range, 0.5 to 7.6%).[14] During storage of livers which were refrigerated 1 to 2 hours after the autopsy and kept at 6 C and a humidity of 96%, the mean weight loss was 3.5% of the original fresh liver weight after 2 days and 7.2% after 5 days.[19]

Lungs

The combined lungs weigh approximately 1% of the body weight.[5] The mean weight of the right lung is 450 gm (range, 360 to 570 gm); the mean weight of the left lung is 375 gm (range, 325 to 480 gm).[15] Whimster[16] found mean weights of 385 gm (SD 97) for the left lung and 456 gm (SD 117) for the right lung in men and 342 gm (SD 91) for the left lung and 405 gm (SD 99) for the right lung in women; this study was based on 350 normal lungs.

On fixation with formalin solution by penetration there may be a weight increase or a weight loss. The mean weight change is 6.6% (range, 0.4 to 17.1%).[14]

Ovaries

The combined weight after pregnancy is 14 gm. The size of one ovary is 2.7 to 4.1 by 1.5 by 0.8 cm; the size in a virgin is 4.1 to 5.2 by 2.0 to 2.7 by 1.0 to 1.1.[15]

Pancreas

The weight of the pancreas is approximately 0.1% of the body weight.[5] The mean weight is 110 gm (range, 60 to 135 gm). The size is 23 by 4.5 by 3.8 cm.[15]

Parathyroid Glands

The combined weight of the parathyroid glands ranges from 0.12 to 0.18 gm.[15] The lower glands normally are larger.

Pineal Gland

The weight ranges from 0.1 to 0.18 gm. The size is 0.5 to 0.9 by 0.3 to 0.6 by 0.3 to 0.5 cm.[17]

Pituitary Gland

The average weight is 0.56 gm in persons 10 to 20 years old and 0.61 gm in persons 20 to 70 years old. The average size is 2.1 by 1.4 by 0.5 cm. In pregnant women the average weight is 0.95 gm (range, 0.84 to 1.06 gm).[15]

Placenta

The average weight is 500 gm; the average size is 16 to 20 by 2.5 to 3.0 cm. On fixation with formalin solution by penetration there is a mean weight increase of 9.9% (range, 0.7 to 23.0%).[14]

Prostate

The average weight is 5.1 gm at age 15 years, 6.1 gm at age 16, 11.4 gm at age 17, 17.9 gm at ages 21 to 25, 20 gm at ages 51 to 60, and 40 gm at ages 71 to 80. The average size of the prostate is 3.6 by 2.8 by 1.9 cm.[15]

Seminal Vesicles

The average size is 4.1 to 4.5 by 1.6 to 1.8 by 0.9.[15]

Skeletal Muscle

The weight of the skeletal musculature is approximately 28.7% of the body weight.[5] On fixation with formalin solution by penetration there is a mean weight loss of 7.0% (range, 0.8 to 13.3%).[7]

Small Intestine

The length is 550 to 650 cm.[15]

Spleen

The weight of the spleen is approximately 0.16% of the body weight. The spleen weight is less in females than in males at all ages.[2]

PERCENTILES OF WEIGHTS OF NORMAL SPLEEN*

Age (yr)	N	Max. weight (gm)	Percentiles of weight (gm) 97.5	90	75	50	25	10	2.5	Min. weight (gm)
Males										
20–29	38	400	364	318	250	194	144	116	96	90
30–39	54	360	356	281	220	172	131	106	86	75
40–49	58	400	327	234	187	144	112	86	65	75
50–59	39	280	285	229	172	135	108	84	61	25
60–69	37	225	243	205	147	113	94	74	61	60
70–79	13	255	234	188	136	108	90	74	66	65
Females										
20–29	19	300	300	255	205	165	130	95	65	65
30–39	14	420	310	258	200	162	118	85	63	55
40–49	11	325	293	252	195	142	102	80	65	80
50–59	11	250	273	227	182	135	95	77	67	75
60–69	13	284	230	198	160	113	87	78	68	61
70–79	5	175	195	175	140	110	95	78	70	90

* From Boyd E: Normal variability in weight of the adult human liver and spleen. Arch Pathol *16*:350–372, 1933. By permission of the American Medical Association.

DeLand[2] recently published tables relating spleen weights to age, body height, body weight, and body surface. This study was based on 440 normal cases and revealed a spleen weight decrease from 20 to 29 years of age and above 60 years of age.

On fixation with formalin solution by penetration there may be a weight increase or a weight loss. The mean weight change is 2.1% (range, 0.1 to 6.2%).[14] During storage of unfixed spleens which were refrigerated 1 to 2 hours after the autopsy and kept at 6 C and a humidity of 96%, the mean weight loss was 5.0% of the original fresh spleen weight after 2 days and 12.1% after 5 days.[19]

Spinal Cord

The mean weight is 27 gm, and the mean length is 45 cm.[15] Sunderman and Boerner[15] also give the frontal and sagittal dimensions of the cervical, thoracic, and lumbar portions of the spinal cord.

Testes

The mean weight of one testis is 25 gm (range, 20 to 27 gm). The average size is 4 to 5 by 2.5 to 3.5 by 2.0 to 2.7 cm.[15] On fixation with formalin solution by penetration there may be a weight increase or a weight loss. The mean weight change is 3.2% (range, 0.0 to 8.8%).[14]

Thymus

The average weight is 25 gm at ages 6 to 25 years, 20 gm at ages 26 to 35, 16 gm at ages 36 to 65, and 6 gm in persons over 65 years.[15]

Thyroid Gland

The mean weight is 40 gm (range, 30 to 70 gm). The size is 5 to 7 by 3 to 4 by 1.5 to 2.5 cm.[15] On fixation with formalin solution by penetration there is a mean weight increase of 14.8% (range, 6.2 to 34.0%).[14]

Uterus

The mean weight after pregnancy is 110 gm (range, 102 to 117 gm). The size is 8.7 to 9.4 by 5.4 to 6.1 by 3.2 to 3.6 cm. The mean weight in virgins is 35 gm (range, 33 to 41 gm); the size is 7.8 to 8.1 by 3.4 to 4.5 by 1.8 to 2.7 cm.[15]

REFERENCES

1. Bloodworth JMB Jr: The adrenal. *In* Pathology Annual 1966. Edited by SC Sommers. New York, Appleton-Century-Crofts, Inc., 1966, pp 172–192.
2. DeLand FH: Normal spleen size. Radiology 97:589–592, 1970.
3. Eckner FAO, Brown BW, Davidson DL, Glagov S: Dimensions of normal human hearts: after standard fixation by controlled pressure coronary perfusion. Arch Pathol 88:497–507, 1969.
4. Faulkner WR, King JW, Damm HC: Handbook of Clinical Laboratory Data. Second edition. Cleveland, Ohio, The Chemical Rubber Co., 1968.
5. Furbank RA: Conversion data, normal values, nomograms and other standards. *In* Modern Trends in Forensic Medicine. Vol 2. Edited by K Simpson. New York, Appleton-Century-Crofts, Inc., 1967, pp 344–364.
6. Hudson REB: Cardiovascular Pathology. London, Edward Arnold (Publishers), Ltd., 1965.
7. Kissane JM, Smith MG: Pathology of Infancy and Childhood. St. Louis, C. V. Mosby Company, 1967.
8. Ludwig J: Unpublished data.
9. Masshoff W, Scheidt D, Reimers HF: Quantitative Bestimmung des Fett- und Myokardgewebes im Leichenherzen. Virchows Arch [Pathol Anat] 342:184–189, 1967.
10. Minckler TM, Boyd E: Physical growth of the nervous system and its coverings. *In* Pathology of the Nervous System. Vol 1. Edited by J Minckler. New York, McGraw-Hill Book Company, Inc., 1968, pp 120–137.
11. Nichols J: Adrenal cortex. *In* Endocrine Pathology. Edited by JMB Bloodworth Jr. Baltimore, Williams & Wilkins Company, 1968, pp 224–255.
12. Reiner L: Gross examination of the heart. *In* Pathology of the Heart and Blood Vessels. Third edition. Edited by SE Gould. Springfield, Illinois, Charles C Thomas, Publisher, 1968, pp 1111–1149.
13. Rössle R, Roulet F: Mass und Zahl in der Pathologie. Berlin, Springer Verlag, Inc., 1932.
14. Schremmer C-N: Gewichtsänderungen verschiedener Gewebe nach Formalinfixierung. Frankfurt Z Pathol 77:299–304, 1967.
15. Sunderman FW, Boerner F: Normal Values in Clinical Medicine. Philadelphia, W. B. Saunders Company, 1949.
16. Whimster WF: Normal lung weights in Jamaicans. Am Rev Resp Dis 103:85–90, 1971.
17. Wurtman RJ: The pineal gland. *In* Endocrine Pathology. Edited by JMB Bloodworth Jr. Baltimore, Williams & Wilkins Company, 1968, pp 117–132.
18. Zeek PM: Heart weight. I. The weight of the normal human heart. Arch Pathol 34:820–832, 1942.
19. Zschoch H, Wunderlich C: Über Gewichtsveränderungen von Leichenorganen bei der Lagerung. Zentralbl Allg Pathol 112:418–420, 1969.

INDEX

Boldface folios in the index indicate main discussion in text.

A

Abortion, 13, **19,** 20, 22, 298, 305
Abscess, brain, 13, 39, 209, **213**
Accidents
  aircraft, 20
  death certificate, 267
  and medicolegal autopsies, 298
  vehicular, 19
Actinomyces israeli, 215
Adhesions, 5
Adipocere, 18
Admissibility, autopsy documents, 303
Adrenal glands, weights
    adults, 335
    fetuses, 317
    infants, 317, 318
Adulterants, drugs, 38
Aerosol, bronchodilators, 41
Afterfixation, lungs, 101
Age determination, **15,** 30
Air content, lungs, 121
Air embolism, 4, 19, **20,** 84
Air in abdomen, 8
Airway obstruction, 24
Alcohol
  and accidents, 20
  and barbiturates, 44
  in blood, 41
  and drowning, 26
  and drug addicts, 39
  elimination, 42
  in embalming fluid, 18
  and exposure to cold, 27
  fixative, 233, 240
  and gunshot injuries, 28
  interpretation, 41
  mounting medium, 254
  proof, 43
  sampling, 34, 35

Alcohol (*continued*)
  toxicologic request, 31
  in vitreous humor, 34, 35, 42
Alcoholism, 270, 272
Alizarin, 259
Alkaloids, 36
Alveolar ducts, 106
Amino acids, 17, 221
Ammonium, 221
Amphetamines, 40
Amyloid, 216, **230**
Anemia, hemolytic, 197
Anesthesia, 13, **24,** 39, 44
Aneurysm
  aorta, 3, 82
  internal carotid artery, 169
Angiitis, 39
Angiography
  brain, 188
  heart, 61, **68,** 82
  intestinal tract, 137, 139
  kidneys, 149
  liver, **142,** 143, 151
  lower extremities, 82, 84
  lungs, 97, **113,** 114, 116, 117, 120
  lymphatic vessels, 88
  mesentery, 137
  pelvic organs, 153
  placenta, 154
  spleen, 147
  stomach, 134
  vena cava, 84
Anticholinergics, 40
Antiformin, **202,** 258
Antifreeze, 36
Aorta
  aneurysm, 3, 82
  dissection, 82
  grading of atherosclerosis, 83
  measurements, 336

349

Aortic isthmus stenosis, 54, 82
Aortic valve homografts, 65, 66
Arcon, 76, 151
Arm, 6
Arnold-Chiari malformation, 162, 169
Arsenic, 32, 36
Arteries. See also *Angiography*
　aorta and major branches, 82
　carotid arteries, 190
　coronary arteries, 53
　fibromuscular dysplasia, 82
　vertebral arteries, 190
Arteriography. See *Angiography*
Arterioles, 76, 114. See also *Angiography*
Arthritis, 198
Asbestos bodies, 124
Asphyxia, 15, 26, 29, 222. See also *Hypoxia*
Aspiration, 24, 93
Assault, 20, 25
Asthma, 41
Atherosclerosis. See *Arteries* and
　　Angiography
Attorneys, 298
Autopsy
　diagnoses, 263, 272, 289
　disclosure of findings, 304
　face sheets, 288
　financing, 312
　functions, 307
　medicolegal, 11
　microbiology, 207
　permission. See *Autopsy authorization*
　protocols, **264**, 303
　rates, 309, **311**, 312
　service organization, 277
　technicians, 276, 311
　tissue storage, 282
　toxicology, 31
Autopsy authorization
　forms, 300, 302
　medicolegal, 298
　organs, tissues, 225, 302
　relatives and others, 272, 273, **299**
　restrictions, 5, 225, 301
　by statute, 299
　verification, 297
Autopsy room
　accidents and infections, 276
　maintenance, 275
　roentgen facilities, 224
Autopsy techniques. See also names of re-
　　spective organs
　adults, 2
　arm, hand, and face lesions, 6, 301
　fetuses and infants, 3, 153
　films, 1
　forensic, 18
　legal restrictions, 5, 225, 301
　postoperative, 4, 134
　radioactive bodies, 248
　references, 1
Autoradiography, 231
Azotemia, 17

B

Bags. See *Plastic bags*
Barbiturates, 32, 34, 35, 36, 40, **43**
Barium sulfate
　impregnation, 109
　radiopaque mixtures, 256
Basal ganglia, 36, 39
Battered child, 30
Beneke technique, 3, 160
Benign prostatic hyperplasia, 153
Benzene, 41
Bile, 24, 33, **34,** 36, 39
Bilirubin, 221
Blood
　alcohol, 41. See also *Alcohol*
　chemistry, 17, 26, 219, 221
　coagulation factors, 222
　content, lungs, 121
　microbiology, 210
　sampling, 34
　volume, 121, 336
Body surface
　adults, 337
　infants, 323, 324
Body weight and length
　adults, 338, 339
　fetuses and newborns, 316
　infant boys, 319, 321
　infant girls, 320, 322
Bone
　aseptic necrosis, 25
　decalcification, 199
　maceration, 201
　microbiology, 214
　prostheses, 199
　sampling, 196
　staining, 259
　undecalcified sections, 201
　weight, 340
Bone marrow
　Helly's fixative, 235
　sections and smears, 198
Bouin's fixative, 154, 233
Brain
　abscess, 13, 39, 209, **213**
　angiography, 188
　chemistry, 177
　dissection, 171
　edema, 25
　fixation, 173
　histochemistry, 231
　ischemic lesions, 185
　microbiology, 177, 213
　removal, 157, 160
　sampling, 184
　storage, 281, 282
　ventriculography, 189
Brain weight
　adults, 340
　fetuses, 317
　infants, 325
Bromides, 36

Bronchi, 93, 106, 112, 119, 123
Bronchiectases, 123
Bronchography, **117,** 120, 258
Buckets, 173, 278. See also *Containers*
Bullets, 14, 27, 28
Burial, 265, 299, 300, 304
Burning, 13, 20

C

Calcium, 36, 221, 230
Capillaries, 76, 117. See also *Angiography*
Carbon dioxide, blood, 221
Carbon monoxide, 20, 32, 35, **36,** 37, 44, 239, 242
Carbon tetrachloride, 32, 35
Carcinoid tumors, 220
Carmine-gelatin, 142
Carnoy's fixative, 233
Cartilage, staining, 259
Caskets, 304, 305
Casts, 6, 14, 120, 258. See also *Angiography* and *Bronchography*
Catheterization, veins, 20
Cephalin flocculation, 223
Cerebral. See *Brain*
Cerebrospinal fluid
  chemistry, 17, 219, 221
  microbiology, 213
  removal, 34
Character reader, optical, 291
Chemistry, 177, **219,** 277. See also *Histochemistry*
Chloride, 44, 221. See also *Drowning*
Chloroform, 32
Chloroma, 240
Cholangiograms, 142, 143
Cholesterol, 221, 223
Choriocarcinoma, 220
Chromosomes, 217
Cinefluorobronchograms, 120
Cirrhosis, liver, 133, 139, 144
Claimant, 301
Classifications, 286
Cleaning, 275
Cleaning fluid, 41
Clearing, tissues, 129, 136, 139, 142, 254, **258**
Cocaine, 40
Coding, 286
Colon, 340
Color preservation, **236,** 253
Computer, 14, 264, 286, 292, 310
Cones, graded, 53
Confidentiality, 287
Congenital malformations
  Arnold-Chiari, 162, 169
  and chromosomes, 217
  encephalocele, 162
  of heart and great vessels, 54, 76, 82, 308
  meningocele, 162, 167
  of veins, 3, 54
Congestion, lungs, 25
Containers, 14, 31, 39, **241,** 249, **254,** 279, **281**

Contaminated specimens, 208
Contrast media, 4, 69, **70,** 71, 72, 76, 82, 88, 115, 116, 120, 142, 188, 231, 256, 257
Conversion factors, 315
Coproporphyrin, 40
Coronary arteries
  angiography, 61, **68,** 82
  atherosclerosis, 53, 83
  insufficiency, 69
  occlusion, 20
Coronary veins, 73, 76
Coroners, 298
Corrosion, 73, 76, **121, 142,** 147, 148, 153, 201, 253, 256, **257**
Cortisol, 221
Creatine, 17, 221
Creatinine, 221, 223
Cremation, 247, 251, 298, 305
Crib death, 272
Crime investigators, 311
Cross references, 286
Crush injuries, 20
Crystals, 124
Culture media, 215, 310
Custody, **14,** 28, 33, 299, 300, 301, 304
Cutis anserina, 27
Cyanide, 18, 32, 38

D

Data, 12, 14, 265, **283**
Daylight saving time, 270
Death
  certificates, **265,** 287, 303, 309
  drug-associated, 44
  estimation of time, 15
  nonviolent, 13
  scene investigation, 12
  signs, 12
  sudden and unexplained, 298
  violent, 11, 12
Decomposition gas, 22
Decompression, 20, **25**
Decontamination, radioactivity, 250
Depressants, 38
Diabetes mellitus, 222
Dialysis fluids, 33
Diaphragm, 133
Diatoms, 26
Diazo print technique, 112
Digitalis, 36
Disinterment, 305. See also *Exhumation*
Disposal, 275, 281
Documentation, 284, 311
Donation, organs, 302
Drag marks, 19
Drains, 4, 28
Driving, 41
Drowning, 20, **25,** 28, 34, 44, 93
Drugs, 13, 24, 27, 28, 36, 40, 43, 270
Dry preservation
  heart, 76
  intestine, 136
  lungs, 101, 106

Duodenum, 340
Dura mater, 169, 310

E

Ear, 171
Edema, lung, 26, 96, 233
Education, 307
Effusion, 210
Electron microscopy, 19, 125, 154, **216,** 235
Embalming, 18, 37, 207, 247, **251,** 301, 304, 305, 312
Embolism, 4, 19, 25, 82, 96
Emphysema
  artifact, **106**
  grading, 111
  of lungs, 109, 123
  subcutaneous, 8
En bloc removal, organs, 2, 5, 84, 88, 139
En masse removal, organs, 2, 3, 82, 84, 88, 139
Encephalocele, 162
Endocarditis, 39, 53, 211
Enterotome, 134
Enzymes, 134, 220, 221, 233
Epidemiology, 309, 310
Esophagus, 129, 133, 340
Ethiodol, 4, 88, 142, 257
Ethylene glycol, 36
Evidence, 14, 242, 303
Exhumation, 31, 203, 305
Expiratory collapse, 120
Exposure dose rates, 247, 249, 250
Exposure to cold, 27
Eye, 12, 171, 173, 301, 302

F

Face lesions, 6
Fat tissue
  fixation and weight, 340
  necroses, 147
  staining, 229
Fatty acids, 221
Femoral vessels, 84, 86
Fetuses, 267, 316, 317
Fiber teasing, 186
Fibrinolysis, 222
Fibrosis, lungs, 13, 106
File cards, 279, 290, **292**
Film strip mounting, 111
Fingerprints, 14, 27, 306
Fistulas, 4, 13, 93
Fixation, organs
  brain, 173
  gallbladder, 146, 240
  heart, 77
  intestine, 135
  kidney, 149
  liver, 139
  lung, 95, 97, 101, 105, 106
  pelvic organs, 153
  spleen, 147
Fixation mixtures, 232
Florence test, 30

Fluoride, 32, 38
Foreign bodies, 13, 14, 19, 28
Formalin, effect on organ weights. See
  weight tables (Appendix)
Formalin solutions, 101, 102, 142, **234**
Forms
  autopsy authorization, 300
  autopsy protocol, 266
  death certificates, 267, 268, 269
  donation, organs, 302, 303
  forensic protocol, 14 (no illustration)
  international shipment, 305
  radioactivity, 245 (no illustration)
  toxicologic request, 32
Fractures, 13
Freezing, tissues, 106, 109, 110, 153, 220, 277
Freons, 41
Fright, 13
Function studies
  liver, 223
  lungs, 123
Funeral directors, 245, 247, 270, 277, 301, 306, 311

G

Gallbladder
  dissection, 146
  fixation, 146, 240
  stones, 146
  storage, 277
Gargoylism, 3
Gases, 22, 39, 41
Gasoline, 41
Gasserian ganglia, 169
Gelatin, 255, 257
Genetics, 217, 273, 309
Gettler test, 26
Ghon technique, 2
Globus pallidus, necrosis, 39
Glomeruli, 149
Glomerulonephritis, 151
Glucose, 221, 223
Glue sniffing, 41
Glutaraldehyde, 235
Glycogen, 221, 231, 233
Glycol, 36
Gough technique, 110
Gout, 198, 240
Grading, 83, 111
Granulomas, 39
Grid methods, 111
Gunshot, 27, 29

H

Hair, 28, 35
Hallucinogens, 38, 40
Hand lesions, 6
Hashish, 38, 40
Head, 319, 320
Heart
  angiography, **68,** 76, 82
  conduction system, 59
  dissection, 51, 54, 58, 78

Heart (*continued*)
  dry preservation, 54, **76**
  histochemistry, 63, 230
  infarcts, 53, 61, 231
  microbiology, 211
  potassium-sodium ratio, 63
  sampling, 64
  staining, 61
  valves, 53, 65, 310
Heart weights and measurements
  adults, 341
  boys, 326
  determination, 53, 58
  fat tissue, 341, 342
  fetuses, 317
  girls, 327
  myocardium, 341
Heat fixation, 236
Heavy metal poisoning, 13, 33, 40
Helly's fixative, 235
Hematoxylin, 136
Hemochromatosis, 142, 230
Hemorrhage
  brain and meninges, 13, 15
  lungs, 27
  middle ear, 27
Hemosiderin, 140, 230
Hepatitis, 39
Hepatoduodenal ligament, 139
Hernias, 5
Heroin, 38, 40
Histochemistry, 63, 230
Histocytosis, 197
Histologic sampling
  bone, 196
  brain, 184
  heart, 64
  nerves, 185
  skeletal muscle, 187
Homicide, 20, 33, 220, 267, 270, 298, 305
Homografts, **65,** 310
Hoppe-Seyler test, 37
Hormones, 170, 220, 310
Hydrocarbons, 41
Hydrocyanic acid, 38
Hydrogen peroxide inflation, 88
Hydronephrosis, 258
Hydrostatic lung test, 29
Hypaque, 4, 257
Hyperglycemia, 28, 222
Hyperventilation, 28
Hypnotics, 40
Hypoglycemia, 222
Hypothalamus, 169
Hypothermia, 27
Hypoxanthine, 17, 221
Hypoxia, 20, **28,** 35, 242

I

Identification, **14,** 18, 20, 27
Ileus, 27
Immunofluorescence, **151,** 154
Incineration, 125

Indemnity, 301
India ink, 139, 142, **257**
Industrial commission, 299
Infant, disposition of body, 302
Infanticide, 29
Infarcts
  in decompression sickness, 25
  myocardial, 53, 61, 231
  pontine, 173
Infections
  autopsy room, 276
  microbiology, 207
Infiltration techniques, 260
Injection techniques, 256. See also
    Angiography
Inositol, 221
Insecticides, 38, 270, 310
Insects, 17
Insulin, 220
Insurance, 263, 265, 299, 301, 304, 305, 309,
    312
Interview, **272,** 304
Intestinal tract, 34, **134,** 210
Intravascular coagulation, 38, 222
Isotopes. See *Radioactivity*

J

Jars, 254, 279. See also *Containers*
Joints, 93, **197,** 214
Jores' solution, 237
Judges, 298

K

Kaiserling's solutions, 237
Karyotypes, 219
Kernohan's technique, 162, 164
Kerosene, 32
Ketones, 221
Kidney, 3, **148,** 209, 231, 258
Kidney weights and measurements
  adults, 343
  fetuses, 317
  infants, 328

L

Labels, 33, 241, 242, 256, 277, 281
Lactic acid, 28, 221, 242
Lactose, 38
Larynx, 93
Latex, 73, 121, 139, 143
Lavage fluid, 33
Lead, 32, 33, **40**
Lead particle coating, 118
Legal. See *Medicolegal*
Letulle technique, 2
Leukemia, 218
Light absorption, lungs, 112
Lighter fluid, 41
Lipids, 221
Liver, 25, 108, **139,** 209, 223, 231
Liver weights and measurements
  adults, 343, 344

Liver weights & measurements (*continued*)
  fetuses, 317
  infants, 329
Livor mortis, 17
LSD (d-lysergic acid diethylamide), 39
Lung, 13, 26, 39, **93,** 209
Lung weights
  adults, 344
  fetuses, 317
  infants, 330
Lymph nodes, 210
Lymphangiography, 88
Lymphatic vessels, 86

M

Maceration. See *Corrosion*
Maggots, 17
Magnesium, 26, 38, 221
Maintenance, 275
Malaria, 39
Malformations. See *Congenital malformations*
Malpractice, 305, 309
Mannitol, 38
Manpower, 311
Maple syrup urine disease, 220
Marihuana, 38
Mastoid, 27. See also *Middle ear*
Medical examiners, 298
Medicolegal, **11,** 242, 267, **297**
Melanotic tissue, 240
Meningitis, 13, 39, 213, 214
Meningomyelocele, 162, 167
Mercury, 32, 135, 310
Mesentery, 136
Mesothelioma, 13
Methanol, 32, 36
Microbiology, 4, 18, 19, 22, 30, 177, **207,** 243. See also names of respective organs
Microdissection, 148
Microfil, 89
Microradiography, lungs, 113
Microvasculature. See *Angiography*
Middle ear, 27, 29, 171, 214
Models, organs, 143, 147, 260
Moritz, temperature formula, 15
Morphine, 32, 39
Morticians. See *Funeral Directors*
Mosaicism, 219
Mounting, 254
Mummies, 31
Mummification, 260. See also *Dry preservation*
Mutilation, 301
Mycobacterium tuberculosis, 215, 216
Myelin, 229
Myelitis, 39
Myeloma, 197
Myocardium. See *Heart*

N

Narcotics, 38
Nasopharynx, 170

Necroses, 25, 36, 39, 147
Needle autopsies, 5
Needle marks, 39
Negligence, 297, 305
Neoprene latex, 73, 258
Nephrons, 148
Newborns, 153, 316, 317
Nicotine, 32
Nitro-BT dye test, 61
Nitrogen, 221
Nocardia asteroides, 215
Nomenclature, 286

O

Ochronosis, 197
Ophthalmoscopy, 21
Organization, autopsy service, 276, 277
Osteomyelitis, 214
Otitis media, 214
Ovary, 331, 344

P

Pancreas, 147
Pancreas weights and measurements
  adults, 344
  fetuses, 317
  infants, 331
Pancreatitis, 27, 222
Paper-mounted sections, 110
Paraproteins, 220
Parathyroid glands, 345
Particle identification, 124
Pathology assistants, 311
Pelvic organs, 153
Penis, 153
Permount, 132
Personnel, 282, 283
Petrous bone, 27, 214
Phenol, 32
Phlebography. See *Angiography*
Phosphatase, stomach, 134
Phosphatides, 221
Phospholipids, 234
Phosphorus, 17, 32, 35, 221
Photographs, 4, 12, 14, 20, 27, 30, 139, 253, 263, 284, 306
Pineal gland, 345
Pituitary gland, **169,** 310, 332, 345
Placenta, 3, 153, 345
Planimetry, 112
Plastic bags, 33, 254, **280**
Plastic casts, 120, 151, 257. See also *Angiography*
Plastic jars, 254
Plastic mounting media, 256
Pleural effusion, 25
Pneumoconiosis, 13
Pneumocystis carinii, 96
Pneumoencephalography, 189
Pneumomediastinum, 8, 13, 224
Pneumoperitoneum, 224
Pneumothorax, 3, 4, **7,** 13, 20
Poisoning, 13, 305. See also *Toxicology*

Police officers, 301, 311
Pollution, 310
Polyethylene, 33
Polylite, 76, 151
Polyvinyl chloride, 120
Popliteal vessels, 84
Portacaval shunt, 139
Portal vein thrombosis, 139
Postmortem changes, 15, 17, 216, 219, 221
Postmortem function, 123
Postmortem interval, 12, 15, 218, 230
Postoperative. See *Autopsy techniques*
Potassium, 17, 221
Prague powder, 239, 254
Pregnancy, 153
Preservative, 25, 34, 42
Prisons, 298, 299
Procaine, 38
Propellants, 41
Prostate, 153, 332, 345
Prostheses, 6, 173, 199, 310
Protein, 220
Protocols, 4, 12, **264**, 303
Pseudogout, 198
Psychomimetics, 40
Public health, 263, 283, 309
Pulmonary. See *Lung*
Punch cards, 290, 291
Putrefaction, 17, 22, 26, 29, 84, 135
Pyrogallol, 22

Q

Quinine, 38

R

Radiation absorption, lung, 113
Radioactivity, 231, **245**
Radiopaque. See *Contrast media*
Rape, 28, **30**
Refrigerants, 41
Regaud's fixative, 235
Rejuvenation, tissues, 239
Replication technique, 125
Reports, toxicologic, 41
Requests, toxicologic, 31, 32
Research, 308, 310
Respiratory distress, 154
Reticulum, spleen, 147
Retrieval systems, autopsy data, 283, 291
Rheomacrodex, 115
Rickettsiae, 235
Rigor mortis, 17
Roentgenograms
    air embolism, 21
    battered child, 30
    blood vessels and lymphatic vessels. See
        Angiography
    bronchi, 119
    decompression sickness, 25
    esophagus, 133
    fistulas, 4
    foreign bodies, 28
    free air, 8

Roentgenograms (*continued*)
    gunshot injuries, 27
    identification of bodies, 14, 20
    lungs, 106, 225
    pneumomediastinum, 7, **8,** 13
    pneumothorax, 7
    stereoscopic, 70, 72
    subcutaneous emphysema, 7, 8
Roentgenography, facilities, 224
Rokitansky technique, 2, 51
Ryder grid, 111

S

Safety officer, radiation, 245
Salicylates, 32
Sarcomas, 217
Saws, 158, 162, 165, 167, 171, **195,** 196
Schatzki rings, 133
Sealing, plastic bags, 280
Seminal vesicles, 332, 345
Sepsis, 39
Serum. See *Blood*
Sex chromatin, 154, 218
Sex determination, 15
Shipping, 28, **241**
Shock, 13, 28
Silicone, 256
Sinuses, 169, 170
Size, 14, 264. See also names of respective
    organs
Skeletal muscle, 187, 345
Skin, 35
Skull fracture, 169
Slang terms, drugs, 40
Slicing, 108, 139
Small intestine, 345
Sniffing, 41
Sodium chloride, 26, 44, 221
Sodium fluoride, 25, 42
Sound transmission, lung, 113
Space requirements, 282
Spalteholz technique, 258
Spermatic fluid, 30
Spermatozoa, 30
Spinal column, 301. See also *Spinal cord*
Spinal cord, 162, 184, 214, 346
Spinal fluid. See *Cerebrospinal fluid*
Spleen, **147,** 209
Spleen weights and measurements
    adults, 345, 346
    fetuses, 317
    infants, 333
Spondylitis, 197
Spray death, 41
Staining, gross organs and tissues
    amyloid, 230
    bone and cartilage, 259
    calcium, 230
    cleared specimens, 259
    fat and lipoid, 83, 136, 229
    gastric mucosa, 134
    glycogen, 60
    intestinal mucosa, 136

Staining, gross organs & tissues *(continued)*
  iron (hemosiderin), 140, 230
  left bundle-branch radiation, 60
  liver, 140
  mesentery, 136
  myelin, 229
  myocardium, 61
Statistics, 309
Stature, 15
Stereomicroangiography, 116
Sterilization, homografts, 65
Stimulants, 38
Stomach, 133
Stomach contents, 26, 34, 36
Storage, 110, 248, **249,** 254, 277, **279**
Strangling, 19, 27
Strychnine, 32, 38
Sucrose, 38
Suffocation, 13, 28
Suicide, 20, 267, 270, 272, 298, 305
Sulfate, 223
Sulfonamides, 41
Sural nerve, 186
Surfactant, 125
Syndromes, 3, 217
Synovial fluid, 198

T

Tags, 241, 245, 249, 275, 277, **281**
Talc granulomas, 39
Tape, 291
Tardieu's spots, 25, 28
Temperature, 15, 315
Temporal bone, 171
Terminology, 286
Testes, 334, 346
Tests
  air vs. decomposition gas, 22
  carbon monoxide, 36
  diatom detection, 26
  drowning, 26
  myocardial infarcts, 61
  pulmonary function, 123
  seminal stains, 30
  stillbirth vs. live baby, 29
Tetanus, 39
Thebesian veins, 76
Thoracic duct, 87
Thorotrast, 231
Thrombocytopenia, 38
Thrombophlebitis, 39
Thromboses, 82, 84, 139
Thymus, 317, 334, 346
Thyroid gland, 317, 347
Time of death, 15
Tissue culture, 217, 310
Tissue registry, 277, **279**
Toluene, 41
Toxicology, 14, 18, **31,** 241
Trachea, 93

Tracheoesophageal fistula, 93, 129
Transfusion, 20, 310
Transplantation, 302, 310
Transportation, bodies, 304
Trauma, 13
Trichloroacetic acid, 236
Trichloroethane, 41
Triglycerides, 221
Triphenyltetrazolium chloride (TTC) test, 62
Tuberculosis, 215, 216, 276, 309
Tumors, intestinal, 134

U

Ulcer, stomach, 133, 134
Umbilical cord, 3, 154
Uniform Anatomical Gift Act, 303
Urates, 233, 240
Urea, 221
Uremia, 223
Ureters, 148
Urethra, 153
Uric acid, 221
Urinary bladder, 153, 210
Urine, 33, **35,** 36, 39, 40, 42, 153, 210, 221
Urobilin, 221
Urobilinogen, 221
Urography, 149
Urokon, 149
Uterus, 153, 335, 347

V

Valve homografts, 65
Varices, esophagus, 129
Vasovagal attacks, 13
Veins, 76, 84. See also names of respective
  organs and *Angiography*
Ventriculography, 189
Vinylite, 257
Virchow's technique, 2, 19, 52, 177
Virtual cooling time, 16
Virus, 216, 276, 310
Vital Statistics Office, 270
Vitreous humor, 17, **18,** 34, 35, 42, 221, 223
Volume determination, 4, 111, 121, 341
Vomitus, 36

W

Weights, 14, 264. See also names of respective organs
Wood's metal, 121, 258
Workman's compensation, 276, 299, 305, 309
Wounds, 4, 19, 20, 25, 27, 28

X

Xanthine, 17, 221

Z

Zenker's fixative, 101, 198, **236**